HUMAN BLOOD COAGULATION

BOERHAAVE SERIES
FOR POSTGRADUATE
MEDICAL EDUCATION

PROCEEDINGS OF THE BOERHAAVE COURSES
ORGANIZED BY
THE FACULTY OF MEDICINE, UNIVERSITY OF LEIDEN,
THE NETHERLANDS

HUMAN BLOOD COAGULATION

BIOCHEMISTRY, CLINICAL INVESTIGATION AND THERAPY

EDITED BY

H. C. HEMKER, M.D., E. A. LOELIGER, M.D., AND
J. J. VELTKAMP, M.D.

WKAP ARCHIEF

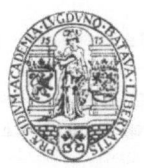

LEIDEN UNIVERSITY PRESS
1969

Reprinted 1970

ISBN-13:978-94-010-3425-8   e-ISBN-13:978-94-010-3423-4

DOI: 10.1007/978-94-010-3423-4

Jacket design: E. Wijnans

© 1969 Leiden University Press, Leiden, The Netherlands

Softcover reprint of the hardcover 1st edition 1969

PREFACE

Since 1952, postgraduate courses for practising physicians and specialists have been given by the Medical Faculty of the University of Leiden in the Boerhaave Quarter, in which most of its clinics and laboratories are located. During these years, recent advances in a wide variety of medical fields and subjects have been discussed by distinguished speakers from many countries. The steadily increasing attendance has shown that, as could be expected from the rapid progress of modern medicine, there is a widely felt need for this form of postgraduate study. In 1957, therefore, the Leiden Medical Faculty appointed a permanent committee for the organization of postgraduate medical education.

Of the courses given since then, certain material proved to have sufficient immediate scientific value to justify publication, and it now gives the Committee great pleasure to announce that in collaboration with the Leiden University Press it will publish the *Boerhaave Series for Postgraduate Medical Education*. The first volume of this new series is the product of the course on Human Blood Coagulation given in November 1968.

It is our hope that this book will prove valuable not only to those who participated in the course but also to many others working in this and associated fields.

For the Committee:

Professor J. Dankmeijer, M. D., President
M. W. Jongsma, M. D., Honorary Secretary

V

INTRODUCTION

Blood coagulation in medicine and biochemistry 1
H. C. HEMKER, E. A. LOELIGER, J. J. VELTKAMP

CHAPTER I

REACTION MECHANISM OF BLOOD COAGULATION

The formation of the fibrin clot from fibrinogen 7
B. BLOMBÄCK, MARGARETA BLOMBÄCK (Stockholm)

Discussion: F. Duckert (The role of factor XIII), Margareta Blombäck 13

On the structure of thrombin and prothrombin 18
S. MAGNUSSON (Cambridge)

Discussion: E. Högenauer (Protein chemistry of factors VII and X) . 22

The interaction of prothrombin and factors V and X with phospholipids
and calcium ions 24
D. J. HANAHAN, P. G. BARTON, A. COX (Tucson)

Discussion: M. J. P. Kahn (On the influence of monoinositol-phospho-
lipid on prothrombinase generation), K. Denson, H. C. Hemker. . 37

The nature of prothrombinase 40
M. P. ESNOUF (Oxford)

Discussion: C. R. M. Prentice (Present concept of prothrombinase) 45

The interaction of factors VII, IX, and X 48
K. DENSON (Oxford)

Discussion: H. C. Hemker, K. Denson, C. Deggeller, C. R. M.
Prentice 54

The nature of the factor IX activating principle 58
C. HAANEN (Nijmegen)

Discussion: L. Vroman (Adsorption of fibrinogen at interfaces, its relation to contact activation and platelet stickiness), S. Magnusson 73

The possible role of factor VII in the intrinsic system 77
F. JOSSO (Paris)

Discussion: H. C. Hemker, F. Josso, K. Denson 82

Factor VII and tissue thromboplastin 83
H. PRYDZ (Oslo)

Discussion: P. M. van der Plas (The use of filipin as a tool in coagulation research), E. Deutsch, M. P. Esnouf, H. Prydz 89

Enzyme systems triggered by the contact factors 94
C. R. M. PRENTICE

Discussion: K. Pondman (The complement system, its relations to other triggered enzyme systems in the blood plasma), C. R. M. Prentice, J. J. Vreeken, L. Vroman 99

Enzyme kinetic evaluation of coagulation systems 104
H. C. HEMKER (Leiden)

Discussion: C. Deggeller, H. C. Hemker, K. Denson, M. P. Esnouf 111

ROUND TABLE DISCUSSION 117
Chairman: E. Deutsch (Vienna)

CHAPTER II

PHYSIOPATHOLOGY

The mechanism of haemostasis 143
E. A. LOELIGER (Leiden)

Morphology of the process of haemostasis 148
J. J. SIXMA (Utrecht)

Laboratory investigation

Indication, assay procedures, diagnosis, and advice 152
J. J. VELTKAMP, ANNEMARIE D. MULLER, E. A. LOELIGER
(Leiden)

Defibrination syndrome

The role of the degradation products of fibrinogen and fibrin in the
blood 224
H. SCHRIJVER (The Hague)

Quantification of split products 228
N. FEKKES (Leiden)

Treatment of haemorrhagic diathesis

General considerations concerning the treatment of haemorrhagic
diathesis 236
E. A. LOELIGER (Leiden)

Platelet transfusion in patients with platelet isoantibodies 242
J. G. EERNISSE (Leiden)

Purification and clinical application of the four factors of the prothrombin
complex 251
P. F. BRUNING (Leiden)

Four clotting factors concentrate 257
J. J. VREEKEN (Amsterdam)

Preparation and clinical application of cryoprecipitate. 260
KLAZINA MEIJER (Leiden)

Some remarks concerning the production and administration of cryoprecipitates 270
J.J. VREEKEN (Amsterdam)

Genetic counselling in haemostatic disorders 274
J.J. VELTKAMP (Leiden)

CHAPTER III

BLOOD COAGULATION CONTROL IN ORAL
ANTICOAGULANT TREATMENT

General considerations on coumarin-induced hypocoagulability and
its control 283
E. A. LOELIGER (Leiden)

The Netherlands Thrombosis Service 286
F. L. J. JORDAN (Utrecht)

Laboratory tests

Prothrombin time

The Manchester Comparative Reagent. A national reference standard
for anticoagulant therapy 290
L. POLLER, JEAN THOMSON (Manchester)

Discussion: H. Stormorken, J. Thomson, E. A. Loeliger, P. A. Owren . 296

Thrombotest

The history of Thrombotest 300
P. A. OWREN (Oslo)

Quality control of Thrombotest (TT) and Normotest (NT) 309
H. STORMORKEN (Oslo)

Introduction of Thrombotest at the Netherlands Thrombosis Services . 314
S. I. DE VRIES (Amsterdam)

Introduction of Thrombotest at the Amsterdam Thrombosis Service . 318
J. E. JAPIKSE (Amsterdam)

Thrombotest versus conventional thromboplastins 320
E. A. LOELIGER (Leiden)

Discussion: H. L. Booij, H. Stormorken, P. A. Owren, E. A. Loeliger,
F. L. J. Jordan, C. Haanen 325

Therapeutic levels

Thrombotest levels in relation to recurrence and bleeding complications in long-term treatment of patients suffering from coronary heart disease 330
C. A. van Dijk, Wilhelmina B. Dominicus, J. Roos (The Hague)

The Utrecht double-blind trial of long-term anticoagulant treatment after myocardial infarction 336
O. J. A. Th. Meuwissen (Utrecht)

The Leiden double-blind trial of long-term anticoagulant treatment after myocardial infarction 339
E. A. Loeliger (Leiden)

Discussion: J. Roos, P. A. Owren, E. A. Loeliger, J. J. Vreeken, S. I. de Vries 342

Vitamin K_1 therapy 345
J. van der Meer (Leidschendam)

CHAPTER IV

THE ASSESSMENT OF LIVER FUNCTION BY BLOOD COAGULATION TESTS

Blood coagulation and liver function 361
E. A. LOELIGER (Leiden)

The Thrombotest dilution curve and its diagnostic significance . . 365
H. C. HEMKER (Leiden)

Normotest in the evaluation o liver function 369
P. A. OWREN (Oslo)

Clinical experience with Normotest 379
M. FISCHER, H. W. PILGERSTORFER (Vienna)

Preliminary experience with Normotest 381
J. J. VELTKAMP·(Leiden)

Discussion: P.M. Mannucci, P.A. Owren, E.A. Loeliger, H. Stormorken, J. J. Veltkamp, H. C. Hemker 386

Index of subjects 400

ACKNOWLEDGEMENTS

The following societies and firms contributed toward the defrayment of the costs of this course:

Amstel Brouwerij N.V.
J. T. Baker Chemicals N.V.
N.V. Ciba
N.V. Gaba
L.K.B. Producten N.V.
Nutricia N.V.
Pharmachemie N.V.
Philips Duphar N.V.

Propharma N.V.
'Roter' N.V.
Unilever N.V.
Nederlandse Vereniging voor Biochemie
Nederlandse Vereniging voor Cardiologie
Nederlandse Hartstichting
Nederlandse Vereniging voor Haematologie

LIST OF ACTIVE PARTICIPANTS

Margareta Blombäck	Stockholm	S. Magnusson	Cambridge
P. F. Bruning	Leiden	J. van der Meer	Leidschendam
C. Deggeller	Deventer	O. J. A. Th. Meuwissen	Utrecht
K. Denson	Oxford	K. Meyer	Leiden
Wilhelmina B. Dominicus	The Hague	P. A. Owren	Oslo
F. Duckert	Basel	P. van der Plas	Utrecht
Cornelia A. van Dijk	The Hague	L. Poller	Manchester
J. G. Eernisse	Leiden	K. Pondman	Amsterdam
M. P. Esnouf	Oxford	C. R. M. Prentice	Glasgow
N. Fekkes	Leiden	H. Prydz	Oslo
M. Fischer	Vienna	J. Roos	The Hague
C. Haanen	Nijmegen	H. Schrijver	The Hague
D. J. Hanahan	Tucson	J. J. Sixma	Utrecht
H. C. Hemker	Leiden	H. Stormorken	Oslo
J. E. Japikse	Amsterdam	A. C. W. Swart	Leiden
F. Josso	Paris	J. J. Veltkamp	Leiden
F. L. J. Jordan	Utrecht	J. Vreeken	Amsterdam
M. J. P. Kahn	Brussel	S. I. de Vries	Amsterdam
E. A. Loeliger	Leiden	L. Vroman	New York

INTRODUCTION

BLOOD COAGULATION IN MEDICINE AND BIOCHEMISTRY

Although the science of biochemistry has its roots in attempts to apply the knowledge of chemistry to benefit the sick, its evolution has long since brought it to independence, even to the extent that there are biochemists to be found who cannot help regarding with a certain dismay their unfortunate colleagues who have to make a living by working in the esoteric surroundings of a hospital. On the other hand, many a physician is of the opinion that one would have to be a scientist of Boerhaave's stature to master both the practice of medicine and the basic science of biochemistry, and so they devote themselves to clinical medicine, willfully resigning themselves to forgetting every bit of biochemistry that does not directly help to cure patients. Recent progress in the field of biochemistry unquestionably means that a choice must be made, but although it is true that the examples given above illustrate extremes, they are also the choices most commonly made. Yet, in a volume meant to open a series called after the man who was a master in the basic sciences as well as of clinical medicine, we think it might be appropriate to remind ourselves of the benefit still to be derived from close collaboration between clinical medicine and biochemistry.

It is sometimes possible to treat a field of study not on the basis of a discipline but on the basis of a problem, and good fortune sometimes makes it possible to build up an academic team in which birds of a different feather can work together to attack a problem. We consider ourselves most fortunate in having been able to bring together for this conference representatives of such groups working in the field of haemostasis and thrombosis. We hope that it will be evident from this volume that interdisciplinary cooperation is a *conditio sine qua non* for the solution of the pathophysiological problems in this field, but also that both basic biochemistry and the treatment of patients can gain from this kind of joint research in a way that can never be achieved by restriction to either pure biochemistry or applied clinical medicine.

Chapter I of this volume is devoted to the problem of the reaction mechanism of blood coagulation. At the present moment, this sounds like a purely biochemical subject, but a glance at the textbooks of biochemistry will show that until fairly recently it was not considered a subject in which a biochemist could take any interest. And indeed, even a brief glance at an older textbook of medicine shows that this attitude was fair enough. Around 1964, however, with Macfarlane's introduction of his cascade hypothesis, the scene changed, and subsequent biochemical research has made it possible to discern the outlines of the biochemical mechanism underlying blood coagulation. At least, this is what we hope to show in Chapter I. No matter how specifically biochemical this chapter is meant to be, it is well to realize that the work reported in it would have been impossible without help from the wards, were it only for the provision of the reagents with which to perform the tests for the various clotting-factor activities. Conversely, the special field of coagulation biochemistry has been able to make some contributions to general enzymology, such as the concepts concerning an enzyme cascade, the interplay of proteins in establishing enzymatic activity at an interphase, and certain developments in enzyme kinetics.

In Chapter II, recent advances in the diagnosis and treatment of haemostatic disorders are discussed. Here, advanced clinical work benefits from the application of fundamental biochemical knowledge related to procedures such as protein purification and immunological methods.

Chapter III, which deals with the supervision of anticoagulant therapy, shows the most interesting mixture of practical needs and theoretical treatment. The lack of comparability of the results obtained with tests using different thromboplastins has worried practical coagulationists for many years. It was not until after the application of enzyme kinetics to the results obtained with these tests that the protein induced by the absence of vitamin K (PIVKA) could be recognized. This step forward led to the better understanding of the physiological basis of these tests, and formed a basis for comparability. But it also opened the way to the solution of a problem in basic biochemistry, namely the question of the mode of action of vitamin K.

Some of these studies will seem to the biochemist to be almost entirely medical, others will look awkwardly biochemical to the clinician. But the thrill of this kind of research is still that one is suspended between two disciplines, and must remain there in order to solve the problems at hand. It is an essential fact that only by such close conjunction can the clinician profit from biochemical knowledge and the biochemist from the unique situation offered by intensive biochemical study of the patient.

We are grateful that so many leading investigators in the field proved willing to contribute to this conference. A glance at the list of active participants will show that it has been our intention to shift the population of the conference to the younger age-groups. This has been our purpose not only because the views of the older investigators are well known from many other sources but also because we believed that the communications would gain in interest if those who made them were still actively engaged in laboratory work.

The Boerhaave Committee of the Medical Faculty of Leiden University deserves our sincere thanks for making this course possible as one of the many post-graduate courses it excels in organizing. Financial aid from the sources mentioned on page xiv is also gratefully acknowledged.

It is our hope that this volume will illustrate the benefit of interdisciplinary and international collaboration by clearly stating some of the problems in the field of haemostasis and thrombosis, a field which is still all too often considered incomprehensible by outsiders. We also hope that this volume will help to establish the points on which a *communis opinio* can be reached, as well as the points now urgently in need of further investigation.

H. C. HEMKER
E. A. LOELIGER
J. J. VELTKAMP

Translations were provided by Mrs. I. Seeger.

CHAPTER I

THE REACTION MECHANISM OF BLOOD COAGULATION

THE FORMATION OF THE FIBRIN CLOT FROM FIBRINOGEN

THE N-TERMINAL DISULFIDE KNOT OF FIBRINOGEN

B. BLOMBÄCK AND MARGARETA BLOMBÄCK

The formation of fibrin from fibrinogen presents an excellent model of how a biological fibre develops. The initiation of the process leading ultimately to the formation of a fibrin thread is enzymatic in nature. The enzyme in this process is thrombin, which causes a limited proteolysis of the fibrinogen molecule.

Mammalian fibrinogen is built up of three peptide chains, $\alpha(A)$, $\beta(B)$, and γ. The N-terminal ends of the $\alpha(A)$-, $\beta(B)$-, and γ-chains are linked together in a firm disulfide knot. Current data indicate that the molecule is a dimeric unit with the formula: $(\alpha(A), \beta(B), \gamma)_2$. The N-terminal disulfide knots have been obtained in a reasonably pure state by the treatment of fibrinogen with cyanogen bromide, a reagent which cleaves peptide bonds involving methionine residues in the protein. Among the fragments produced by treatment with CNBr is a fragment containing N-terminal portions of the three peptide chains of fibrinogen crosslinked by s-s bridges. This fragment can be purified from the digest by gel filtration on Sephadex G-100 and G-200. Its demonstration during the purification procedure is indirect, and is based on the fact that specific 'fibrinopeptides' are released from the

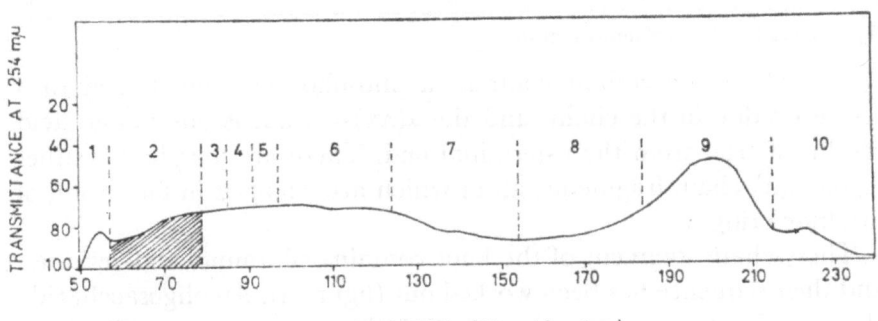

TUBE NUMBER (24.8 ml fractions)

Fig. 1. Chromatogram of CNBr-treated fibrinogen

7

α('A')- and β(B)-chain fragments by digestion with thrombin. As an example, I will take the chromatogram of CNBr-treated fibrinogen on Sephadex G-100 (figure 1). Only from fraction 2 are fibrinopeptides released on digestion with thrombin. This fraction can, as already mentioned, be further purified by gel filtration on Sephadex G-200.

The molecular weight of the disulfide knot is about 26,000. The amino acid sequences of the chain-fragments contained in it have been almost completely elucidated. The α('A')-chain fragment contains 49-50 amino acid residues. It is heterogeneous. Three different types of α('A')-chain can be distinguished (figure 2), *i.e.*, α(A), α(AP), and

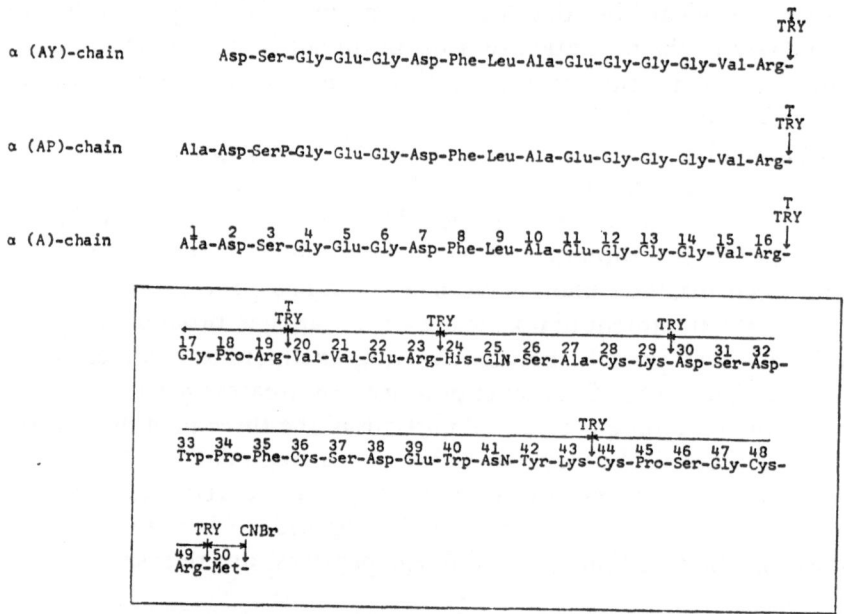

Fig. 2. The α (A) chains of human fibrinogen

α(AY). The α(AP)-variant contains a phosphorous atom linked to a serine residue in the chain, and the α(AY)-variant is one amino acid residue shorter from the N-terminal end. There are four half-cystines in the α(A)-chain fragments, all of which are engaged in formation of disulfide bridges.

The γ-chain fragment of the knot contains 78 amino acid residues, and their sequence has been worked out (figure 3). An oligosaccharide chain of about ten sugar residues is linked to residue no. 52. The fragment contains, like the α(A)-chain fragment, four half-cystines.

The amino acid sequence of the β(B)-chain fragment has not yet been completed. It consists of 63-64 amino residues, including two half-cystine residues.

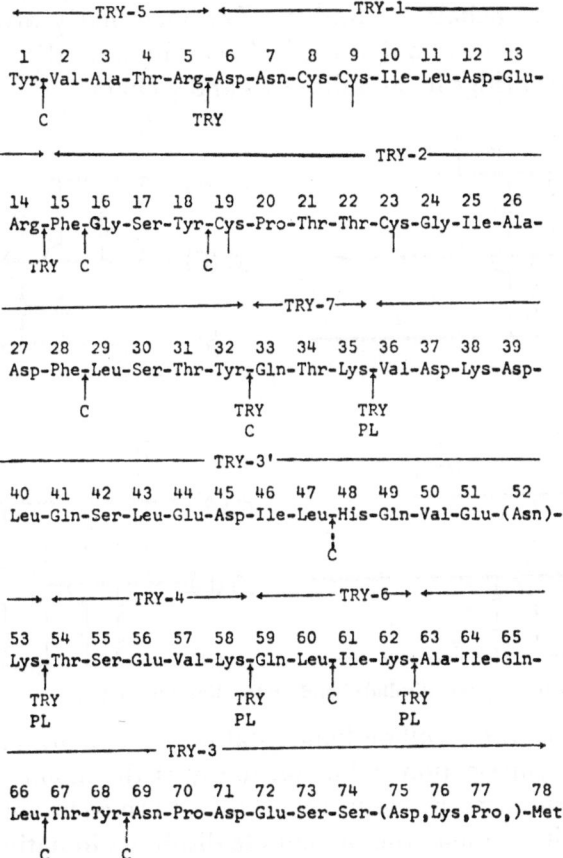

Fig. 3. The γ-chain fragment of the disulfide knot

There are ten half-cystine residues in one N-terminal disulfide knot. Since no free SH-groups can be demonstrated either in fibrinogen or in the knot, the chain fragments must be held together by disulfide bonds. If we assume that all ten half-cystines are involved in the formation of five disulfide bridges, there are in principle four different ways of arranging them (figure 4). Recent limited reduction experiments indicate that there are three interchain and two intrachain disulfide bridges in the disulfide knot. The interchain bonds are more easily reduced than the intrachain bonds with reducing agents such as

dithioecrytrol. Consequently, the intrachain bonds can be specifically labelled after preliminary reduction of all interchain bonds. In
our experiments, 14C-labelled iodacetic acid was used for alkylating
the reduced intrachain s-s bridges. The most likely arrangement of
the disulfides is shown in figure 4 I. As can be seen, there is one intrachain disulfide bridge in both the α(A)- and γ-chain.

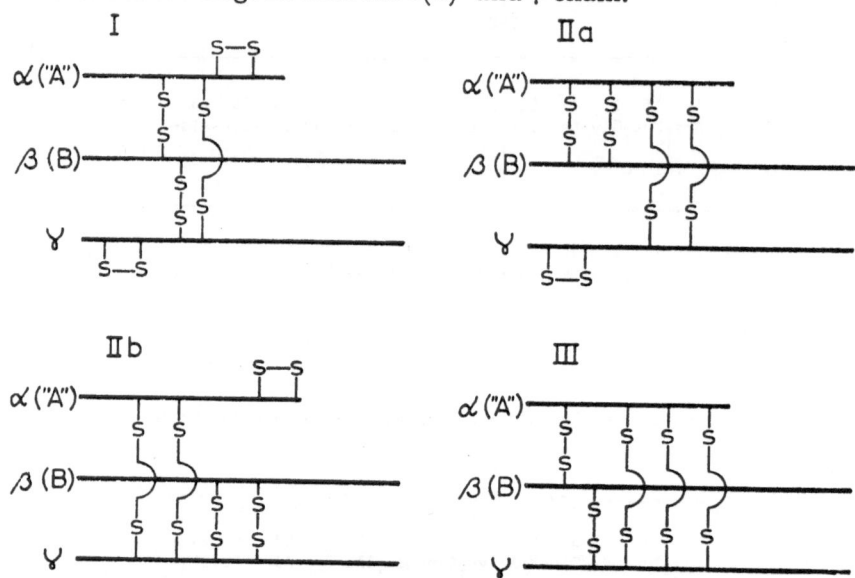

Fig. 4. Possible arangements of disulfide bonds in the disulfide knot

To what extent the disulfide bonds stabilize a conformation suitable
for proper polymerization is difficult to say at the moment. However,
about 4-5 disulfides are easily reduced in fibrinogen without loss of
clotting activity. Among the susceptible disulfides in native fibrinogen
are some of the interchain bonds involved in the N-terminal 'disulfide
knot', at least those between the α('A')-chain fragments, and the other
partners of the knot. It may therefore be said that at least at a pH
around 8, some of the disulfides in the knot have a limited function in
keeping the protein in the right conformation for polymerization.

In a fibrinogen dimer with a molecular weight of 340,000, there are
two in principle identical N-terminal disulfide knots located at opposite
ends of the molecule perpendicular to an axis of symmetry (figure 5).
This symmetrical model for fibrinogen bears some similarity to the divalent symmetrical model proposed for immunoglobulins. The regions
of biological activity for both types of molecules may be presumed to

reside at opposite poles of the molecule. We speculate that in the three-nodule structure of fibrinogen deduced from the electron-microscopic picture by Hall and Slayter, the end nodules contain the N-terminal disulfide knots. The middle nodule in the electron micrographs might represent the region where fibrinogen monomers of 170,000 unit weight are joined together.

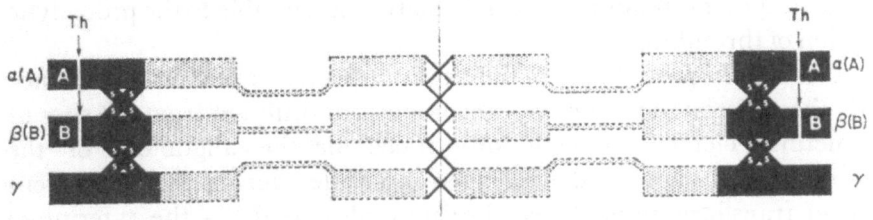

Fig. 5. A model of the fibrinogen molecule

The fibrinogen dimer is activated by thrombin. When trombin acts on fibrinogen, fibrinopeptides are split off from the N-terminal ends of the α'(A')- and β(B)-chain. The peptide split off from the A-chain is denoted as peptide A, and that split off from the B-chain as peptide B. The release of peptide A occurs more rapidly than that of peptide B. In its proteolytic action on fibrinogen, thrombin has a narrow specificity of action. Only a few bonds in the protein are rapidly hydrolyzed. These are the arginyl-glycine bonds linking the fibrinopeptides in fibrinogen to the rest of the fibrinogen molecule. Some other arginyl and possibly also lysyl bonds in fibrinogen are split by the enzyme, but at a much slower rate. It should be mentioned here that in the α('A')-chain fragment as well as in the disulfide knot, thrombin cleaves not only the no. 16 but also the no. 19 arginyl bond (cf. figure 2). The rate of cleavage of the latter bond in the disulfide knot and in the α('A')-chain fragment is, however, quite slow. In native fibrinogen the no. 19 arginyl bond is not split by thrombin to any appreciable extent. The change in substrate specificity indicates that the tertiary structure in the isolated disulfide knot is different from that of the 'disulfide knot', being an integral part of the fibrinogen molecule.

We have suggested that the fibrinopeptides might contain structural features responsible for the narrow specificity of the enzyme. The structures that might favour a rapid association between enzyme and substrate (or possibly activate the enzyme) would be present in the c-terminal part of fibrinopeptide A. This idea has arisen mainly from the fact that this part has remained essentially unchanged during mammalian evolution. However, in a discussion of thrombin action one has to take into consideration not only the fibrinopeptides but also the adjacent structures on the other side of the split bonds, let alone the complex conformation of the whole fibrinogen molecule. So far, we have established that the N-terminal disulfide knot and its isolated chain fragments maintains a conformation susceptible to the proteolytic action of thrombin.

It is highly probable that the sites in fibrinogen having importance for the substrate specificity of thrombin are different from the sites or structural elements having importance for the alignment of the proteolytically activated fibrinogen molecules during the fibrinogen-fibrin transformation. These sites may also reside in the N-terminal portion of the molecule.

In fact, there are observations favouring the view that certain structures in the disulfide knot are directly or indirectly of importance for the polymerization of activated fibrinogen. Thus, in a Detroit Negro family afflicted with a hemorrhagic diathesis, an abnormal fibrinogen has been demonstrated. In this fibrinogen an amino acid substitution (serine for arginine) has occurred in the N-terminal disulfide knot in the vicinity of the bond split by thrombin during normal clotting (no. 19 arginine being replaced by a serine residue). It is extremely unlikely that this mutation is unrelated to the hemorrhagic disorder of the patient. In fibrinogen Detroit the fibrinopeptides have a normal structure and they are released at a normal rate. However, the proteolyzed fibrinogen only forms a clot at an exceedingly slow rate. The reason for the slow aggregation may simply be the change in electric charge due to the replacement of a basic amino acid by a neutral one. It could also be that the conformational change which might follow the release of the fibrinopeptides is different in fibrinogen Detroit from that in normal fibrinogen, resulting in a slow unfolding of reactive sites for polymerization.

DISCUSSION

F. Duckert: The role of factor XIII

When the fibrinopeptides A and B are separated from fibrinogen by the action of thrombin, the fibrin monomers can aggregate and form a three-dimensional network. This aggregation is not the last step of the physiological fibrin formation, since this fibrin is still unable to fulfill its physiological function and is characterized by its solubility in 5 M urea and 1% monochloroacetic acid.

The fibrin aggregate in which the monomers are held together by hydrogen bonds must be further modified, 'stabilized', by the enzymatic action of factor XIII. The fibrin is converted to a polymer insoluble in 5M urea and 1% monochloroactic acid. It then has a normal haemostatic function.

The role of thrombin is a double one: first, it prepares fibrinogen for the reaction with factor XIII, and second, it activates factor XIII itself.

The splitting of the fibrinopeptides is essential for the reaction with factor XIII. Lorand et al. (9) demonstrated that factor XIII incorporates very little glycine-ethylester into fibrinogen, whereas the incorporation into soluble fibrin amounts to a minimum of 4 molecules per fibrinmonomer. These results suggest that the binding sites are more easily available in fibrin than in fibrinogen. Native factor XIII or fibrin-stabilizing factor is unable to convert soluble fibrin into insoluble fibrin. It must be previously activated. The physiological activation is due to a limited proteolytic effect of thrombin, which uncovers new sylfhydryl groups. The activation of factor XIII by thrombin was first demonstrated by Buluk et al. (1) who observed that at constant factor XIII concentration the formation rate of insoluble fibrin depends on the thrombin concentration. These authors also report a transient increase of the free sulfhydryl groups (2). These observations were confirmed by Konishi and Lorand (3). During activation of factor XIII by thrombin, the number of sulfhydryl groups available for titration with p-chloromercuribenzoic acid increases from 3-SH in non-activated factor XIII to 5-6 SH moles per mole of activated factor XIII.

The importance of the thrombin activation is also demonstrated by the inhibition with SH-blocking compounds. The monoiodoacetic acid, for instance, does not inhibit the native factor XIII. It is not yet bound to the SH group, and is easily removed by dialysis with total recovery of the original activity. After activation by thrombin, the inhibition with monoiodoacetic acid is irreversible. Intact sulfhydryl groups are therefore essential for the enzymatic action of factor XIII. They are protected by a thiol compound, such as cysteine.

For the activation of factor XIII, trypsin, reptilase, and papain can replace thrombin, whereas thrombin coagulase is ineffective. The similar action of several proteolytic enzymes confirms the assumption that a limited proteolysis takes place during the activation of factor XIII, with an alteration of the electrophoretic mobility. These data suggest that thrombin may split one or several peptide bonds. This cleavage changes the structure of factor XIII, so that new sulfhydryl groups are exposed. It is not known whether discrete amounts of peptidic material are released during the activation of factor XIII.

The activation of factor XIII and the action of factor XIIIa (activated form) proceed at high velocity and are simultaneous with the formation and aggregation of fibrin monomers.

Various roles have been attributed in the past to factor XIII_a. The more recent findings are now all in agreement. It has been demonstrated by Lorand et al. (8) that some amines, i.e. glycine methyl ester, glycine amide, and above all dansylcadaverine, are very good inhibitors of the formation of insoluble fibrin. They explained these results by a transpeptidation mechanism, leading to the establishment of covalent linkages between fibrin monomers. This hypothesis was modified by Loewy, (4) who found that only NH_3 was released during the reaction: a transamidation.

Factor XIIIa was inhibited not only by amines but also by carbonylamides, especially CBZ-L-asparagine amide, which suggests a participation of the β-aspartyl, possibly of the γ-glutamyl groups (7).

Furthermore, the inhibitors were incorporated into fibrin, and casein, and even in glucagon (5), with the formation of γ-glutamyl glycine peptide bonds. It was then assumed that in the formation of covalent bonds the γ-carbonyl of the glutamyl residue functions as the acceptor. The nature of the donor groups was widely disputed, and was only definitively characterized after the isolation of the actual cross-link in fibrin.

This final demonstration was made at about the same time by three different groups of investigators. Matacic and Loewy (11), Pisano, Finlayson and Peyton (12) and Lorand et al. (6) found that the hydrolysate of insoluble fibrin by pronase and leucine aminopeptidase contained a dipeptide, the ε-(γ-glutamyl)lysine absent in the soluble fibrin. This formation of covalent bonds for the cross-linking of fibrin closely resembles the reaction catalyzed by the tissue transglutaminase (10). In addition, these transglutaminases are also able to convert soluble fibrin into an insoluble product.

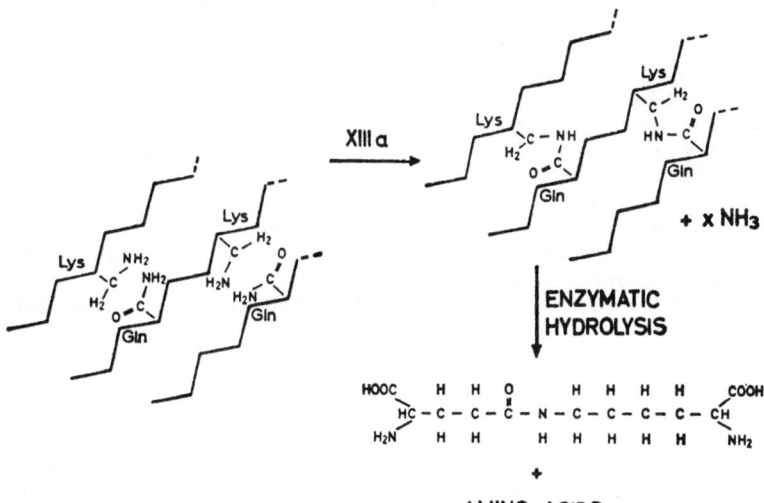

Fig. 1. Action of activated factor XIII (XIIIa) on fibrin with formation of covalent bonds and release of NH₃, followed by degradation of the insoluble fibrin and recovery of unhydrolyzed ε-(γ-glutamyl)lysine.

For its activation and function the enzyme requires the presence of calcium ions. This transglutaminase is more specific than tissue transglutaminases, which work in presence of Sr·· and Mn··. With plasma transglutaminase, these two metal ions can replace Ca·· only in the presence of reducing agents, e.g. cystein. It may therefore be concluded with a high degree of probability that factor XIII is a coagulation factor, circulating in blood as an inactive precursor that can be activated by limited proteolysis into a plasma transglutaminase, which specifically requires calcium ions.

REFERENCES

1. Buluk K., T. Janusko and J. Olbromski, Conversion of fibrin to desmofibrin. *Nature*: 191, 1093-1094 (1961).
2. Buluk K., J. Olbromski, T. Januszko and A. Zuch, Desmofibrin formation and the activity of the fibrin stabilizing factor (FSF) during the cleavage of its SH groups by thrombin. *Thrombos. Diathes. haemorrh.* (Stuttg.): 16, 51-60 (1966).
3. Konishi K., and L. Lorand, *Activation of fibrin stabilizing factor (factor XIII) by thrombin and trypsin.* Abstracts of the 7th Internat. Cong. Biochem. Tokyo J. 381, 1042, (1967).
4. Loewy A., G. Fibrinase (factor XIII). In Fibrinogen and fibrin, Turnover of clotting factors. *Thrombos Diathes. haemorrh.* Suppl. 13, 109-114 (1963).
5. Loewy A. G., S. Matacic and J. H. Darnell, Transamidase activity of the enzyme responsible for insoluble fibrin formation. *Arch. Biochem. Biophys.*: 113, 435-438 (1966).
6. Lorand L., J. Downey, T. Gotoh, A. Jacobsen and S. Tokura. The transpeptidase system which crosslinks fibrin by γ-glutamyl-ε-lysine bonds. *Biochem. Biophys. Res. Comm.*: 31, 222-230 (1968).
7. Lorand L., and A. Jacobsen, Specific inhibitors and the chemistry of fibrin polymerization. *Biochem.*: 3, 1939-1943 (1964).
8. Lorand L., K. Konishi and A. Jacobsen, Transpeptidation mechanism in blood clotting. *Nature*: 194, 1148-1149 (1962).
9. Lorand L. and H. H. Ong, Labelling of amine-acceptor cross-linking sites of fibrin by transpeptidation. *Biochem.*: 5, 1747-1753 (1966).
10. Lorand (Bruner) J., T. Urayama and L. Lorand, Transglutaminase as a blood clotting enzyme. *Biochem. Biophys. Res. Comm.*: 23, 828-834 (1966).
11. Matacic S., and A. G. Loewy, The identification of isopeptide crosslinks in insoluble fibrin. *Biochem. Biophys. Res. Comm.*: 30, 356-362 (1968).
12. Pisano J. J., J. S. Finlayson and M. P. Peyton, Cross-link in Fibrin Polymerized by factor XIII: ε-(γ-glutamyl)lysine. *Science*: 160, 892-893 (1968).

Hemker: At the last F.E.B.S. meeting in Prague (I. Witt, H. Müller, W. Künzer. *F.E.S.B.-abstracts*, 5, 776 (1968)) there was a communication stating that there may be a foetal fibrinogen differing from adult fibrinogen.

M. Blombäck: As yet we have no experience with foetal fibrinogen but we plan to study it in co-operation with Dr. E. Beck.

In this connexion I would like to mention some studies that B. Blombäck and I have made in co-operation with Dr. Mammen and Dr. Prasad on part of the fibrinogen from a Detroit patient, a young girl with a severe hemorrhagic diathesis. There were a total of nine children (of three fathers) in this Negro family. One of the stepsisters also had a severe hemorrhagic diathesis, and the mother and some of the brothers had a mild form. The probandus was found to have a prolonged prothrombin time and an extremely long thrombin time.

The fibrinogen of this patient did slightly inhibit the reaction of thrombin with normal fibrinogen. Fibrinogen could be precipitated just as in normals. Immunoelectrophoretic studies on the patient's fibrinogen indicated a slight divergence from normal. Ultracentrifugation showed a normal sedimentation. Chemical studies of the patient's fibrinogen showed some slight difference in sugar content.

We have examined the tryptic fingerprint of the α(A)-chain fragment (see lecture by B. and M. Blombäck) of the patient's fibrinogen (Fibrinogen Detroit). When we compared the fingerprint with the normal print, we found discrepancies. It was shown that an amino acid substitution (arginine to serine) had occurred at position no. 19 from the N-terminal end.

The tryptic fingerprints of the α(A)-chain fragments of Fibrinogen Paris, Zürich, Baltimore, and Louvain have been investigated. All these fibrinogens appear to contain only normal tryptic fragments.

ON THE STRUCTURE OF THROMBIN AND PROTHROMBIN

S. MAGNUSSON

Eagle and Harris (1) found in 1937 that a clot could be formed from fibrinogen by incubating it with papain. This led them to postulate that the normal fibrinogen-fibrin conversion entails a peptide bond cleavage in fibrinogen and that thrombin is the proteolytic enzyme responsible. Since the previous speakers have dealt in detail with the chemistry of the fibrinogen-fibrin conversion, I shall just briefly summarize the characteristics of thrombin specificity. The synthetic substrates that thrombin has been found to attack most efficiently are arginyl- and lysyl-esters or -amides with a blocked -amino group (2, 3). This predilection for arginyl and lysyl bonds makes the specificity of thrombin appear similar to that of trypsin. In its action on polypeptide and protein substrates, however, thrombin is much more selective than trypsin. In fibrinogen, for example, it splits only four (or eventually six) (4) out of more than a hundred potentially trypsin susceptible bonds. Apart from fibrinogen, only two polypeptide substrates of known structure have been found, namely secretin (5) and cholecystokinin (6). In each case only a single arginyl bond is split.

After it had been shown that thrombin could be inhibited with di-isopropyl phosphorofluoridate (7) (DFP) and that radioactive peptides containing serine could be isolated from a digest of ^{32}P DFP-inhibited thrombin (8), it was clear that thrombin is a serine proteinase like chymotrypsin (9), trypsin (10), and elastase (11). Based on their finding that prothrombin could be activated to thrombin by trypsin, Eagle and Harris (1) also postulated that the activation of prothrombin to thrombin is a proteolytic process.

Bovine prothrombin was found to contain one mole of N-terminal alanine per mole (12, 13). On activation of the prothrombin either in 25% sodium citrate or in the presence of thromboplastin, calcium ions and factor V, a series of new N-terminals appeared in the activation

18

mixture (12). These were mainly isoleucine but also threonine and tyrosine. Their rate of appearance roughly equalled that of thrombin formation (14). When activation mixtures were incubated in the presence of DFP, no thrombin activity and less than ten per cent of the 'normal' amount of N-terminal isoleucine was found (14). Further evidence for the proteolytic nature of prothrombin activation was provided by the finding that carboxpeptidase B could release arginine from thrombin, and arginine and lysine from a thrombinopeptide fraction, whereas no C-terminal amino acid was revealed in prothrombin by either of the carboxypeptidases (15). The finding that bovine thrombin has two N-terminal amino acids, namely isoleucine and threonine (16) strongly indicated that the thrombin structure consists of at least two polypeptide chains.

The first hint of sequence similarities between thrombin and the pancreatic serine proteinases outside the sequence around the active serine was provided by Edman degradation of unmodified human and bovine thrombin. The two thrombins were found to have the sequences Ile-Val-Gly-Gly- and Ile-Val-Glu-Gly-, respectively (17).

Our first step in the investigation of the primary structure of bovine thrombin was to separate the two polypeptide chains after breaking the disulphide bonds by oxidation in performic acid or reduction in mercaptoethanol (18). The A-chain was found to contain 49 amino acid residues and no carbohydrate. Its sequence has been determined by overlapping the sequences found for degradation peptides obtained by chymotryptic and partial or complete tryptic digestion, and is as follows (19):   Thr-Ser-Glu-Asn-His-Phe-Glu-Pro-Phe-Phe-Asx-Glx-Lys-Thr-Phe-Gly-Ala-Gly-Glu-Ala-Asp-Cys-Gly-Leu-Arg-Pro-Leu-Phe-Glu-Lys-Lys-Glu-Val-Glx-Asx-Glx-Thr-Gln-Lys-Glu-Leu-Phe-Glu-Ser-Tyr-Ile-Glu-Gly-Arg. This chain accounts for both the N-terminal threonine and the C-terminal arginine of thrombin. It is quite acidic, having an over-all negative charge of about 4.5 at pH 6.5. It has a very high content of glutamic acid-glutamine (12 residues) and of phenylalanine (6 residues) but completely lacks tryptophan and methionine. The A-chain shows no apparent homology in sequence to the pancreatic serine proteinases.

Evidence for the amino acid sequence of the B-chain has been obtained from tryptic digests of reduced, aminoethylated B-chain (20), and of performic acid oxidised thrombin (20), from a peptic digest of native thrombin (20) and from cyanogen bromide degradation of native thrombin (21).

The B-chain fragments so far account for at least 225 amino acid residues, and extensive sequence homology with chymotrypsin A and trypsin (22, 23), chymotrypsin B (24), and elastase (25) has been found in several areas. The N-terminal is one example of this. If the numbering system for chymotrypsin is used, the B-chain sequence of thrombin from 16 to 32 is as follows:

16   32
Ile- Val- Glu- Gly- Gln- Asp- Ala- Glu- Val- Gly- Leu- Ser- Pro- Trp- Gln-
Gln-Val-Met-

The sequence around the active centre serine (capitalised) is also obviously homologous:

Ile- Thr- Asx- Asx- Met- Phe- Cys- Ala- Gly- Tyr- Lys- Pro- Gly- Glu- Gly-
Lys-Arg- Gly-Asp-Ala- Cys- Glu- Gly-Asp-SER- Gly- Gly- Pro- Phe-Val-
Met-Lys-Ser-Pro-Tyr-Asn-Asn-Arg-Trp-Tyr-Gln-Met-

The C-terminal part of the B-chain has the sequence:
Val-Ile-Asp-Arg-Leu-Gly-Ser.

The N-terminal isoleucine of the B-chain thus accounts for the N-terminal isoleucine found in thrombin (16). The C-terminal serine of the B-chain was not released by carboxypeptidase digestion of thrombin (15). The fact that only one N-terminal alanine could be found in prothrombin (12, 13) indicates that there is probably only one polypeptide chain. Further support for this has been obtained recently. It was found (20) that when bovine prothrombin was subjected to performic acid oxidation and maleylation and then passed through a Sephadex G-200 column, it still emerged with the same effluent volume as native prothrombin and at an approximate molecular weight of 68,000. Therefore, it cannot consist of two disulphide-bridged polypeptide chains. Also, no evidence for dissociation into subunits was found (26) when prothrombin was studied in the ultracentrifuge in 6M guanidine hydrochloride in the presence of 0.5% mercaptoethanol. At the moment therefore, the best guess as to the structure of prothrombin seems to be that it consists of a single polypeptide chain with N-terminal Ala-Asx- (17) containing about 600 residues of which 49 constitute the A-chain of thrombin and about 240 the B-chain, which is probably the C-terminal portion of the zymogen.

REFERENCES

1. Eagle, H., T. N. Harris, *J. gen. Physiol.* 20, 543 (1937).
2. Sherry, S., W. Troll, *J. biol. Chem.* 208, 95 (1954).
3. Elmore, D. T., E. F. Curragh, *Biochem. J.* 86, 9P (1963).
4. Blombäck, B., M. Blombäck, A. Henschen, B. Hessel, S. Iwanaga, K. R. Woods, *Nature*, 218, 130 (1968).
5. Mutt, V., S. Magnusson, E. Jorpes, E. Dahl, *Biochemistry*, 4, 2358 (1965).
6. Mutt, V., *personal communication*.
7. Miller, K. D., M. van Vunakis, *J. biol. Chem.* 223, 227 (1956).
8. Gladner, J. A., K. Laki, *J. Chem. Soc.* 80, 1263 (1958).
9. Brown, J. R., B. S. Hartley, *Biochem. J.* 101, 214 (1966).
10. Walsh, K., H. Neurath, *Proc. Nat. Acad. Sci. U. S.* 52, 884 (1964).
11. Brown, J. R., D. L. Kauffman, B. S. Hartley, *Biochem. J.* 103, 497 (1967).
12. Magnusson, S., *Acta Chem. Scand.* 12, 355 (1958).
13. Miller, K. D., *J. Biol. Chem.* 231, 987 (1958).
14. Magnusson, S., *Arkiv för Kemi*, 23, 271 (1965).
15. Magnusson, S., B. Steele, *Arkiv för Kemi*, 24, 359 (1965).
16. Magnusson, S., *Arkiv för Kemi*, 24, 349 (1965).
17. Magnusson, S., *Arkiv för Kemi*, 24, 375 (1965).
18. Magnusson, S., B. S. Hartley, Unpublished work (1967).
19. Magnusson, S., E. Merler, J. Wootton, B. S. Hartley, Unpublished work (1967).
20. Magnusson, S., B. S. Hartley, Unpublished work (1968).
21. Magnusson, S., K. Simons, B. S. Hartley, Unpublished work (1968).
22. Hartley, B. S., J. R. Brown, D. L. Kauffman, L. B. Smillie, *Nature*, 207, 1157 (1965).
23. Neurath, H., K. A. Walsh, W. P. Winter, *Science*, 158, 1683 (1967).
24. Smillie, L. B., A. Furka, N. Nagabhushan, K. J. Stevenson, C. O. Parkes, *Nature*, 218, 343 (1968).
25. Shotton, D., B. S. Hartley, Unpublished work.
26. Tishkoff, G. H., L. C. Williams, D. M. Brown, *J. biol. Chem.* 243, 4151 (1968).

DISCUSSION

E. Högenauer: Preliminary investigatons on the protein chemistry of factors VII and X.

The impressive results presented by Dr. Magnusson in-dicate that the time is ripe for the application of methods used in molecular biology to solve problems of blood coagulation.

Our group has been engaged in the purification and chemical characterization of the blood-clotting factors VII and X. We felt that this could contribute to the resolution of the unsettled controversy as to whether prothrombin is the common precursor of both these factors.

It is interesting that Dr. Magnusson found that the single peptide chain of prothrombin is changed to a double chain in thrombin. Our findings of two N-terminal amino acids and two C-terminal amino acids in both factor VII and factor X indicates that these factors, too, consist of two polypeptide chains.

We purified both factor VII and factor X by adsorption to $BaSO_4$ and subsequent ion exchange chromatography. In a final purification step, each of the factors was obtained as a homogeneous band by preparative electrophoresis on polyacrylamide gel. Yields, however, were low. For this reason we decided to take advantage of the method described by Gray and Hartley (1) for the determination of terminal amino acids. We found Gly and Ser to be N-terminal amino acids in both factors. By treatment with carboxypeptidase B, the C-terminal amino acids were liberated, labeled with dansyl-Cl, and identified. Ser and Gly proved to be the C-terminal amino acids in both factors. Fingerprints of dansylated tryptic peptides from factors VII and X according to Schmer and Kreil (2) revealed striking similarities (figure 1).

We take this to be preliminary evidence of a close similarity between the primary structures of these two clotting factors. We are quite aware of the fact that our results require supplementation by chemical analysis of factor II before a final answer can be given to the question of whether factors VII and X orginate from prothrombin.

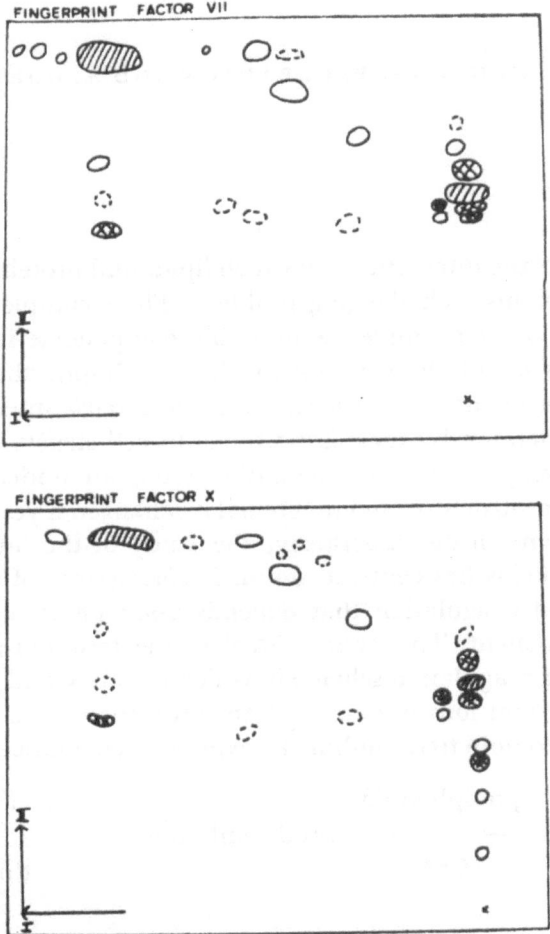

Fig. 1. Fingerprints of dansylated tryptic peptides from factor VII (above) and factor X (below).

REFERENCES

1. W. R. Gray, B. S. Hartley, *Biochem. J.* 89, 379 (1963).
2. G. Schmer, G. Kreil, *J. Chromatog.* 28, 458 (1967).

THE INTERACTIONS OF PROTHROMBIN AND FACTORS V AND X WITH PHOSPHOLIPIDS AND CALCIUM IONS

J. HANAHAN, P. G. BARTON AND A. COX

Clarification of the interactions by which lipids and proteins form large complexes remains a challenging problem. These complexes occur in diverse forms – for example, as insoluble components in cell membranes and as soluble lipoproteins in plasma. Despite the interesting speculation on membrane structure and the intense interest in these complexes generated by their importance to cell structure and function, lipid transport, blood coagulation, etc., an understanding of their formation, structure, and functional mechanism is yet to come.

For some time in our laboratory, the study of the interactions of lipids and proteins has centered on an *in vitro* system of a particular phase of blood coagulation that depends upon phospholipids as an essential component. This system involves the terminal stage of the intrinsic blood coagulation scheme in which factors v and x, phospholipids and calcium ions interact to form prothrombinase, which can convert prothrombin to thrombin. To express it schematically:

$$\left.\begin{array}{l} \text{factor v} \\ \text{factor x} \\ \quad\downarrow \\ \text{factor } x_a \end{array}\right\} \xrightarrow[\quad Ca^{2+}\quad]{\text{phospholipid}} \text{prothrombinase} \rightarrow \begin{array}{c} \text{prothrombin} \\ \downarrow \\ \text{thrombin} \end{array}$$

As indicated above, factor v as isolated from blood plasma can participate in the formation of prothrombinase, but plasma factor x must be converted to an activated form, x_a. This activation can be accomplished *in vivo* by factor viii and *in vitro* by such agents as trypsin or Russell's viper venom. Subsequently, factors v and x_a react with a phospholipid mixture (e.g., phosphatidyl serine and phosphatidyl choline) in the presence of calcium ions to yield a prothrombin activator, prothrombinase. This latter entity, as indicated below, is a large-

24

molecular-weight complex or lipoprotein. It should be emphasized, however, that the system discussed here consists of an *in vitro* (or isolated) reaction sequence and does not necessarily proceed by the exact steps operative in an *in vivo* system where the lipid is furnished by platelets, most probably as a lipoprotein. Nonetheless, the reactions in this experimental system closely mimic the reactions observed *in vivo*. For purposes of defining the various facets of these interactions, it is an excellent system for study.

Evidence was presented some time ago that in the *in vitro* system, factors v and x_a would interact to form an active prothrombinase only if phospholipids and calcium ions were present (1). In addition, the chemical identity of the phospholipid was not quite as important as the surface charge of the cluster that had been added to the reaction mixture. (Since the word 'micelle' connotes structure, whereas none is here implied, 'cluster' or 'aggregate' appear to be better terms.) Thus, a mixture of phosphatidyl choline (PC) and phosphatidyl ethanolamine (PE) or phosphatidyl serine (PS) and PE in the proper ratio, and at the correct pH, was very active in promoting prothrombinase activity. Yet, each of these compounds alone had low activity.

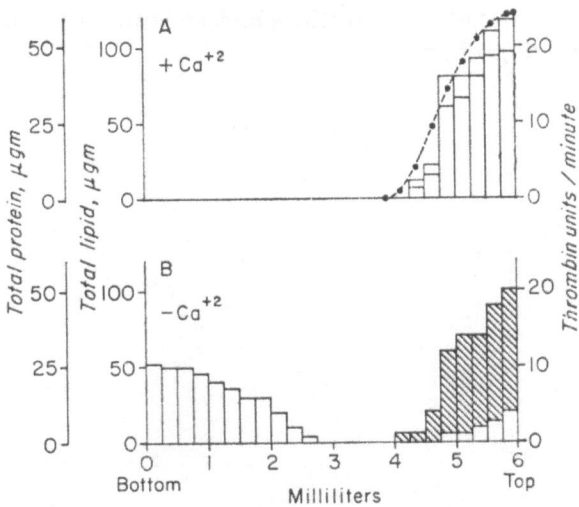

Fig. 1. Adjusted density centrifugation of prothrombin activation mixture in the presence (A) and absence (B) of calcium ions. Fractions of 0.25 ml were analyzed for prothrombin activator (—●—●—), total lipid (hatched bars) and total protein (open bars).

The properties of the prothrombinase were first investigated using purified factors v and x_a, PS and PC, with and without $CaCl_2$. These preparations with their high prothrombinase activity were subjected to adjusted density centrifugation, yielding the data presented in figure 1 (average values from three experiments). When $CaCl_2$ was present in the mixture, all of the prothrombin converting activity, 95% of the phospholipid, and 90% of the protein were recovered in the top 1.5 ml of the tube, indicating that the prothrombinase had a hydrated density of less than 1.04 g/ml under these conditions. Omission of $CaCl_2$ from the medium during centrifugation resulted in total loss of activity in all fractions. Although at least 95% of the lipid remained in the top 1.8 ml, 87% of the protein now sedimented into the bottom half of the tube.

This technique suggests that the complete activator is analogous to a low density lipoprotein that can be dissociated into a low density lipid fraction and high density protein fraction by the removal of calcium ions. A further attempt was made to determine more accurately the hydrated density of the complex through the use of a density gradient technique. In a linear 5-25% sucrose gradient, the complex sedimented to a point about one-third down the tube (figure 2). According to the average of data from six tubes in two centrifugation runs, the density of the sucrose solution at this point was 1.02 ±0.01 g/ml. This corresponds to densities characteristic of S_f class 0—10 or low density β-lipoprotein.

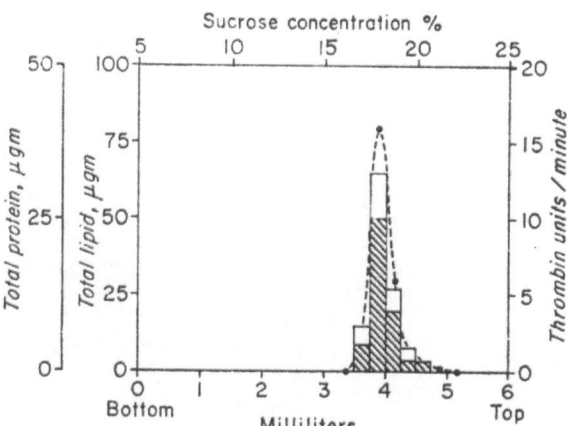

Fig. 2. Density gradient centrifugation of prothrombin activation mixture in a 5-25% sucrose gradient in the presence of calcium ions. Fractions of 0.25 ml were analyzed for prothrombin activator (—●—●—), total lipid (hatched bars) and total protein (open bars).

Dependence of prothrombinase formation upon concentrations of the interacting lipids and proteins (factors v and x_a) has been investigated to some extent. When a series of dilutions of a prothrombinase solution was examined for activity, the activity was found to decrease linearly with increasing dilution, up to a dilution of 20:1. At this point, complete loss of activity which could not be reversed was caused by changing the medium to 0.025 M $CaCl_2$. Activity could be restored by suspending the pellet obtained by centrifuging this diluted solution (15 min at 40,000 rpm in the Spinco Model L, SW 39 rotor) in a minimum volume of 0.025 M $CaCl_2$. Serial dilution of this suspension produced the same effect as before, with total loss of activity at the same critical concentration. Obviously, this relationship is complex, and more evidence must be gathered to affirm the significance of these observations.

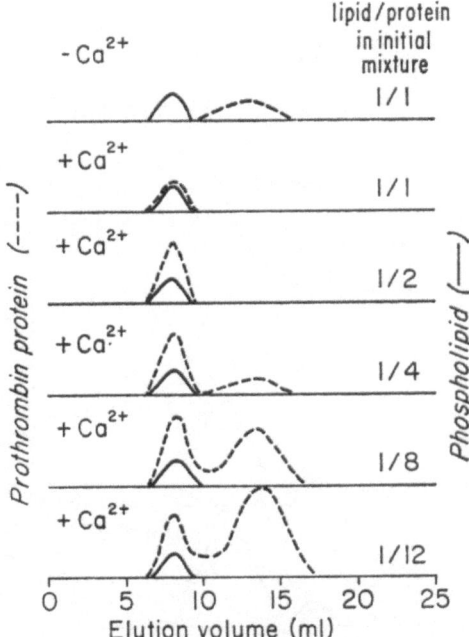

Fig. 3. Stoichiometry of the lipid-protein complex. Samples of 0.5 ml containing 1.0-12 mg/ml prothrombin and 1 mg/ml PS/PC in 0.025 M $CaCl_2$ were incubated 4 minutes prior to chromatography on Sephadex G-200 at room temperature. Elution was carried out with Michaelis buffer containing the same concentration of Ca^{2+}. The distribution of prothrombin between the two components (Ve 7.1-7.2 and Ve 11.7-11.9) was calculatied from areas under the peaks in each experiment.

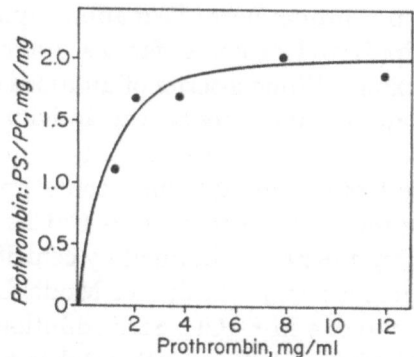

Fig. 4. Adsorption isotherm of prothrombin onto PS/PC constructed from the data in figure 3.

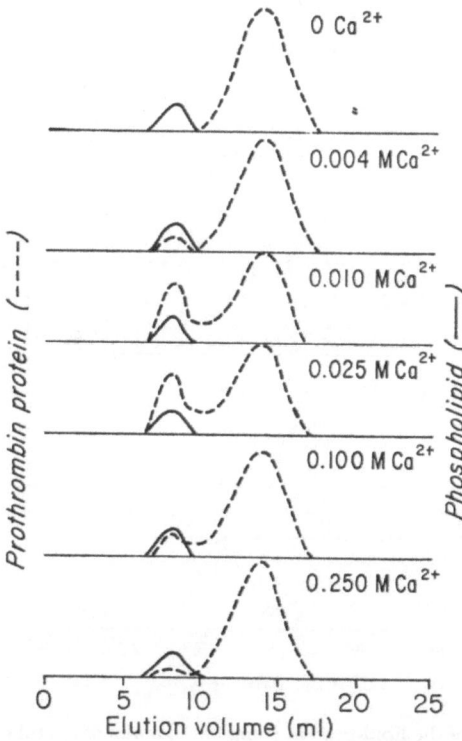

Fig. 5. Effect of CaCl₂ concentration. Samples of o.5 ml containing 12mg/ml prothrombin adn 1 mg/ml PS/PC in buffer (0-0.25 M CaCl₂) were incubated and chromatographed on Sephadex G-200 and the distribution of prothrombin was determined as described for previous experiments.

Factors v and x_a were shown by gel filtration chromatography to be bound to the phospholipid clusters independently, regardless of the presence or absence of the other. Prothrombin was also shown to be bound independently. Figure 3 depicts the chromatographic patterns of prothrombin with varying amounts of a sonicated mixture of PS:PC (50:50 w/w). The ratios of the areas under the peaks representing prothrombin are plotted in figure 4. Clearly, the prothrombin was bound and, whatever the mechanism, the apparent binding constant must be large. The necessity for calcium ions is clarified in figure 5, which shows the chromatographic patterns obtained when calcium ion concentration alone was varied. The order of addition of the components was important; prothrombin had to be added to the phospholipids before calcium ion, or precipitation of the lipids resulted.

The binding of prothrombin to the phospholipid cluster as well as the necessity for calcium ion were also demonstrated in the analytical ultracentrifuge. When prothrombin and a sonicated mixture of phospholipids were centrifuged at 59,000 rpm, the lipid clusters sedimented rapidly to the bottom of the cell – long before the prothrombin (figure 6). When calcium ion was present, however, the prothrombin sedimented along with the lipid clusters. Similar results were obtained by this method for the binding of prothrombin to a sonicated mixture of PE:PC (50:50, w/w).

The interaction of prothrombin with a PS:PC dispersion contrasts with the inability of some other proteins (thrombin, albumin, and α_1-acid-glycoprotein) to form complexes under similar conditions with the same phospholipids (table 1). These observations may indicate the existence of some chemical or physical characteristic peculiar to the prothrombin molecule whereby it can adsorb to the phospholipid cluster. The possibility was considered that complex formation could be due to the presence of specific residues, such as neuraminic acids or uronic acids, having free negatively charged groups. However, neither free neuraminic acids nor an α_1-acid-glycoprotein containing neuraminic acid appear to complex PS:PC under these conditions (2) and uronic acids are reportedly absent from prothrombin (3).

Binding of the various protein factors to the surface of the lipid cluster is the usually accepted concept, although proof has been lacking. Our measurements of the difference spectra of the aromatic absorption region offer evidence that the contact of protein and lipid is limited. Table 2 lists the results of the difference spectroscopy ex-

Table 1. Chromatography on sephadex G-200 in veronal acetate, pH 7.35; PS/PS, 50/50, (w/w).

Sample	Ca^{2+} in eluting buffer and sample	Ve
Dextran Blue 2000	—	7.1 — 7.2
Sucrose	—	18.6
Phosphatidyl serine (PS)/Phosphatidyl choline (PC)	±	7.1 — 7.2
Prothrombin		
a. alone	±	11.7 — 11.9
b. plus PS/PC*	—	7.1 — 7.2
		11.7 — 11.9
c. plus PS/PC*	+	7.1 — 7.2
Thrombin		
a. alone	±	13.8 — 14.1
b. plus PS/PC*	±	7.1 — 7.2
		13.9 — 14.1
Albumin		
a. alone	±	12.5 — 12.6
b. plus PS/PC*	±	7.1 — 7.2
		12.5 — 12.6
α-Acid Glycoprotein		
a. alone	±	12.5 — 12.8
b. plus PS/PC*	±	7.1 — 7.2
		12.5 — 12.8

* Mixtures incubated at 37° for 4 minutes prior to chromatography.

Table 2. Difference spectra of prothrombin

Solvent	% residues perturbed*		Light scattering
	Tyr	*Trp*	
0.001 M CaCl$_2$	0	0	+
0.001 M CaCl$_2$ plus 1% PS/PC	0	0	—
20% v/v DMSO	25	25	0
20% v/v Glycerol	25	25	0

* The % residue values perturbed by dimethylsulfoxide and glycerol were estimated from the perturbation of model compounds by dimethylsulfoxide and glycol, respectively (unpubl. data A. C. Cox).

periments. A difference spectrum was obtained with glycerol and with dimethylsulfoxide in 20% v/v concentration which were typical of those of solvent perturbation of tyrosyl and tryptophyl residues located at the surface of proteins (4). (The difference spectra of solvent perturbation arise from the slight shifting of the absorption band by a change in the polarizability of the environment of these residues.) Calcium ions with or without a PS:PC dispersion did not induce a perturbation of these residues. Therefore, the calcium ions are not linked directly to these residues or even bound in close proximity to them.

Furthermore, the lipid cluster must not replace the solvent that is in contact with these residues. The binding of prothrombin in a lipid matrix, as is graphically represented in figure 7b, is excluded since the solvent in contact with the residues has been displaced.

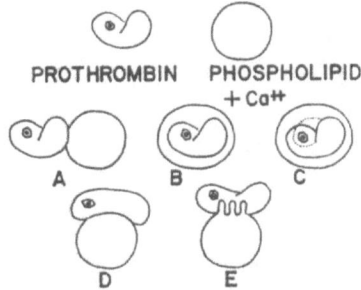

Fig. 7. The possible forms of binding of prothrombin to the phospholipids in the presence of calcium ions. An aromatic amino acid residue is depicted on the surface of the prothrombin. In B the aromatic group is no longer exposed to the solvent and in C the dashed line represents the incorporation of the solvent with the prothrombin within the lipid matrix. The conformations of the depicted prothrombin and phospholipid cluster are not meant to imply the actual conformations of either.

The form of binding represented in figure 7A meets the requirements of the experimental data. However, the type of binding depicted in 7c, where the solvent around these residues is incorporated along with the protein into the lipid matrix, cannot be ruled out. However, even in 7A the contact of lipid with protein has been limited by the presence of this solvent.

The conformational changes of prothrombin on being bound to the phospholipid cluster (as represented by figure 7D and E) are probably limited or absent. Extensive changes should have given rise to a difference spectrum. More convincingly, however, little difference in the optical rotatory dispersion (ORD) of prothrombin in the free or bound state was detectable in the 230—400 m µ wavelength region. This lack of change in the ORD indicates that the conformation does not change and also supports the concept of surface binding, since no apparent solvent effect (on the ORD) was induced by binding of the phospholipid cluster.

Figure 8 shows the ORD curve of prothrombin. The apparent α-helicity of prothrombin is very small, whether estimated from the $[\alpha']_{233}$ (5) or the $b_0 = -21$ obtained from the Yang-Moffit plot (6).

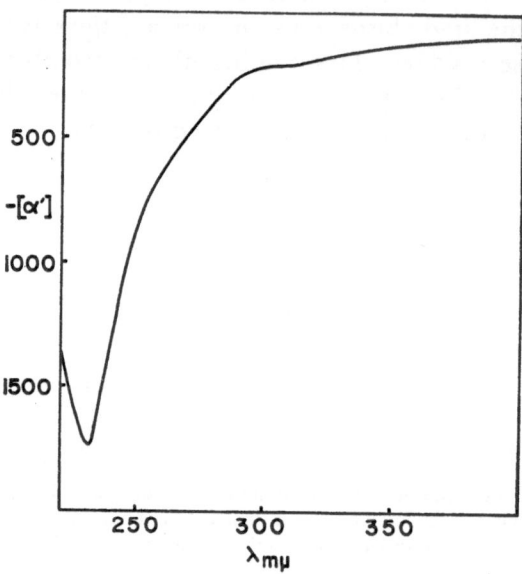

Fig. 8. The optical ratatory dispersion of bovine prothrombin in 0.15 M KCl, pH 7.4 at a concentration of 0.1 - 0.02 g/100 cc.

(The apparent α-helicity is obtained from the linear interpolation between the values for 0 and 100% α-helix, which are for $[\alpha']_{233}$-2000 and -12,000 and for $b_0 = 0$ and -630). The parameter from this plot was -244. The specific rotation at 400 m µ was about 15% less between the measurements on prothrombin solutions of 0.1 g/100cc or less and the 3.8 g/100cc solution used in the measurement of the specific rotation from 400—600 m µ for the Yang-Moffit plot. This difference probably arises from the aggregation of prothrombin at the higher concentration.

As mentioned above, a negative charge on the phospholipids is required for optimum clotting activity. We have studied in more detail

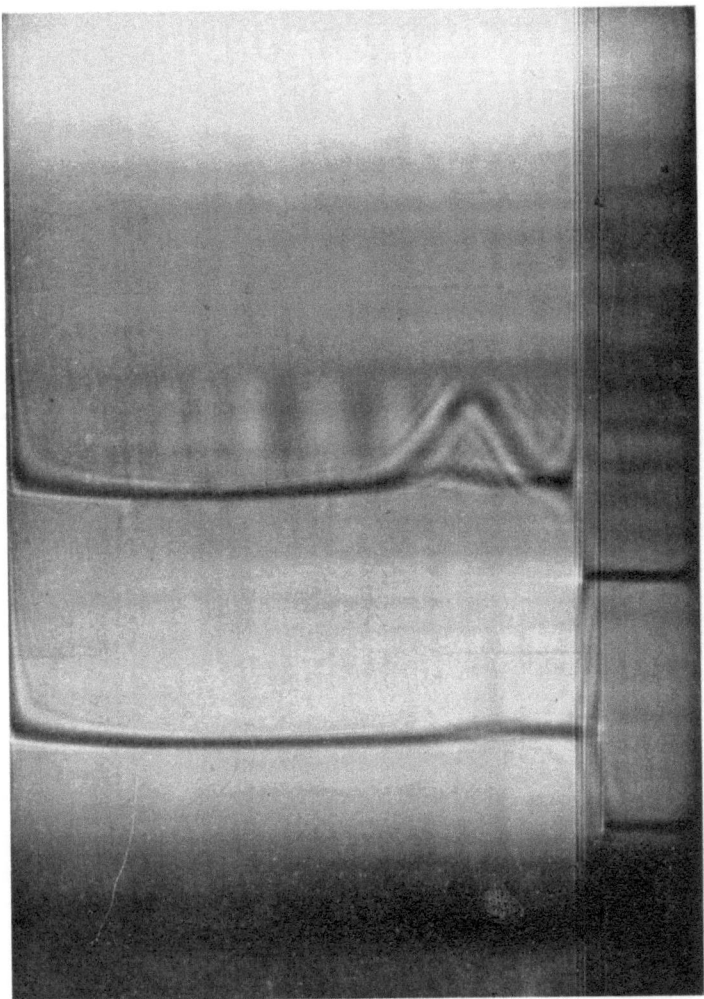

Fig. 6. The schlieren pattern of prothrombin with phospholipids during ultracentrifugation. In the upper pattern, prothrombin sediments alone whereas the lipids had sedimented to the bottom (left) of the cell. This compartment contained no calcium. The base line was the lipid solution without prothrombin and shows that a little lipid sediments with approximately the same rate.

The lower pattern shows that only this lipid or perhaps a little prothrombin sediments at the same rate when calcium is present. The base line was a 0.1 M KCl solution. The concentrations were 0.2 g/100 ml of the sonicated mixture of phosphatidylserine - phosphatidylcholine (50/20 w/w), 0.4 g/100 ml of prothrombin and 0.01 M CaCl$_2$ in each solution containing these compounds.

the calcium ion binding to PE:PC mixtures to determine the importance
of this negative charge on this ion binding. In the case of the sonicated
mixture of PE:PC, however, the origin of the negative charge on the
cluster was not obvious. The apparent pK_a for the amino group of PE
was reported to be 9.1 by Garvin and Karnovsky (7); this value was
measured in 2-ethoxy-ethanol and corrected to a water solution on the
basis of model compounds. We synthesized ethyl-O-phosphoryletha-
nolamine and measured an apparent pK_a of 9.4 for the amino group
in water (figure 9). If the true pK_a for the amino group of PE is 9.4,
little charge would appear on the cluster at pH 7.4 (the usual pH for
clotting assays). The titration curve of the mixed lipid cluster (figure 9)

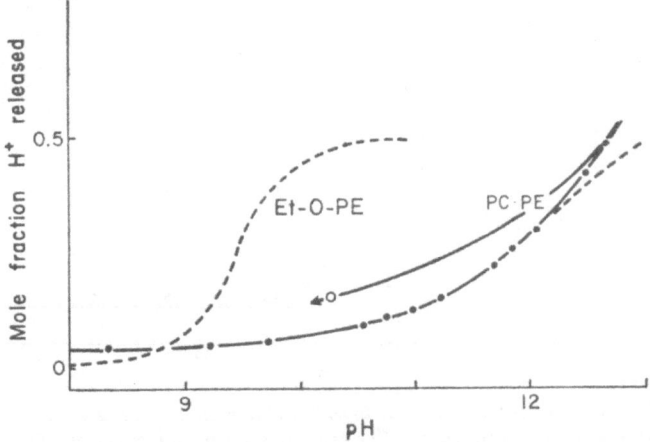

Fig. 9. Hydrogen ion titration curve of a sonicated mixture of phosphatidylethanolamine
(PE) and phosphatidylcholine (PC) (50/50 w/w). The curve does not represent a true equilibrium titration since the titration is not reversible. The equilibrium curve should lie somewhere between the two curves. The ethyl phosphorylethanolamine (ETOPE) curve is plotted
on a scale comparable to the amount of phosphatidylethanolamine present in the mixture.

indicated that a larger fraction of the groups had been titrated at pH
7.4 than would have been expected on the basis of the K_a given for the
amino group. Most of the amino groups titrate at pH values considerably higher than expected on the basis of the pK_a of 9.4. The negative
charge arises from the wide distribution of the apparent pK's of the
amino groups. This wide distribution probably results from a combination of factors.

The binding of calcium ions to the PE:PC mixture (figure 10) was
studied by use of the calcium ion specific electrode (Orion). Very few

or no calcium ions were bound at low calcium ion concentrations. Calcium ions at higher concentrations were bound to the mixed lipid clusters, but were either not bound or were sparsely bound to PC clusters. During the binding of calcium ions to the mixed lipid clusters, a small percentage of hydrogen ions was released with respect to the number of calcium ions bound (measured by the amount of base necessary to restore the pH to its original value prior to the addition of $CaCl_2$). Therefore an increase in pH and in negative charge on the lipid cluster must increase the number of calcium ions bound.

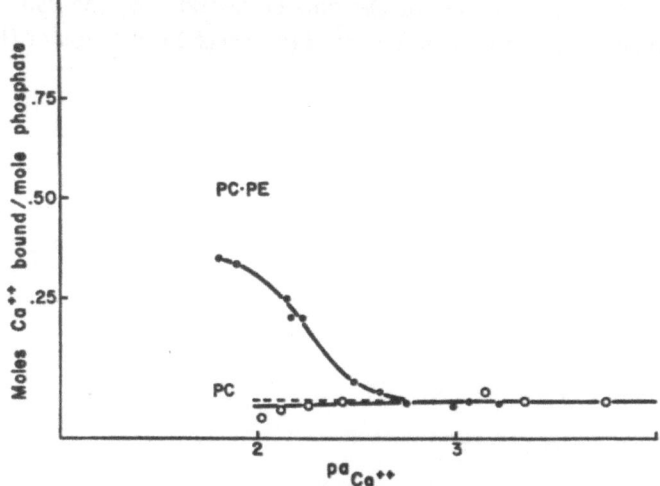

Fig. 10. Calcium ion titration curves of phosphatidylcholine alone and as a (50/50 w/w) mixture of phosphatidylethanolamine. The calcium ion titration curve of ethylphosphoryle-thanolamine was the same as that of the phosphatidylcholine.

Binding of calcium ions to the phospholipid cluster would appear to be a property of the cluster rather than of a group on an individual lipid molecule. As shown in figure 10, the calcium ion activity was not affected by ethylphosphorylethanolamine, which suggests that calcium ions are bound to the cluster because of the proximity of the polar ends of two phospholipid molecules.

The calcium ion titration curve of PE:PC clusters at higher calcium ion concentrations than in figure 10 shows a break indicating that the titration is biphasic. If the curve expected for the titration of one phase is subtracted from the other, then the first phase represents the binding of one calcium ion for each four phospholipid molecules, or perhaps one calcium ion for each two PE molecules.

The negative charge on the phospholipid cluster is necessary for optimum performance in the clotting system because of the effect of this charge on calcium ion binding. The increase of calcium ion binding with increased charge on the PE:PC cluster has been shown above. Recently, Barton (8) has reported electrophoretic measurements indicating the charge to be reversed by calcium ion binding for mixtures of PS:PC and PC with phosphatidic acid. Both of these mixed phospholipid dispersions have been shown to be active in the clotting assay. Therefore, a negative charge on the lipid cluster would not appear to be important for binding of the proteins *per se*.

Prothrombin activation by factor x_a is greatly accelerated by adding phospholipids, factor v, and calcium ions. Neither the phospholipids nor the factor v alone, however, can activate prothrombin; they only increase the rate of conversion (9). Factor x_a presumably activates prothrombin by proteolytic cleavage of specific, susceptible bonds. One explanation for the effect of phospholipid clusters on the generation of thrombin could be that the prothrombin structure is modified in such a way as to effect greater exposure of susceptible bonds. However, the gross structure of prothrombin appears unaltered when bound to the surface of the phospholipid cluster, since no difference spectrum or change in ORD occurred.

That the gross conformation remains unchanged by the binding of prothrombin implies that no part of the lipids has become inserted into prothrombin. If, for example, part of the binding force were derived from insertion of hydrocarbon tails of the fatty acyl residues of the phospholipids into prothrombin, the gross structure would have to expand to accommodate these residues (figure 7E). Also, because prothrombin cannot be unfolded and spread on the surface of the lipid cluster, a rather limited area must be involved in the binding – perhaps even a specific site and therefore a specific orientation.

The binding of prothrombin to prothrombinase in a specific orientation could explain the effect of phospholipid on the rate of thrombin generation, but it adds little to our understanding of the role of factor v in this process. Recently, Hemker et al. (10) reported kinetic experiments which suggest that no interaction occurs between the protein factors that would increase the binding constants of any of the factors. This would also appear to rule out factor v as causing a conformational change in either factor x_a or prothrombin. In fact, it is difficult to imagine what factor v does to accelerate thrombin generation. For this reason, the continued study of the gross conformations of the factors as affected by their binding, separately and together, on the phospholipid clusters will be actively pursued.

REFERENCES

1. Papahadjopoulos, D., D. J. Hanahan, *Biochem. Biophys. Acta* 90, 346 (1964).
2. Schultze, H. E., *Deutsche Med. Wochschr.* 83, 1742 (1958).
3. Hjort, P. F., *Scand. J. Clin. Lab. Invest.* 9, suppl. 27, 1 (1957).
4. Herskovits, T. T., M. Laskowski, *J. Biol. Chem.* 237, 2481 (1962).
5. Simmons, N. S., C. Cohen, A. G. Szent-Gyorgyi, D. E. Wetlaufer, E. R. Blout, *J. Amer. Chem. Soc.* 83, 4766 (1961).
6. Moffit, W., J. T. Yang, *Proc. Nat. Acad. Sci.* 42, 596 (1956).
7. Garvin, J. E., M. L. Karnovsky, *J. Biol. Chem.* 221, 211 (1956).
8. Barton, P. G., *J. Biol. Chem.* 243, 3884 (1968).
9. Barton, P. G., C. Jackson, D. J. Hanahan, *Nature* 214, 923 (1967).
10. Hemker, H. C., M. P. Esnouf, P. W. Hemker, A. C. W. Swart and R. G. MacFarlane, *Nature* 215, 248 (1967).

DISCUSSION

M. J. P. Kahn: On the influence of monoinositolphospholipid on prothrombinase generation

I would like to present some data concerning factors influencing the activity of prothrombinase. Prothrombinase activity very probably results from the adsorption of factor v and factor x_a on a phospholipid cluster in the presence of Ca-ions. High Ca-ion concentrations inhibit factor v adsorption but enhance the adsorption of factor x_a. In the presence of monoinositolphospolipid (MPI) prepared from beef brain, the adsorption of the factors v and x_a on phospholipid clusters is very much disturbed. Previous experimental data (Kahn and Bourgain) have demonstrated that the anticoagulant action of MPI was due to the inhibition of the prothrombin-thrombin conversion. Furthermore, it was found that as soon as prothrombinase had gained its full activity, no inhibition by MPI could be elicited. It seems possible that the anticoagulant activity of MPI goes hand in hand with the disturbance of the adsorption of factor v and x_a on phospholipid clusters caused by MPI.

We have studied the adsorption of factors v and x_a from fractions that were not pure (e.g. from $BaSO_4$-adsorbed plasma and from serum). This has the additional advantage that the conditions in the test are closer to physiological conditions. In this type of experiment, the formation of small amounts of thrombin from residual serum-prothrombin or prothrombin still present in $BaSO_4$-adsorbed plasma is possible. For this reason, a small amount of hirudin was added, which specifically neutralizes the thrombin that may be generated in the test. The reaction mixture consists of $BaSO_4$-adsorbed plasma, phospholipid, Ca^{++} and hirudin or of a mixture of serum, phospholipid, Ca^{++} and hirudin. The mixture is first incubated at 37°C for 9 minutes. Half the volume of the mixture is kept at 4°C after addition of 0.1 ml veronal acetate buffer (pH 7.35). The other half is centrifuged at

37

100,000 g. for 35 minutes at 4°C. The supernatant is decanted and 0.1 ml of a phospholipid suspension added so as to restore the original concentration of phospholipid. The barely visible sediment is resuspended in veronal acetate buffer (pH 7.35) containing the same concentration of hirudin and calcium as the original incubation mixture. The testing of serial dilutions of non-centrifuged incubation mixture provides a reference curve. The factor v and factor x_a activities of the supernatant and the resuspended sediment are indicated in table I as a percentage of that of the noncentrifuged mixture. Identical experiments were also performed in the presence of MPI. In the presence of

Table 1

Ca ion concentration (mM)	Percentage of clotting factor activity adsorbed			
	factor v		factor x	
	without MPI	with MPI	without MPI	with MPI
0	82	72	34	90
40	64	74	50	96
90	1	76	85	94

Ca ion concentration (mM)	Percentage of clotting factor activity found on sediment			
	factor v		factor x	
	without MPI	with MPI	without MPI	with MPI
0	18	0.8	1	0.1
40	4	2	2.5	0.01
90	0.5	0.05	5	0.01

The final concentration of MPI was 40 mcg/ml.
The figures give the mean of five different experiments.
In each experiment each determination was carried out eight times.
The percentage adsorbed is calculated as the amount that disappeared from the supernatant.
All concentrations are expressed as a percentage of the non-centrifuged control.

the MPI there was an increased adsorption of factors v and x_a on the phospholipid cluster. Furthermore, the adsorption was no longer dependent upon the calcium ion concentration. Factor v and x_a activity was lower in the sediment in the presence of MPI. We concluded that the presence of MPI leads to a disturbance of the way in which factor v and x_a are adsorbed on the phospholipid cluster and therefore inhibits the activation of factor II by this complex.

A possible mechanism could be a modification in the electrostatic properties of the lipoprotein moiety by addition of MPI. Indeed, Abramson (1968) has described strong surface-charges for MPI at pH values between 6.5 and 7.5. The pH of our reaction mixture lay in this range. When the physicochemical characteristics of purified factor v and x_a are more clearly understood, they may provide support for this hypothesis.

Denson: I would like to ask Dr. Hemker wether he thinks that the adsorption in the presence of very high levels of calcium ions has any physiologic significance, since the physiologic calcium concentrations are only between 1 and 2 millimolar?

Hemker: The advantage in doing adsorptions over a wide range of calcium concentrations lies in the possibility it offers to differentiate between the adsorption of factors v and x, because these adsorptions are influenced by calcium ions in an opposite way.

High calcium ion concentrations prevent the adsorption of factor v and favour the binding of factor x. Low calcium ion concentrations do just the opposite. The physiological calcium concentration is somewhere at a point where both factors v and x are adsorbed, as might of course be expected. Every experimental situation is an artefact, and good experiments are useful artefacts. I feel that changing the calcium concentration in adsorption experiments is useful.

THE NATURE OF PROTHROMBINASE

M. P. ESNOUF

Although Morawitz postulated in 1905 that thrombin was derived from an inactive precursor, prothrombin, which is present in plasma, it is only comparatively recently that the mechanism by which this conversion takes place is becoming understood. One of the difficulties in understanding this process has been the change made by Dr. Seegers and his colleagues in the definition of prothrombin as envisaged by Morawitz; that is, that thrombin is the unique derivative of prothrombin. Throughout this paper, prothrombin is referred to in its original sense.

It is now becoming clear that the physiological conversion of prothrombin requires two coagulation factors, factor x_a and factor v, in addition to bivalent metal ions and phospholipid. Before describing what is known of the interaction of the proteins, a brief resumé of the properties of the individual components will be given.

ACTIVATED FACTOR X (x_a)

Factor x_a can be derived by the interaction of the components of the extrinsic clotting system (1, 2, 3) or by the intrinsic system after the contact of blood with a foreign surface (4, 5).

x_a can also be obtained by incubating factor x with trypsin (6) or with the coagulant protein from Russell's viper venom (7). There is no evidence at present to suggest that x_a produced by the various activating systems is chemically similar however, although the biological properties are the same.

Most workers would agree that x_a (autoprothrombin C), is an enzyme which has a molecular weight on the order of 24,000 (8).

Besides coagulant activity, x_a has esterolytic activity on those synthetic ester substrates that contain arginine (7, 9). Both the esterolytic activity and the coagulant activity of x_a are inhibited by plasma antithrombin (10) and by soya bean trypsin inhibitor but not by pancreatic trypsin inhibitor (7, 11). x_a is also inhibited by 2,3 dimercapto-propan (12, 13). Diisopropyl fluorophosphate (DFP) inhibits both the coagulant and esterolytic activity of x_a (13) but not as rapidly as does phenyl methyl sulphonyl fluoride (14).

Recently, Leveson (13) isolated serine O.^{32}P after hydrolysis of x_a previously reacted with DF^{32}P. x_a slowly converts factor II to thrombin (II_a), a reaction which is independent of calcium ions (11, 15, 16). x_a will also activate chymotrypsinogen (17) but has little caseinolytic activity (18).

FACTOR V

Until recently, attempts at purification were hampered by the instability of the preparations. However, stable preparations of bovine factor v are now available. The amino acid composition has been determined, and only 75 per cent of the weight of the protein appears to be due to its amino acid content (11). These authors obtained a molecular weight of 291,000 from sedimentation studies; Barton and Hanahan (19) obtained two components, both having biological activity, with molecular weights of 350,000 and 70,000 as obtained from gel filtration experiments. Other authors using different preparations have given values of 180,000 from sedimentation data (20), 200,000 based on gel filtration experiments (21), and 98,000 calculated from amino acid analysis (22). The electrophoretic mobility of factor v in 0.1 M sodium phosphate buffer at pH 7.0 was found to be 3.3 $\times$ 10^{-5}v/cm^2/sec (11).

The factors influencing the instability of factor v preparations have been investigated (11, 19, 23, 24); it has been concluded that the decay of factor v activity is a physical process and that Ca^{++} ions are an important factor in stabilizing factor v in the high molecular weight form. The inactivation of the protein found on prolonged storage in 0.1 M phosphate is accompanied by a slight change in the tertiary structure (11).

The mechanism by which thrombin increases the reactivity of factor v preparations, mentioned in a previous section, is not understood. Esnouf & Jobin (11), were not able to find any increase in activity in the presence of thrombin, but rather a progressive loss in activity was observed, although the activity of impure preparations was stimulated by the addition of thrombin. Barton & Hanahan (19), on the other hand, obtained a spontaneous increase in activity of about threefold on adding thrombin, and Papahadjopoulos, Hougie & Hanahan (21) found a considerably greater activation by thrombin, which increased over a period of 5 minutes and was accompanied by a reduction in the molecular weight of the factor v, to 150,000 as judged by gel filtration.

PROTHROMBIN

The literature contains descriptions of several methods for the preparation of prothrombin, the type of preparation depends on whether the particular group of workers accepts the prothrombin complex to be prothrombin or whether the aim has been to obtain the unique zymogen of thrombin (factor II).

The other problem which arises and is reflected in the nature of the final product is the cleanness and rapidity with which the blood is collected and mixed with anticoagulant. Lamy and Waugh (25) give a molecular weight of 69,000 for the complex, which is in good agreement with that of 70,500 obtained by Tishkoff et al. (26). The latter authors showed that whereas this preparation appeared homogeneous as regards M_w, it was heterogeneous when examined by disc electrophoresis, and further that the other components of the complex could be partially separated by gel filtration.

The amino acid composition of the bovine prothrombin complex has been determined (27), as has that of prothrombin (28), the significant differences between the results of the analysis by the different authors probably being due to differences in the material analysed. Prothrombin complex and prothrombin contain carbohydrate, which includes hexoseamine and sialic acid (27, 29) and evidence has been obtained that the carbohydrate is terminated by sialic acid (26).

PROTHROMBIN ACTIVATION

The principal chemical difference between the preparations of prothrombin complex and prothrombin, is that prothrombin complex is slowly converted to thrombin on incubation with 25 per cent sodium citrate (30), while prothrombin is unaffected by citrate (28, 31). The latter authors suggest that the citrate activation of the prothrombin complex is due to the factor x present in the complex. The prothrombin complex is also converted slowly to thrombin on standing with the synthetic polycations poly L-lysine, poly L-ornithine, and protamine (32).

The N-terminal amino acid of bovine prothrombin complex and

prothromin is alanine (28, 33). On citrate activation several new N-terminal acids appeared, which, expressed as moles/mole of original N-terminal alanine, were isoleucine 2.20: glycine 0.95; glutamine 0.7; small amounts of phenylalanine, aspartic acid, and threonine were also found. Biological activation yielded essentially the same N-terminal amino acids, except that 1 mole of N-terminal threonine was found. The yield of N-terminal amino acids was depressed by the addition of DFP (28). These results are consistent with the idea that in both activation systems, prothrombin is cleaved in the same way. In the original cascade hypothesis put forward by Macfarlane (34), it was suggested that x_a converted factor v to an enzyme, which in turn converted factor II to thrombin. However, Papahadjopoulos and Hanahan (35), Barton et al. (16), Jobin and Esnouf (11), Hemker et al. (36) and Baker and Seegers (37), using purified reagents, synthetic substrates, and from kinetic studies, have come to the conclusion that factor v_a is not formed. Instead, factor v appears to accelerate the rate of thrombin formation when added to mixtures of x_a and factor II in the presence of metal ions. Factor v can, therefore, be considered as a high molecular weight cofactor for x_a. So far, the mechanism by which factor v acts is not clear, although it has been found that the esterase activity of x_a is unaffected by the addition of factor v. It may be that either factor v increases the affinity of the enzyme (x_a) for the substrate (factor II) or that the conformation of substrate is modified by factor v, rendering it more susceptible to the action of x_a.

REFERENCES

1. Williams, W. J., D. G. Norris, *J. Biol. Chem.* 241, 1847 (1966).
2. Nemerson, Y., *Biochemistry* 5, 601 (1966).
3. Denson, K. W. E., *The use of antibodies in the study of blood coagulation* (1967) Blackwells, Oxford.
4. MacFarlane, R. G., R. Biggs, B. J. Ash, K. W. E. Denson, *Brit. J. Haematol.* 10, 530 (1964).
5. Lundblad, R. L., E. W. Davie, *Biochemistry* 4, 113 (1965).
6. Hanahan, D. J., D. Papahadjopoulos, *Thromb. Diathes haemorrhag.* suppl. 17, 71 (1965).
7. Williams, W. J., M. P. Esnouf, *Biochem. J.* 84, 52 (1962).
8. Seegers, W. H., E. R. Cole, C. R. Harmison, E. Marciniak, *Can. J. Biochem. Physiol.* 41 1047 (1963).
9. Milstone, J. H., *Proc. Soc. Exptl. Biol. Med.* 103, 361 (1960).
10. Seegers, W. H., E. R. Cole, C. R. Harmison, E. Monkhouse, *Can. J. Biochem.* 42, 359 (1964).
11. Jobin, F., M. P. Esnouf, *Biochem. J.* 102, 666 (1967).

12. Caldwell, M. J., W. H. Seegers, *Thromb. Diathes. haemorrhag.* 13, 373 (1965).
13. Leveson, J., unpublished observations (1967).
14. Davey. J. J., M. P. Esnouf, unpublished observations (1967).
15. Milstone, J. H., *Fed. Proc.* 23, 742 (1964).
16. Barton ,P. G., M. G. Jackson, D. J. Hanahan, *Nature*, 214, 923 (1967).
17. Milstone, J. H., V. K. Milstone, *Proc. Soc. Exptl. Biol. Med.* 290, 117 (1964).
18. Milstone, J. H., N. Oulianoff, V. K. Milstone, *J. Gen. Physiol.* 47, 315 (1963).
19. Barton, P. G., D. J. Hanahan, *Biochem. Biophys. Acta.* 138, 506 (1967).
20. Hussain, Q. Z., T. F. Newcombe, *Ann. Biochem. Exptl. Med.* 23, 569 (1963).
21. Papahadjopoulos, D., C. Hougie, D. J. Hanahan, *Biochem. Biophys. Acta.* 90, 436 (1964).
22. Aoki, N., C. R. Harmison, W. H. Seegers, *Can. J. Biochem. Physiol.* 41, 2409 (1963).
23. Blombäck, B., M. Blombäck, *Nature* 198, 886 (1963).
24. Leikin, S., S. P. Bessman, *Blood* 11, 916 (1956).
25. Lamy, F., D. H. Waugh, *Thromb. Diathes. haemorrhag.* 2, 188 (1958).
26. Tishkoff, G. H., L. C. Williams, D. M. Brown, *J. Biol. Chem.* 2443, 4151 (1968).
27. Laki, K., D. R. Kominz, P. Symonds, L. Lorand, W. H. Seegers, *Arch. Biochem.* 49, 276 (1954).
28. Magnusson, S., *Arkiv Kemi* 22, 271 (1965).
29. Magnusson, S., *Arkiv Kemi* 23, 285 (1965).
30. Seegers, W. H., *Prothrombin* (1962). Harvard University Press.
31. Lechner, K., E. Deutsch, *Tromb. Diathes. haemorrhag.* 13, 314 (1965).
32. Miller, K. D., W. H. Copeland, J. F. MacGarrahan, *Proc. Soc. Exptl. Biol. Med.* 108, 117 (1961).
33. Thomas, W. R., W. H. Seegers, *Biochem. Biophys. Acta.* 42, 556 (1960).
34. MacFarlane, R. G., *Nature* 202, 498 (1964).
35. Papahadjopoulos, D., D. J. Hanahan, *Biochem. Biophys. Acta*, 90, 436 (1964).
36. Hemker, H. C., M. P. Esnouf, P. W. Hemker, A. C. W. Swart, R. G. MacFarlane, *Nature* 215, 248 (1967).
37. Baker, W. J., W. H. Seegers, *Thromb. Diathes. haemorrhag.* 17, 205 (1967).

DISCUSSION

C. R. M. Prentice: The present status of the prothrombinase concept.

I would like to congratulate Dr. Esnouf on his studies in this area of coagulation. Most investigators agree that the conversion of prothrombin to thrombin is probably achieved enzymatically by factor x_a and that factor v, in a reactive form, acts as some sort of co-factor or accelerator. Dr. Breckenridge and Dr. Ratnoff originally suggested that activated factor v was the final prothrombin converting principle. They found that when they incubated factor x, activated by Russell's viper venom, phospholipid, calcium, and factor v, there was a time-consuming reaction when increasing activity of the pro-thrombin converting principle was generated (figure 1, line A). They concluded that factor x_a was activating factor v.

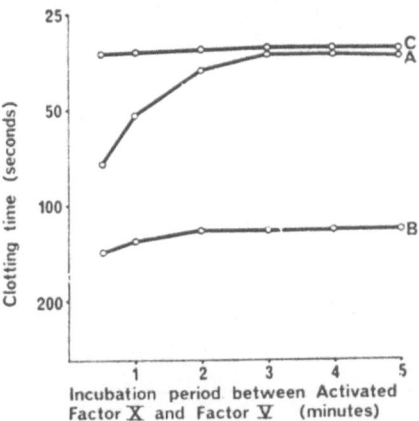

Fig. 1. Yield of prothrombin converting principle formed by incubation of factor x_a, calcium, phospholipid, and factor v. In line A, the Russell's viper venom, used to activate factor x, was not neutralized. In B, factor x_a was pre-incubated with venom antiserum. In C, factor v was pre-treated with venom before addition to factor x_a. The prothrombin converting principle was assayed on a substrate containing prothrombin and fibrinogen.

45

However, further studies done when I was working with Dr. Ratnoff suggested that factor x_a might not have an action on factor v. We repeated the first experiment with the difference that factor x_a was pre-incubated with a specific antiserum against Russell's viper venom. In this case only a very slight increase in the activity of the prothrombin converting principle was found (figure 1, line B). It seemed that it was the venom that caused the increased activity of the principle rather than factor x_a. When factor v was pre-incubated with the venom, maximum activity of the principle was immediately present (figure 1, line C). Apparently, the venom had an action on factor v as well as factor x.

It is extremely interesting to find that factor v prepared by chromatography by Dr. Esnouf is fully reactive in that it does not develop increased activity on incubation with thrombin. Our human factor v preparation needed thrombin or Russell's viper venom to make it fully reactive. This was shown by studying the initial rate of thrombin for-

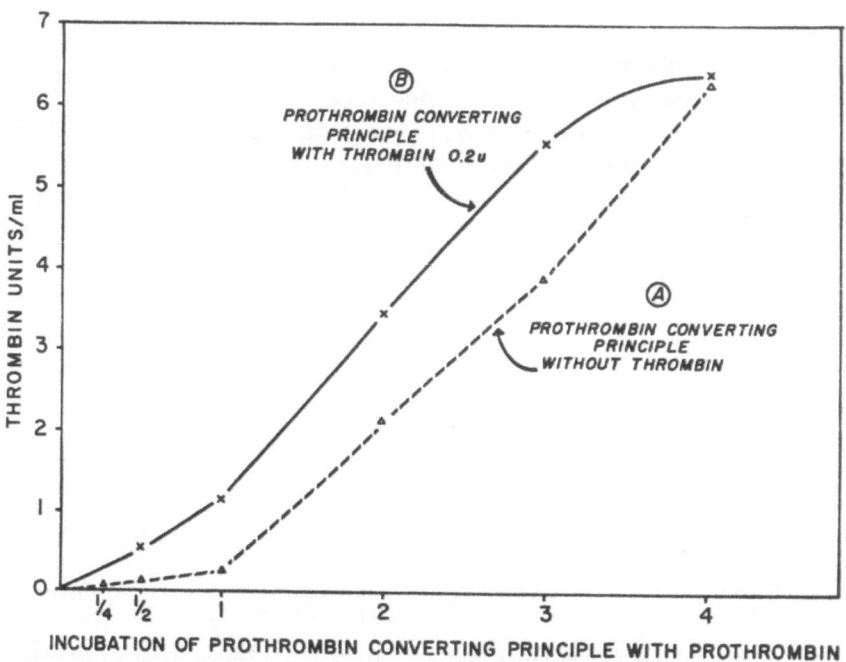

Fig. 2. Rate of thrombin formation on addition of the prothrombin converting principle to prothrombin. In the presence of a trace of pre-formed thrombin, the initial lagphase is abolished.

mation, when the prothrombin converting principle was incubated with prothrombin (figure 2). When the prothrombin converting principle contained untreated factor v, there was a distinct lag phase before thrombin generation started. In the presence of a trace of preformed thrombin, or venom, the reaction proceeded immediately. Further studies showed that both thrombin and venom increased the activity of the factor v preparation.

Apparently, there are important differences between the factor v preparations used by different investigators. Dr. Esnouf with his highly purified factor v possibly removed some co-factor or impurity that is sensitive to the action of thrombin and Russell's viper venom. Alternatively, one may be seeing a species difference, in that bovine and human factor v have different properties. One obvious difference is that bovine factor v is present in serum, whereas human factor v is absent. We found that human factor v deteriorated shortly after a trace of thrombin was added to it. Certainly it seems that, in man, there is an interaction between factor v and thrombin.

THE INTERACTION OF FACTORS VIII, IX, AND X

K. DENSON

It has been shown by Macfarlane, Biggs, Ash and Denson (1) and Biggs, Macfarlane, Denson and Ash (2) that factors VIII and IX$_a$ react in the presence of calcium chloride and traces of thrombin to form factor X activator (factor VIIIa) (figure 1). The curves shown in figure 1 were obtained using a one-stage method for following the development of factor X activator activity, and a two-stage assay method to follow the destruction of factor VIII when mixtures of factor VIII, IX$_a$, thrombin, and calcium chloride were pre-incubated. It can be seen that coincident with the disappearance or consumption of factor VIII in figure 1, there is development of an activator of factor X. It appeared

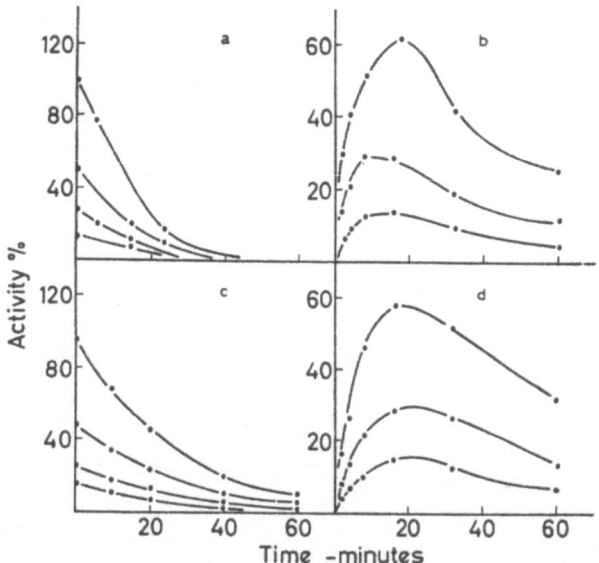

Fig. 1. Mixtures of factor IX$_a$, thrombin, calcium chloride, and different levels of factor VIII were incubated. In *a* the curves show the disappearance of factor VIII with time, and in *b* the curves show the appearance of factor X activator, *c* and *d* are theoretical curves.

48

that factor VIII was a substrate in this reaction, and that formation of the factor X activator was *catalysed by both activated factor* IX (factor IXa) and *thrombin*. The effect of thrombin was unmistakebly clearcut. There

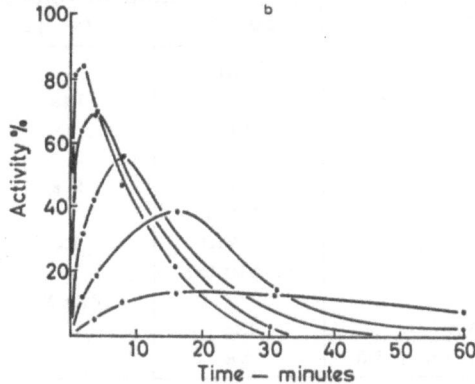

Fig. 2. The curves show the development of factor x activator in mixtures of factor IXₐ, factor VIII, calcium chloride, and different levels of thrombin.

appeared to be little doubt that even traces of thrombin had a powerful effect on factor VIII alone, at first activating it and subsequently destroying it. Acceleration in the rate of formation of the factor x activator by different concentrations of thrombin is shown in figure 2. The overall reaction was depicted by the following equations

$$VIII \xrightarrow{\text{Thrombin}} VIII^* \xrightarrow{\text{IX}_a} VIIIa \text{ (x-activator)}$$

$$\downarrow \qquad\qquad\qquad \downarrow$$

$$\text{unstable} \qquad\qquad \text{unstable}$$

Fig. 3. The formation of factor x activator from thrombin-activated factor VIII and factor IXₐ.

In these experiments, the observed activity, which was attributed to the formation of VIIIₐ, could equally well have been due to contaminating amounts of factor x in the various preparations of factor IX used. This could have resulted in the formation of small amounts of activated factor x (factor Xₐ), and the amount formed would have been related to the amount of factor IX used in the mixtures. Thus, these experimental results may suggest that an intermediate factor VIIIₐ is formed, but do not provide unequivocal evidence for its existence.

Later, Hougie, Denson and Biggs (3) studied the gel filtration of mixtures of factors VIII, IXₐ, X, calcium chloride, and phospholipid on Sephadex G 200. A schematic pattern of the results obtained when

Table 1. The elution pattern of various mixtures of clotting factors during Sephadex filtration

Mixture	Effluent volume (ml)		
	20 – 21	40 – 42	46 – 50
VIII	VIII		
IXa		IXa	
PL	PL		
IXa + Ca			IXa
IXa + PL	PL	IXa	
IXa + PL + Ca	PL IXa		
IXa + VIII + PL	PL VIII	IXa	
IXa + VIII + PL + Ca	PL VIII IXa		
IXa + X + PL		IXa X	
IXa + X + PL + Ca	IXa		X
IXa + X + VIIIa + PL + Ca	Xa		Xa

PL = phospholipid, IX_a = activated factor IX, VIII = factor VIII, X = factor X, X_a = activated factor X.

different combinations of these five substances were passed through a Sephadex G 200 column, is given in table 1. This shows that factor VIII and phospholipid are totally excluded, with a distribution coefficient of zero. Activated factor IX complexes with phospholipid when calcium is present in the eluting buffer. Since factor VIII has the same distribution coefficient as phospholipid, it was not possible to establish whether factor VIII complexed with phospholipid. A mixture of factors VIII and IX_a, phospholipid, and calcium produced peak activity with a distribution coefficient of zero, as also did a mixture of factors VIII, IX, and X with phospholipid and calcium. These results suggest that complex formation between factors VIII and IX might occur in the presence of phospholipid.

The interaction of purified clotting factors in the presence of various antibodies has been studied by Denson (4). A mixture of factor VIII, factor IX, and calcium chloride was able to shorten the partial thromboplastin time of either factor VIII or factor IX deficient substrate plasma. *When specific antisera to either factor VIII or factor IX were added after pre-incubation of the constituents, the activity was completely neutralized* (table 2). Activity resulting from contaminating traces of factor X in the mixture was also neutralized by an antiserum to factor X (table 3). Thus, these results suggest that no molecular change in factor VIII occurs when factors VIII and IX_a and calcium chloride are allowed to interact,

Table 2. Mixtures of factors IX and VIII, contact product, and calcium chloride were pre-incubated, and either normal rabbit serum or antisera to factor VIII or IX added, and the mixtures subsampled into calcium chloride, phospholipid, and either factor VIII deficient or factor IX deficient plasma.

Reaction	Substrate plasma	Incubation time in minutes before adding to substrate plasma			
		0	5	10	20
		Clotting times in seconds of substrate plasma			
IX + CP + Ca + VIII + NRS	VIII deficient	121	81	75	68
	IX deficient	139	85	79	69
IX + CP + Ca + NRS (no VII)	VIII deficient	243	240	220	221
	IX deficient	147	118	92	100
CP + Ca + VIII + NRS (no IX)	VIII deficient	110	94	93	—
	IX deficient	303	287	294	—
CP + IX + VIII + Ca	VIII deficient	102	74	75	—
15 minutes and then anti IX	IX deficient	476	420	425	—
CP + IX + Ca + VIII	VIII deficient	83	130	167	180
15 minutes and then anti VIII	IX deficient	83	93	93	97

Table 3. The neutralization of activated factor X in a mixture of factors VIII and IX$_a$

Addition	Clotting times in seconds	
	Not preincubated	Preincubated
Normal rabbit serum	73	23
Factor X antiserum	75	56
Factor V antiserum	87	24

although complex formation may occur when phospholipid is involved, and it is only when factor X is present that factors VIII, IX$_a$ and X interact together with the formation of factor X$_a$. Hemker and Kahn (5) have demonstrated the similarity in behaviour between factor V and factor VIII, and between factor X$_a$ and factor IX$_a$ in their absorption to phospholipid in the presence of various amounts of calcium ions. At a concentration of 100 mM, calcium ions, factor V and factor VIII are not absorbed, whereas factor IX and factor X show maximum adsorption.

The exact mode of interaction of factor VIII, IX and X, remains ill defined, but according to the experimental evidence so far available, it seems likely that the reaction may be similar to the reaction involving factors x_a, V, II, phospholipid, and calcium chloride.

Hemker (1967) (6) has suggested that in the reaction between factors x_a, V, prothrombin, phospholipid, and calcium chloride a complex is formed which converts prothrombin into thrombin.

$$\text{II} \xrightarrow{\quad x_a \qquad v \qquad \text{phospholipid} \qquad \text{calcium chloride} \quad} \text{II}_a$$

and that similar complex formation could be envisaged for factors VIII, IXa, phospholipid, and calcium chloride

$$\text{X} \xrightarrow{\quad \text{IX}_a \qquad \text{VIII} \qquad \text{phospholipid} \qquad \text{calcium chloride} \quad} x_a$$

An alternative to the 'enzyme cascade' hypothesis based on the results with antisera and modelled on the most fundamental reaction in clotting, namely the conversion of fibrinogen into fibrin polymer, is shown in figure 4. In these reactions, only four substrates are involved, fibri-

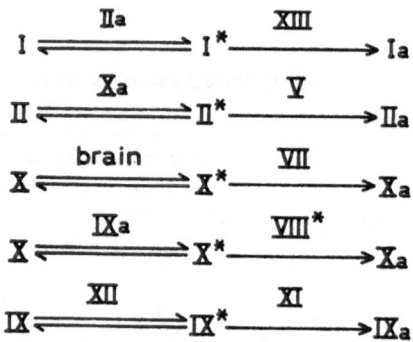

Fig. 4. Proposed reaction sequences in blood coagulation.

nogen, factor X, prothrombin, and factor IX, and the yield of activated factor in each case is governed by the concentration of the substrate, the remaining factors behaving as enzymes in the over-all reactions. Factor x_a is able to convert prothrombin to thrombin directly but slowly in the complete absence of factor V, and brain extract is able to convert factor X to x_a directly but slowly in the absence of factor VII. It seems likely that two consecutive enzyme substrate reactions may be involved, the product for the first becoming the substrate for the second. Thus, factor IX_a could convert factor x into a product, which becomes a substrate for the reaction involving factor VIII with the formation of factor X_a. This hypothesis is as good as any on the basis or the experimental evidence to date, and it is offered in the hope that it will at least give rise to further experiments.

REFERENCES

1. MacFarlane, R. G., R. Biggs, B. J. Ash, K. W. E. Denson, The interaction of factors VIII and IX. *Brit. J. Haemat.* 10, 530 (1964).
2. Biggs R., R. G. MacFarlane, K. W. E. Denson, B.J. Ash, Thrombin and the interaction of factors VIII and IX, *Brit. J. Haemat.* II, 276 (1965).
3. Hougie C., K. W. E. Denson, R. Biggs, A study of the reaction product of factor VIII and factor IX by gel filtration. *Thromb. Diath. haem.* 18, 211 (1967).
4. Denson K. W. E., *The use of antibodies in the study of blood coagulation.* D. Phil. Thesis. University of Oxford (1966).
5. Hemker H. C., M. J. P. Kahn, Reaction sequence of blood coagulation. *Nature* 215, 1201 (1967).
6. Hemker H. C., The pathways of blood coagulation. *Folia Med. Neerl.* 10, 102 (1967).

DISCUSSION

Hemker: There is very little disagreement between what Dr. Denson has said and our findings. There are three possible mechanisms, the first of which is the original cascade in which IX_a activates VIII into VIII_a and VIII_a is a factor x activator. Does Dr. Denson agree that this is not a very probable reaction mechanism; and does he agree that the kinetic experiments that have been performed by Macfarlane, Biggs, Denson and Ash on basis of which a cascade mechanism for the interaction of these factors was proposed, can be explained by an alternative mechanism in which factors IX_a and VIII_a react stoichiometrically as proposed by us?

Denson: Yes, I think that it is a possible explanation, but I do not think that you can entirely exclude the cascade, because it is not possible to isolate factor VIII_a. The rate of formation of factor VIII_a might be very low, so that there are only minimal amounts of VIII_a present at any time.

Hemker: I agree that we cannot differentiate on basis of the kinetics or because we cannot find a factor VIII_a that activates factor x, but we still have the absorption experiments, which are strongly in favour of a parallelism between x_a and IX_a and between v_a and VIII_a. Now, the adsorption of factors x_a and v_a onto phospholipid has been shown to be the essential mechanism in forming prothrombinase. When we see that IX_a and VIII_a adsorb in just the same way, this in my opinion is very suggestive indeed for the reaction

$$VIII_a + IX_a + Ca^{++} + phospholipid \longrightarrow factor\ x\ activator$$

Denson: I agree that it is quite likely. On the other hand, I do not think that you can satisfactorily dispose of the third hypothesis, i.e. that an intermediate form of x is formed by the action of IX_a and that this is then acted upon by VIII to produce activated factor x. I don't think even that you have exact evidence that when you react x_a, v and prothrombin you don't get an intermediate prothrombin formed which is then converted by factor v to thrombin.

Hemker: You proposed the reactions

$$x \; \underset{\longrightarrow}{\overset{IX_a}{\rightleftharpoons}} \; x^* \; \xrightarrow{VIII_a} \; x_a \;\; \text{and}$$

$$II \; \underset{\longrightarrow}{\overset{X_a}{\rightleftharpoons}} \; II^* \; \xrightarrow{V_a} \; \text{thrombin}$$

I do think that there is a lot of very convincing kinetic evidence that these cannot be operative. In the first place, I should like to ask why you consider these reactions reversible?

Denson: When the equilibrium in these reactions is to the left, only very small amounts of the intermediates would be formed at any one time. It is interesting that in all of these reactions, v, VIII (and also XIII) are activated by thrombin and then are subsequently destroyed by high levels of thrombin. In the case of x_a and II_a there are natural inhibitors so that during the clotting v_a and VIII_a are rapidly disposed off and then x_a and IX_a slowly desappear from the circulation. Therefore, if you have the reaction going completely to the right in the first case, you would have a very lethal intermediate present.

Hemker: There seems no harm in postulating an intermediate even if you cannot find it, and I see that you think it a logical consequence of your postulate to have the first reaction reversible; still, I think reversibility in this type of reaction is highly improbable. When you work out the kinetics of a system like this, they do not agree with the observed facts. I wonder if Dr. Deggeler could perhaps explain the reasons for this.

Deggeller: When we assume that the first reaction is reversible – which, I too do not think very probable – then the amount of enzyme catalizing this reaction would not influence the state of the equilibrium, but only the time necessary for the equilibrium to be attained. If the equilibrium were reached quickly enough, variations in the concentration of x_a would no longer cause variations in the velocity of thrombin formation. This is not found. When the equilibrium is not reached during the experiment there is no essential difference with a reaction mechanism that is not reversible, because the reverse reaction $II^* \longrightarrow II$ will only cause a certain proportion of II^* not to be converted into II_a. In other words, reversibility in this case only leads to an apparent decrease of the reaction constant of $II^* \longrightarrow II_a$. Reversibility of course provides a convenient way out of the difficulty of not finding II^* when x_a is added to prothrombin, but it has no major kinetic consequences when the equilibrium occurs too slowly to be attained.

Now, a mechanism of the type $II \;\overset{x_a}{\underset{v_1}{\longrightarrow}}\; II^* \;\overset{v_a}{\underset{v_2}{\longrightarrow}}\; II_a$ is not consistent with the kinetics, because either $v_1 > v_2$, and then the reaction velocity is dependent only on the concentration of v_a; *or* $v_2 > v_1$, and then the reaction velocity is dependent only on the amount of x_a present. This obviously has not been found, either by Hemker, Esnouf, Hemker, Swart, and Macfarlane for bovine material, or for human material by myself.

Prentice: I too should like to challenge the model that II goes to II^* and then to thrombin. One can incubate prothrombin with activated factor x, lipid, and calcium, and then add an antiserum to activated factor x to knock it out. Then, on addition of factor v, if the model is correct, you should still get thrombin. In fact, if you carry out this experiment, you don't get thrombin, suggesting that all three factors, i.e. II, x_a, and v, are working together at one stage rather than sequentially as suggested by the model.

Denson: I've done that same experiment and can confirm your results. Still, I think the outcome of the experiment depends upon how much of the II^* you get, which might be minimal. I wish to point out, though, that I do not consider my proposition as a final hypothesis, but just as a very attractive one. If anyone can tell me of any analogous biochemical system in which three proteins react together simultaneously and only in the presence of a phospholipid surface and a metallic ion activator, I would be delighted to hear about it. There is an analogy to my hypothesis in the fibrinogen to fibrin conversion.

Hemker: There certainly are other biochemical systems of this kind.

This type of reaction is encountered at least twice in the reaction mechanism that causes cell lysis by the complement system. It also very probably occurs in oxidative phosphorylation, as can be deduced from the experiments of Racker and his group.

THE NATURE OF THE FACTOR IX
ACTIVATING PRINCIPLE

C. HAANEN

INTRODUCTION

When blood or plasma is brought into contact with certain surfaces, such as glass, kaolin, and celite, it acquires the capacity to accelerate clotting. This surface activation does not occur in the blood of patients with deficiency of Hageman factor (factor XII) or plasma thromboplastin antecedent (factor XI).

Factor XI can be absorbed from plasma by many insoluble substances and afterwards eluted. If the plasma used for adsorption contains factor XII, the factor XI that is eluted is in an activated, clot-promoting form. This and many other observations (9, 17, 24) give evidence that first factor XII is activated by contact with a suitable surface and that activated factor XII then in turn converts factor XI into a clot-promoting substance. The mechanism of this surface activation and the nature of the evolving clot promoting principle is not yet clarified.

This paper presents circumstantial evidence that activation of factor XI by factor XII consists of the formation of a complex between these two factors, which takes place in the presence of a suitable surface. This complex formation explains many otherwise conflicting and puzzling observations and sheds soms light upon the mechanism of clotting-factor consumption during coagulation.

MATERIAL AND METHODS

Factor XII activity

Factor XII activity was tested as described elsewhere (7). The clotting mixture consisted of 0.1 ml factor XII-deficient plasma; 0.1 ml test substance in barbiturate buffer (pH: 7.35- I.: 0.15) and 0.1 ml 'cephalin'-kaolin suspension. After incubation at 37°C for 6 min, 0.1 ml 0.033 M $CaCl_2$ was added and the clotting time was measured. The clotting times obtained with various dilutions of purified factor XII, plotted against the corresponding dilutions on a log-log scale, gave a straight line. Arbitrarily, one factor XII unit (HFU) was defined as the quantity of active material that shortens the clotting time of the test system from its zero value of more than 300 seconds to 112 seconds (figure 1).

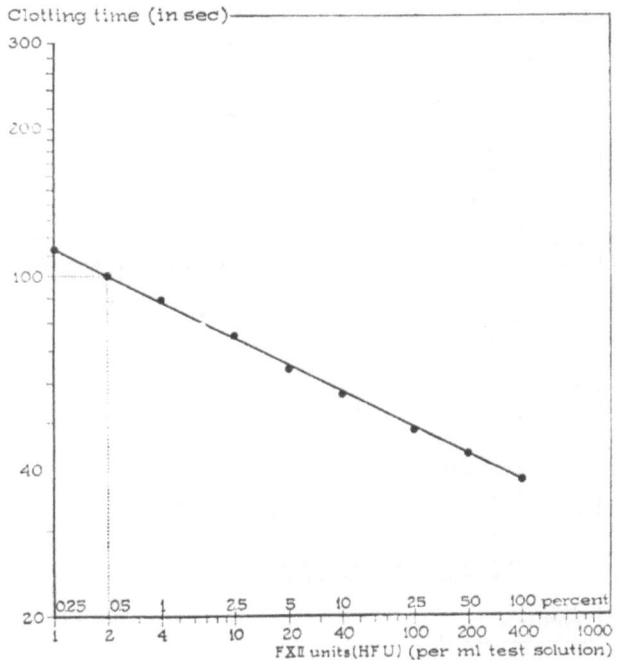

Fig. 1. Reference curve for factor XII assay. Test system: 0.1 ml factor XII-deficient plasma + 0.1 ml purified factor XII in various dilutions + 0,1 ml 'cephalin'-kaolin suspension were incubated for 6 min at 37°C. After incubation, 0.1 ml 0.033 M CaCl was added and the clotting tine was measured. One factor XII unit (HFU) is defined as the quantity of active material that shortens the clotting time of the test system from its zero value of more than 300 seconds to 112 seconds.

Purification of factor XII
The experiments on the nature of contact activation were done with a highly purified bovine factor XII preparation made by Schoenmakers et al. (23). The purification was carried out in the following steps: Al $(OH)_3$- adsorbed citrated plasma was adsorbed onto a glass powder column and, after washing with saline, factor XII was eluted from the column with 1 M NaCl, buffered at pH 9.6. The eluate was further purified by Cohn fractionation, zinc precipitation, and chro-

matography on DEAE sephadex and CM cellulose (5, 20, 23). The entire procedure is shown in figure 2.

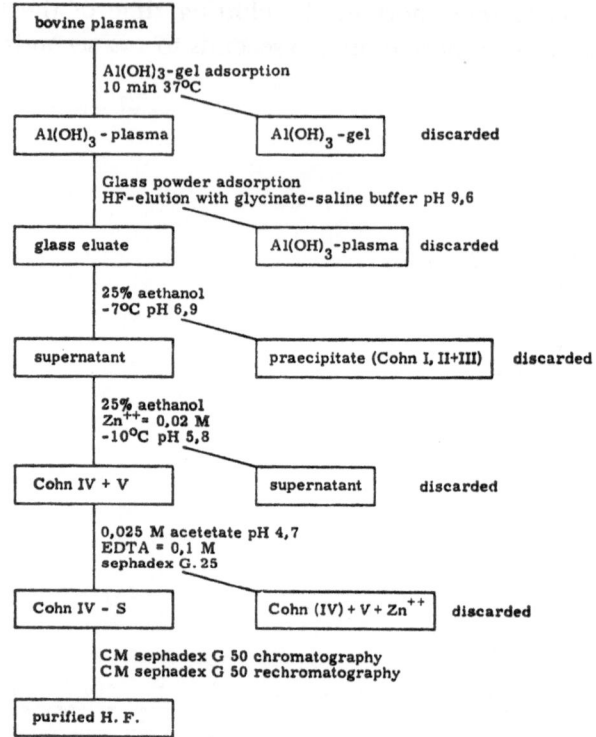

Fig. 2. Purification procedure for factor XII from bovine citrated plasma.

EXPERIMENTS

Pseudo-reversibility of factor XII activation

The purified factor XII could be expected to be completely activated by this procedure. Surprisingly, a given quantity of this purified, activated factor XII gave much shorter clotting times in factor XII assays when tested in the presence of glass or kaolin, as is shown in table 1.

To collect more information about this unexpected finding, the interaction of factor XII, factor XI, and surface was studied in the following experiment. Mixtures lacking one of the three components essential for activation product formation (factor XII, factor XI, or surface) were incubated together at 37°C for various periods. After 0, 2, 6 and 10 minutes incubation, the missing component was reconstituted and the

Table 1. The effect of glass on the activity of a purified factor XII preparation, 0.1 ml factor XII- deficient plasma + 0.1 ml cephalin suspension + 0.1 ml purified factor XII were incubated with and without surface contact. After incubation for 6 min at 37°C, 0.1 ml 0.033 M CaCl₂ was added.

Clotting test carried out in ·	clotting time in seconds	factor XII U/mg protein
Plastic tube	140	32
Glass tube	70	2500
Glass tube together with kaolin susp. 005 ml	59	6000

mixture was recalcified. Maximal clot-promoting activity proved to evolve only when factor XII and factor XI (factor XII-deficient plasma) were incubated together with kaolin. Incubation of purified factor XII with surface alone gave no increase in clot-promoting activity. The differences in factor XII activity found when the same quantity of purified XII was used in the various procedures, are shown in figure 3. The unexpected finding that the purified, already completely activated, factor XII can be activated anew, and that this activation only takes

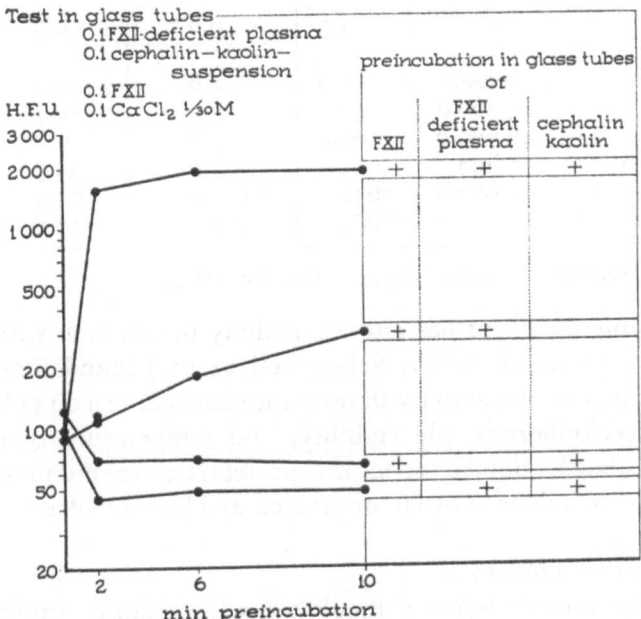

Fig. 3. Influence of factor XI and surface contact on the activity of purified factor XII.

place when factor XII is incubated with kaolin in the presence of factor XI, gives some insight into the phenomenon of surface activation. The shortening of the recalcification time, which occurs only when factor XII and surface are incubated in the presence of factor XI, seems not to be caused by an alteration of factor XII itself but by the catalyzing action of surface on the interaction between factor XII and factor XI, possibly by preferential adsorption of these two factors.

Proteolytic properties of purified bovine factor XII

There are a great many observations suggesting that purified factor XII has proteolytic activaties. In high concentrations, factor XII causes fibrinolysis of ^{131}iodine-labeled fibrin clots and of unheated fibrin plates (table 2), as though factor XII were an activator of plasminogen.

Table 2. Factor XII esterase and activities and fibrinolytic properties of various fractions during purification of bovine factor XII.

	Factor XII activity (F. XII U/mg)	Esterase activity	131 I-fibrinolysis (in %)[*]	Fibrin plate lysis (in sq. mm) unheated	heated
Al (OH)₃- plasma	—	1.5	0.0	0.0	0.0
Glasspowder - eluate	2300.0	80.0	1.8	12.3	0.0
Cohn II + III	160.0	48.0	13.2	14.4	0.0
Cohn IV – S	2.900.0	90.0	3.8	0.0	0.0
CM-Sephadex I	5.200.0	244.0	73.0	39.7	0.0
CM-Sephadex II	10.000.0	1630.0	100.0	162.5	0.0
DEAE-Sephadex	44.000.0	6680.0	100.0	347.8	0.0

[*] Plasminogen-rich fibrin clots; Alkjaersig (1) — Dudok de Wit (4).

Purified bovine factor XII has esterase activity in common with other proteases (3,21,27). Moreover, Schoenmakers (22) found that factor XII activity and esterase activity showed the same pattern on polyacrylamidegel electrophoresis, pH stability, and temperature sensitivity. The finding that bovine factor XII is a proteolytic enzyme may imply that activation of factor XI by factor XII is caused by proteolysis.

The mode of action of factor XII

When normal intact plasma is incubated with celite or kaolin, consumption of factor XI occurs. As is shown in figure 4, this consumption is more complete and more rapid when the plasma is exposed to larger quantities of active surface. While factor XI progressively disappears with increasing exposure to contact surface, factor XII shows no decrease, even after 24 hours incubation. If we assume that the presence of increasing amounts of contact surface promotes the interaction of factor XII with factor XI, then the progressive consumption of the latter supports the hypothesis that degradation of activated factor XI is due to a proteolytic action of factor XII.

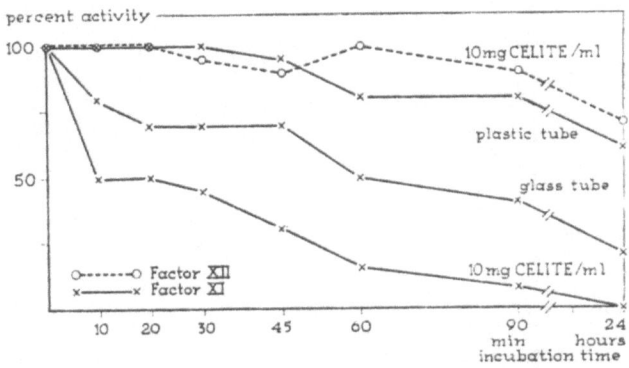

Fig. 4. Factor XII and factor XI content of normal plasma after incubation for various periods with and without surface contact. The factor XII and factor XI activities are expressed in per cent activity read from a reference curve made with various dilutions of the same intact plasma.

The interaction of factor XII *and factor* XI

The assumption that activation of clotting factors is caused by proteolytic action of the foregoing factor does not explain why, in the case of factor XI activation, consumption of this factor only occurs in the presence of sufficient contact surface and why factor XI is still present in outdated plasma or in serum.

To collect more information about the reaction kinetics between factor XII and factor XI, the following experiments were done. Various amounts of factor XII were incubated at 37°C with factor XII-deficient plasma in the presence of kaolin. After various intervals, 0.1 ml $CaCl_2$ 0.033 M was added to 0.3 ml of the incubation mixture, and the clotting time was measured.

As is shown by figure 5 the maximal activity of activation product depended on the quantity of factor XII added. When the development of activation product had stopped, re-addition of factor XII restarted

the process of activator production (figure 6). The observed shortening
of clotting times must actually have been caused by activator production, because the purified factor xii did not contain even traces of factor
xi and activation of other clotting factors requires the presence of
calcium ions, which were not present during incubation.

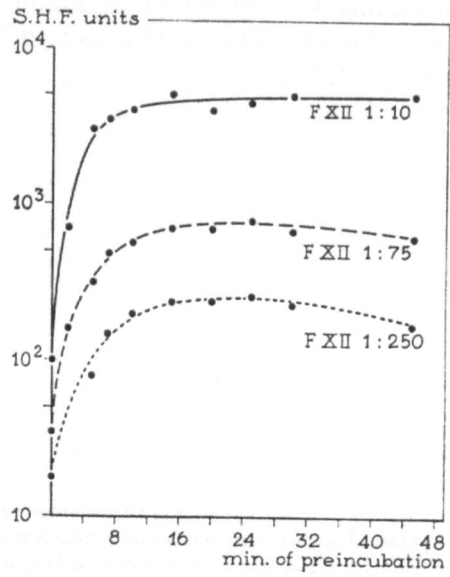

Fig. 5. Corrective effect of purified factor xii on the clotting time of factor xii-deficient plasma
after pre-incubation for various intervals. Equal volumes of purified factor xii, 'cephalin'-
kaolin suspension and factor xii-deficent plasma were incubated at 37°C. After various periods
0.3 ml of the mixture was recalcified with 0.1 ml. 0.033 M CaCl₂. The clotting times obtained are expressed in factor xii units per mg protein (HFU).

These findings demonstrate that activation of factor xi by factor xii in
the presence of a suitable surface does not follow zero-order reaction
kinetics, for in that case the amount of factor xii added would only
determine the rate of activator production and not the magnitude of
which is formed. If we accept that factor xi is a substrate of activated
factor xii in the formation of activation product, as shown by Ratnoff
et al. (18) and Nossel (12), we must presume the existence of some
complicating mechanism in the activation system that could account
for the observed phenomenon:

1. The assumption of an inhibitor against factor xii-activation does
not explain the observed reaction kinetics, because such an inhibitor

would only influence the rate of activator production and not the magnitude of its formation.

2. The assumption of an inhibitor against activated factor XII is also unlikely because, as is shown in figure 6, minute amounts of activated factor XII shorten the clotting time of plasma deficient in this substance.

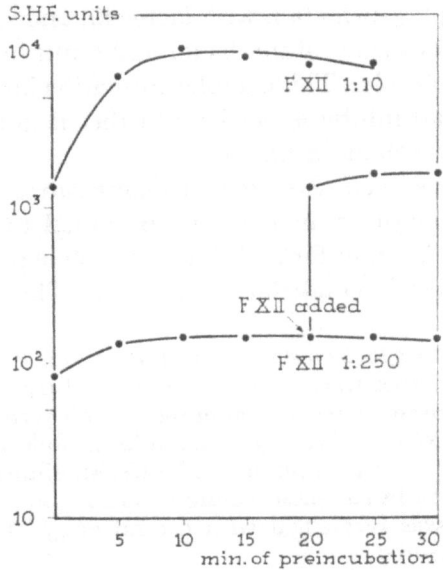

Fig. 6. Effect of re-addition of purified factor XII on activator production in a plasma sample with a low factor XII content. Factor XII-deficient plasma was incubated at 37°C with 'cephalin'-kaolin suspension together with a small quantity of purified factor XII. After various intervals, 0.3 ml of the mixture was recalcified with 0.1 ml 0.033 M CaCl₂. The clotting times obtained are expressed in factor XII units (HFU).

3. Extreme lability of activated factor XII is excluded as the explanation for the observed kinetics because, as shown by Schoenmakers, (22) the highly purified factor XII used in these experiments is stable and does not lose its activity even after 15 minutes of incubation at 50°C.

4. The limitation of maximal activation production by the amount of factor XII present in the incubation mixture could be caused by an equilibrium between formation and deterioration of a labile activation product. Such a mechanism would mean a continuous consumption of factor XI. Although there seems to be no doubt about the lability of

activation product (11,12,13,15,29), this presumption of continuous consumption of factor XI is not in accordance with the presence of this factor in out-dated plasma.

5. The formation of a factor XII-factor XI complex could explain the observed limitation of activator production, and is not in contradiction with other observed properties of factor XII and XI. Factor XI is activated during this complex formation with factor XII and sticking to factor XII it covers the active centre of this factor and limits further activation of other factor XI molecules. This complex formation has the same effect as the presence of an inhibitor blocking further factor XII activity as long as the complex remains in existence.

After factor XI has been activated, it deteriorates. The amount of factor XI left in the plasma is inversely proportional to the amount of activation product initially formed. This was shown by Nossel (12) and also by the experimental date in figure 4. The consumption of

Table 3. The effect of surface contact on factor XII and factor XI activities. Factor XII and XI activities were measured in normal plasma and in factor XII-deficient plasma, immediately and after incubation at room temperature. Factor XII and factor XI assays were carried out in the following manner: 0.1 ml deficient plasma*) + 0.1 ml plasma to be tested, diluted 1:10 in barbiturate + 0.1 ml cephalin-kaolin suspension were incubated for 6 min. at 37°C. The mixture was recalcified with 0.1 ml 0033 M CaCl₂ and the clotting time was measured.

	Incubation in plastic tubes, together with celite (10 mg/ml plasma)	
	Clotting times (in seconds)	
	factor XII assay	factor XI assay
Normal plasma		
after 5 min	241 sec	262 sec
after 90 min	260 sec	298 sec
after 24 hr	261 sec	421 sec
F XII-defic. plasma		
after 5 min	> 2700 sec	263 sec
after 90 min	> 2700 sec	244 sec
after 24 hr	> 2700 sec	248 sec

* Substrate plasma for factor XI assay, derived from a case of severe congenital factor XI deficieny, was kindly supplied by Dr. S. I. de Vries, Amsterdam.

factor xi by contact takes place only when factor xii is simultaneously present, as shown by table 3. The assumption that factor xii forms a complex with factor xi and that this complex continues to exist even after factor xi has deteriorated, suggests a mechanism that could explain not only the limited activation of factor xi but also the factor xi activity that can still be found in out-dated plasma or serum. A plasma sample taken from the middle of the contents of a glass tube in which surface contact has taken place, shows a distinct clot-promoting activity for some time, thus indicating that at least a part of the factor xii-xi complex is released from the surface. This release from the surface gives rise to the question why these vacated surface places do not give rise to further factor xii activation and subsequent complete deterioration of factor xi. The following experiments possibly explain this discrepancy. Thromboplastin screening tests were carried out according to Hardisty and Margolis (9), using as a substrate factor xii-deficient plasma. The incubation tubes were coated with normal

Table 4. Thromboplastin screening tests of factor xii-deficient plasma in uncoated tubes and in tubes coated with normal plasma for three days or 10 min. with the plasma sample used for this three-day incubation. Coating was done by filling a tube with normal plasma. After three days the plasma was brought in to a second tube for 10 min. The incubation tubes were emptied and rinsed with 20 changes of 0.9% saline. In each of the tubes 0.9 ml saline + 0.1 ml factor xii deficient plasma + 0.1 ml cephalin suspension were incubated at 37°C. The mixtures were recalcified with 0.1 ml of 0.025 M $CaCl_2$. At various intervals, 0.1 ml incubation mixture was added together with 0.1 ml 0025 M $CaCl_2$ to 0.1 ml normal plasma and the clotting time was recorded in (seconds).

	minutes after recalcification diluted factor xii-deficient plasma					
	1	3	5	7	9	11
normal glass tube	80	76	40	35	34	32
glass tube coated with normal plasma for three days, then rinsed	60	32	21	24	27	32
glass tube coated for 10 min with plasma from tube 2, then rinsed	34	12	9	11	13	15

plasma and then rinsed with ten changes of 0.9% saline as described elsewhere (6). When the incubation tubes had been coated with normal plasma for 3 days at room temperature, thromboplastin generation of factor XII-deficient plasma in these coated tubes was poor. When fresh incubation tubes were coated with the same normal plasma previously incubated in glass for 3 days but this time the tubes had been exposed to plasma for only 10 minutes, thromboplastin generation of factor XII-deficient plasma was completely normal (table 4). Therefore, the plasma sample, which had so poorly coated the incubation tubes with factor XII during prolonged contact, still possessed enough factor XII to coat other glass tubes very well in 10 minutes.

It is unlikely that factor XII itself is inactivated *in situ* upon the glass surface, because it is possible to purify factor XII by glass-powder adsorption (5, 20, 23) and subsequent elution. Another explanation of the observed phenomenon must be that the surface places that come vacant after loosening of the factor XII-factor XI complexes are filled not only by new factor XII molecules but also by other proteins with affinity for glass surface. The presence of these proteins was proposed earlier by Haanen et al. (5) and has recently been described by Didisheim (3) and Vroman (28). After some time, the whole surface is occupied by factor XII molecules blocked by factor XI sticking to them and by other proteins with glass affinity and without clotting activity. The factor XII and factor XI molecules left in the plasma cannot be activated further and remain unaltered. The effect of complex formation and of other proteins with glass-affinity on the mechanism of factor XII activation is shown in the following diagram:

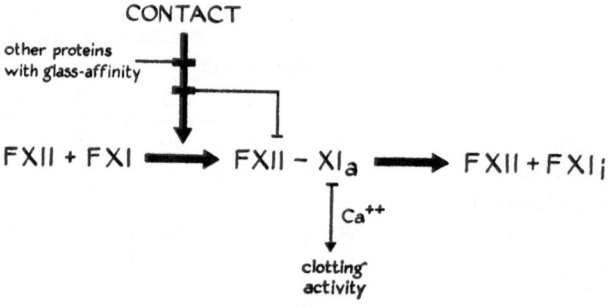

DISCUSSION

The following observations, which till now have been conflicting, can be explained completely by the suggested mechanism of factor XII activation and complex formation of factor XII with factor XI:

1. *The limited activation and consumption of factor* XI *by factor* XII, *such as appears from the presence of this factor in out-dated plasma and from the experimental results shown in figures 3, 4, and 6.*

The presumption that factor XII in the adsorbed state forms a complex with factor XI, implies that factor XI exerts an inhibiting effect on further factor XII activity, comparable with the antithrombin activity of fibrin brought about by complex formation with thrombin. When the available contact surface is limited, the process of activation of factor XI soon comes to an end because the surface is covered both by factor XII molecules, that have been blocked by factor XI and by other inert proteins having an affinity for glass-surface.

2. *The complete consumption of factor* XI *when plasma is exposed to celite, as described by Soulier and Prou-Wartelle (26) and Horowitz et al. (10).*

From the suggested mechanism concerning the role of factor XII it can be concluded that factor XI activation continues as long as there is enough surface area free and there are factor XII molecules in the plasma to adsorb to it. It has been recognized (11, 12, 15, 29) that the activation product developing after contact activation is unstable. As shown by Nossel (12) and by the experimental results shown in figure 3, the amount of factor XI left in the plasma is inversely proportional to the amount of activation product initially formed. When plasma is exposed to a large surface area the interference with adsorption by other molecules having glass affinity is excluded and all factor XII molecules from the plasma can be adsorbed, thus giving rise to maximal activation product formation after which all factor XI is consumed.

3. *The limited activation (and consumption) of factor* XI *when there are few factor* XII *molecules present, as appeared from the experimental results shown in table 2 and in figures 4 and 5.*

The suggested mechanism concerning the interaction of factor XII and factor XI carries the implication that intact factor XI combines with factor XII when this factor is in the adsorbed state and that this complex continues to exist even after factor XI has been activated and consumed. This mechanism not only provides an explanation for the limitation of the magnitude of contact product formation when there is little factor XII present but is also compatible with the observations of Ratnoff (18) and Nossel (12) that the amount of factor XII determines the rate of activator production.

4. *The conflicting findings with respect to the presence of an inhibitor of factor* XII *activity (16, 25) and the accelerating effect of minute amounts of factor* XII *on the clotting time.*

The suggested complex formation between factor XII and factor XI implies that activation of factor XI also means inhibition of further factor XII activity.

5. *The observation made by Ratnoff and Crum (19) and Haanen et al. (8) and shown in table I, i.e. that purified factor* XII *occurred almost entirely in the inactive form, contrary to what had been expected from the maximal activition that must have taken place during the purification procedure.*

The assumption that the reaction between factor XII and factor XI must take place in the adsorbed state whether or not factor XII has been activated previously, could explain the observations made by Ratnoff and Crum (19) and Haanen et al. (8), shown in figure 3, that formation of contact product by surface or ellagic acid evolves only when factor XII and factor XI are present simultaneously.

6. *The suggested mechanism concerning the action of factor* XII *would explain the limited action of this factor upon factor* XI *even if the action of factor* XII *is enzymatic.*

A similar mechanism of limited proteolysis could be present at other stages of coagulation, thus explaining the incomplete consumption of clotting factors in deficient plasma and the complete consumption after supplying an excess of the foregoing factor (2, 14).

This discussion has purposely given only indirect evidence for the suggested mechanism of the action of factor XII and its interaction with factor XI. A more exact and meaningful analysis of this interaction would be possible if pure factor XI could be prepared.

SUMMARY

The activity of highly purified factor XII depends on the test conditions.

The highest activity develops when a suitable contact surface and factor XI are present simultaneously during incubation. Arguments are given for the supposition that factor XII forms a complex with factor XI, a complex which is unstable and probably identical with the so-called activation product. The instability is caused by deterioration of factor XI while factor XII remains. The process of contact activation stops because further factor XII activity is blocked by factor XI, which sticks to factor XII even after it has deteriorated. Under normal circumstances, not all the factor XII molecules are adsorbed to a surface, due to the competing effect of other proteins in the plasma having glass affinity. The exposure of plasma to a large surface causes complete adsorption of all factor XII molecules and in this way leads to complete consumption of factor XI. The proposed complex formation between factor XII and factor XI could explain many otherwise conflicting observations.

REFERENCES

1. Alkjaersig, N., A. P. Fletcher, S. Sherry, The mechanism of clot dissolution by plasmin. *J. clin. Invest.* 38, 1086 (1959).
2. Biggs, R., A. A. Sharp, J. Margolis, R. M. Hardisty, J. Stewart, W. M. Davidson, Defects in the early stages of blood coagulation A report of four cases. *Brit. J. Haemat.* 4, 177 (1958).
3. Didisheim, P., Panel Discussion. *Xth Congress of the International Society of Haematology*, Stockholm (1964).
4. Dudok de Wit, C., H. W. Krijnen, G. J. H. den Ottolander, The measurement of fibrinolytic activity with ^{131}J labeled clots. I: Methods. *Thrombos. Diathes. haemorrh.* (Stuttg.) 8, 315 (1962).
5. Haanen, C., F. Hommes, H. Benraad, G. Morselt, A case of Hageman factor deficiency and a method to purify the factor. *Thrombos. Diathes. haemorrh.* (Stuttg.) 5, 201 (1960).
6. Haanen, C., F. Hommes, G. Morselt, Some observations on the role of Hageman factor in blood coagulation. *Thrombos. Diathes. haemorrh.* (Stuttg.) 6, 261 (1961).
7. Haanen, C., J. G. G. Schoenmakers, One-stage assay for Hageman factor (factor XII). Further studies on the role of Hageman factor in blood coagulation. *Thrombos. Diathes. haemorrh.* (Stuttg.) 9, 557 (1963).
8. Haanen, C., G. Morselt and J. Schoenmakers, Contact activation of Hageman factor and the interaction of Hageman factor and plasma thromboplastin antecedent. *Thrombos. Diathes. haemorrh.* (Stuttg.) 17, 307 (1967).
9. Hardisty, R. M., J. Margolis, The role of Hageman factor in the initiation of blood coagulation *Brit. J. Haemat.* 5, 203 (1959).
10. Horowitz. H. I., W. P. Wilcox, M. M. Fujimoto, The use of artificially depleted normal plasma for the assay of factor XI (PTA). *Fed. Proc.* 22, 162 (1963).
11. Margolis, J., Initiation of blood coagulation by glass and related surfaces. *J. Physiol.* 137, 95 (1957).
12. Nossel, H. L., *The contact phase of blood coagulation.* Blackwell Scientific Publications, Oxford (1964).

13. Nossel, H. L., J. Niemetz, The contact product inhibitor. *Clin. Res.* 12, 228 (1964).
14. Nossel, H. L., Differential consumption of coagulation factors resulting from activation of the extrinsic (tissue thromboplastin) or the intrinsic (foreign surface contact) pathways. *Blood*, 29, 331 (1967).
15. Ratnoff, D. D., An enzyme in plasma inactivating Hageman factor. *J. Clin. Invest.* 37, 923 (1958).
16. Ratnoff, O. D., J. M. Rosenblum, Role of Hageman factor in the initiation of clotting by glass: Evidence that glass frees Hageman factor from inhibition. *Amer. J. Med.* 25, 160 (1958).
17. Ratnoff, O. D., Hageman trait. *Thrombos. Diathes. haemorrh.* 4, Suppl., 116 (1960).
18. Ratnoff, O. D., E. W. Davie, D. L. Mallet, Studies on the action of Hageman factor: Evidence that activated Hageman factor in turn activates plasma thromboplastin antecedent. *J. Clin. Invest.* 40, 803 (1961).
19. Ratnoff, O. D., J. D. Crum, Activation of Hageman factor by solutions of ellagic acid. *J. lab. clin. Med.* 63, 359 (1964).
20. Schoenmakers, J. G. G., R. M. Kurstjens, C. Haanen, F. Zilliken, Purification of activated bovine Hageman factor. *Thrombos. Diathes. haemorrh.* (Stuttg.) 9, 546 (1963).
21. Schoenmakers, J., R. Matze, C. Haanen, F. Zilliken, Proteolytic activity of purified bovine Hageman factor. *Biochim. biophys. Acta* (Amst.) 93, 433 (1964).
22. Schoenmakers, J. G. G., *Purification and properties of Hageman factor*. Thesis, University of Nijmegen (1965).
23. Schoenmakers, J. G. G., R. Matze, C. Haanen, F. Zilliken, Hageman factor, a novel sialoglycoprotein with esterase activity. *Biochem. biophys. Acta* (Amst.) 101, 166 (1965).
24. Soulier, J. P., O. Wartelle, D. Ménaché, Caractères différentiels des facteurs Hageman et PTA; rôle du contact dans la phase initiale de la coagulation. *Rev. franc. Etud. Clin. Biol.* 3, 263 (1958).
25. Soulier, J. P., O. Wartelle, D. Ménaché, Hageman trait and PTA deficiency: The role of contact of blood with glass. *Brit. J. Haemat.* 5, 121 (1959).
26. Soulier, J. P., O. Prou-Wartelle, New data on Hageman factor and plasma thromboplastin antecedent: The role of 'contact' in the initial phase of blood coagulation. *Brit. J. Haemat.* 6, 88 (1960).
27. Speer, R. J., H. Ridgway, J. M. Hill, Activated human Hageman factor. *Thrombos. Diathes. haemorrh.* (Stuttg.) 14, 1 (1965).
28. Vroman, L., *Behavior of coagulation factors at interfaces. Biophysical mechanism in vascular homeostasis and intravascular thrombosis.* p. 81. Ed. P. N. Sawyer, Appleton-Century-Crofts, New York (1965).
29. Waaler, B. A., Contact activation in the intrinsic blood clotting system. *Scand. J. clin. lab. Invest.* 11 suppl., 37 (1959).

DISCUSSION

L. Vroman: Adsorption of fibrinogen at interfaces, its relation to contact activation and platelet stickiness.

Imagine, with appropriate difficulty, that you have a recording ellipsometer. This is a machine that can record changes in optical thickness occurring at reflecting solid/liquid and other interfaces. For example, a polished slice of a silicon crystal with an oxidized surface can provide the reflecting substrate. If it sits in the path of plane-polarized light while submerged in buffer solution maintained at, let us say, 37°C, the crystal will give a certain elliptical movement to the light it reflects; then, after some plasma is added to the buffer, the tilt and flatness of the reflected ellipse will change, so that a quarter wave plate and analyzer will pass more or less of this light. After proper measurements and control experiments for calibration have been carried out, the recorded curve of light passed can be interpreted as a change in optical thickness of the solid surface caused by its adsorption of matter from the plasma. You will then realize that this adsorption occurs within seconds. If the added plasma had been intact and contained factor XII, you would have seen that adsorption is followed by some desorption, and your premature conclusion may have been that the ellipsometer recorded for you the adsorption of factors XI and XII and the desorption of activation product. However, we found that the very first material deposited by plasma on these glass-like solids was able to adsorb large amounts of matter, presumably antibody, specifically out of anti-human fibrinogen sera, and very little out of other antisera to human plasma proteins. The ability of the fresh film to attract anti-fibrinogen is destroyed by the plasma in less than 10 seconds at room temperature, more slowly with higher plasma dilutions and more rapidly at 37°C. I am calling this loss of reactivity with anti-fibrinogen 'conversion' of the fibrinogen film. Activated plasma converts its films more slowly, but factor XII-deficient plasma converts its films like normal plasma. Desorption occurs a little later and does require the presence of factor XII in plasma.

How much of the unconverted film is fibrinogen? We compared the ability of pre-formed fibrinogen films and of unconverted plasma films to attract antifibrinogen, and we found that both the rate of adsorption and ultimate thickness of the antifibrinogen were the same for purified fibrinogen films and plasma films, as if no room would be left for factor XII or XI. Some of a preformed fibrinogen film will be removed when exposed to intact plasma, provided it contains factor XII.

All this was shown with ellipsometry. Now let us turn to similar information obtained more cheaply, by a method that has been available to anyone and that should have been applied by us much sooner. A typical experiment with this method is the following. Clean a glass plate with detergent and water, dry, flame briefly, let cool. Pour some fibrinogen solution over one area of it, rinse off with buffer and then with water, and allow to drip dry. Then put small drops of various antisera on the dried surface. Rinse again after one minute and drip dry. Now put some water of about 40-60°C in a dark container, and place the glass plate on it as a well-sealing lid, with the treated surface facing down. Water will condense onto the glass in drops that are rounder and therefore scatter more light, creating a whiter area where the surface is more hydrophobic. In this experiment, the fibrinogen adsorbed onto the glass will turn white while the (wettable) glass remains black against the black background; the only spot on the fibrinogen that turns black is the one that had been occupied by the anti-fibrinogen serum on top of the fibrinogen. You can block this 'wetting action' of the matching antiserum by premixing it with some antigen, to show it is a specific effect. Well, using this new application of a very old method, we found that normal intact plasma deposits fibrinogen onto glass, and then converts it, as it appears to do on other surfaces in the ellipsometer. I had good reason to be happy about this, because it was already known that platelets in afibrinogenemic plasma do not stick to glass unless a dash of fibrinogen is added to the plasma. To me, this always suggested that platelets will not stick to glass unless fibrinogen is adsorbed on it first. Will they also stick to a film of 'converted' fibrinogen? To find out, Marjorie B. Zucker and I did a series of experiments, for example as follows. A drop of intact citrated normal plasma is placed on a carefully cleaned glass slide. After two minutes, the slide is picked up with clean forceps and tilted so that the drop runs off, leaving a wet track. Within two to five seconds, the drop site, the track, and finally the entire slide are rinsed with buffered saline followed by large amounts of distilled water, then drip dried, or merely rinsed with buffered saline and left wet. The slide is then covered with normal platelets that have been washed and suspended in a fibrinogen-free medium (such as serum or afibrinogenemia plasma). The covered slide is left in a moist chamber for about thirty minutes then rinsed with buffered saline, followed by a fixative such as formaline, rinsed again and observed dry with phase contrast, or left wet and stained before observation. We will see that on the circular spot where the platelet-poor plasma had been sitting for two minutes, the platelet suspension left only very few platelets; but the track where the plasma had been in contact with the glass surface for only a few seconds, has become very attractive to platelets; the whole picture is one of a rather clear disc with a plateletrich tail. I presume that the area of the disc has converted fibrinogen on it, while the fibrinogen deposited on the tailing track had no chance of being converted.

If you now remember that we found activated plasma much less able to convert its own fibrinogen deposit, then you must anticipate a complex of changes that decide whether or not platelets will stick when intact whole blood touches glass. Depending, for example, on flow, the plasma may deposit fibrinogen and convert it before platelets have a chance to come near; or the plasma may be converted somewhere and then flow on to deposit unconvertible fibrinogen, and platelets will stick to that area rather than to the region of glass that activated the plasma. Where does activation fit in? We have looked for some interaction between fibrinogen and factor XII adsorption and found none. For example, we tried to detect how fast afibrinogenemia plasma deposits a film that can correct factor XII deficient clotting; we had hoped that normal plasma, which may have to deposit fibrinogen first, would be slower. However, both plasmas were faster than we are, leaving factor XII activity on the glass within seconds. In short, we may have found some explanation of one phenomenon while destroying the explanation of another.

Magnusson: In this context it may be interesting to mention an experiment I did with Dr. Birger Blombäck in 1960. We wanted to see

whether the Hageman factor had any proteolytic activity on fibrinogen.

We took normal plasma, adsorbed it on glass beads, rinsed the beads
thoroughly, and then incubated them under sterile conditions with
fibrinogen. We also incubated fibrinogen with glass beads that had
been rinsed with physiological saline and also with glass beads that
had been permitted to adsorb whatever they could from Hageman
deficient plasma. We found that fibrinogen with normal plasma glass
beads coagulated in about 3 days and it had N-terminal glycine-like
fibrin clotted with thrombin. There was no fibrin formed in either of
the other tubes – neither the one with the Hageman glass beads nor the
one with the glass beads rinsed with physiological saline.

THE POSSIBLE ROLE OF FACTOR VII IN THE INTRINSIC SYSTEM

F. JOSSO AND S. BEGUIN

In previous work (9) we have shown that, under certain circumstances, tissue thromboplastin in the presence of factor VII may activate factor IX in the same way as 'contact product' does in the intrinsic system. These data agree with the results obtained by Biggs and Nossel (4) and later extended by Nossel (10). This theory is consistent with the clinical observation that factor XII deficiency does not produce any significant bleeding tendency, whereas factor VII deficiency often results in a severe haemorrhagic disease. This theory also explains the experimental fact observed by Rapaport et al. (13) that factor IX is consumed 'in vivo' by the infusion of tissue thromboplastin.

Thus it appears that, in the absence of contact with glass, tissue thromboplastin and factor VII may replace the contact product formed by the interaction between factor XI and activated factor XII. In the intrinsic system however, factor VII, although not necessary for normal coagulation, is nevertheless involved in the clotting process. Many investigations have demonstrated that factor VII is found in activated form in serum (1, 7, 12). Soulier and Prou-Wartelle have shown that factor XII is necessary for this activation (17).

The possibility that factor VII may play a role in the intrinsic system is apparently confirmed by our observation that, in the three severely factor VII-deficient patients we have studied, residual serum prothrombin was particularly low.

The kinetics of prothrombin consumption in these patients show that, in the absence of factor VII, prothrombin is consumed much more rapidly than in control subjects; moreover, the consumption is nearly complete in systems where residual prothrombin is high in the control (figure 1).

We have speculated that factor VII activation in normal subjects and high prothrombin consumption in factor VII-deficient patients are perhaps linked. To test this hypothesis, we allowed factor VII-deficient plasma to clot in the presence of purified factor VII.

Human factor VII was prepared either from plasma (plasma factor VII) or from serum (serum factor VII). The starting material was in the first case the plasma PPSB fraction (II, VII, X, IX), in the latter case, the serum CSB fraction (VII, X, IX) prepared at the Centre National de Transfusion Sanguine (16). Factor VII was purified by column chromatography on DEAE-Sephadex, using a step-wise elution by increasing molarity of the buffer (3).

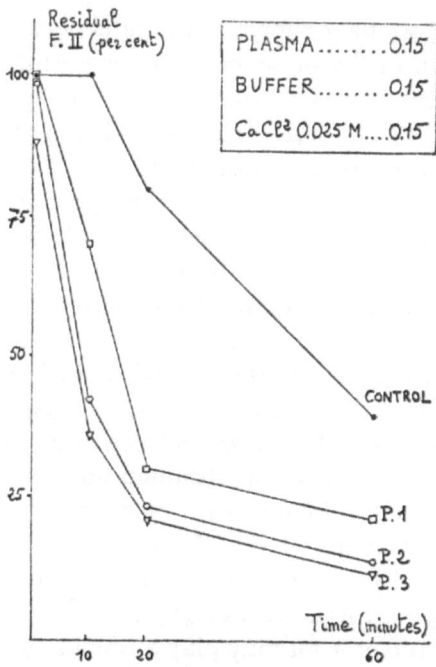

Fig. 1. Prothrombin consumption in three patients with severe factor VII deficiency. System: citrated plasma 0.15 ml; buffer 0.15 ml; CaCl₂ 0.025 M 0.15 ml.

Factor VII-deficient plasma was allowed to clot in the presence of plasma factor VII in such an amount as to bring its concentration to a nearly normal level. Prothrombin consumption was greatly decreased and factor VII was activated (figure 2 A). In the presence of serum factor VII no modification of prothrombin consumption was observed and factor VII activity was not modified by clotting (figure 2 B). These data suggest that factor VII acts as a competitive inhibitor of prothrombin consumption. More precisely, factor VII seems to act as a competitive substrate in the reactions leading to prothrombin activation in the intrinsic system.

To try to pinpoint the exact site of factor VII activation, we studied this phenomenon in plasma deficient in various blood coagulation factors (figure 3). Factor VII activation normally occurs in patients deficient in factor II, V, X, or VIII (three cases). We found virtually no activation in factor IX (two cases), factor XI or factor XII deficiencies.

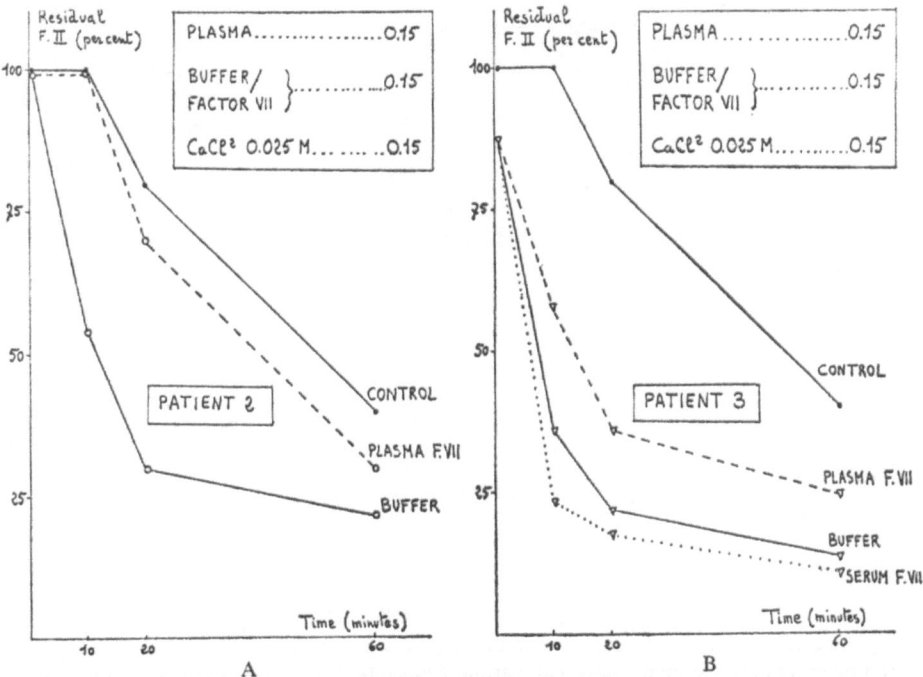

Fig. 2. Prothrombin consumption in patients with factor VII deficiency: effect of the addition of purified factor VII obtained from plasma (plasma factor VII) or from serum (serum factor VII). A: Patient 2. B: Patient 3. System: citrated plasma 0.15 ml; buffer or factor VII (for 100% level in plasma) 0.15 ml; CaCl$_2$ 0.025 M 0.15 ml.

These data suggest that factor VII activation by glass involves factors XII, XI, and IX. Shanberge and Matsuoka (14) arrived at the same conclusion in their study regarding the effect of contact on the one-stage prothrombin time determination. This opinion was also shared by Verstraete and Vermylen in order to explain the apparent factor VII deficiency in cases of hemophilia B (18). However, these results contradict those obtained by Altman and Hemker (2), who studied the shortening by glass contact of the 'thrombotest' clotting time of various deficient plasmas.

In fact, it is clear that factor IX is, like factor X, a meeting point of the so-called intrinsic and extrinsic systems. Recent data reported by Nossel (11) show that tissue thromboplastin decreases the consumption of factors IX and XI produced by celite. All happens as if a competition existed between tissue thromboplastin (or VIIa) and contact product at the level of factor IX activation.

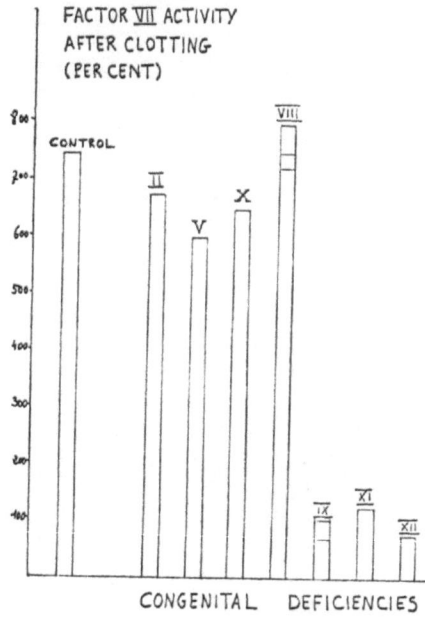

Fig. 3. Factor VII activity (by reference to initial plasma level) after clotting of control plasma and plasma samples from patients with various congenital deficiencies. System: citrate plasma 0.3 ml; kaolin (5 mg/ml) 0.15 ml; cephalin in $CaCl_2$ 0.5 M 0.15 ml.

The discrepancies between the results obtained by various investigations concerning the role of factor IX in factor VII activation could be explained by recent findings regarding hemophilia B. At least two molecular varieties of hemophilia B are now recognized: in some families factor IX is apparently not synthesized; in others an abnormal biologically inactive molecule is present (5, 8, 15) and competes with the extrinsic system. (8) Perhaps the discrepancy between data obtained on factor VII activation in hemophilia B is due to the fact that the investigations were dealing with different kinds of factor IX abnormalities. Everybody now accepts that molecular complexes are formed during the reaction sequence of blood coagulation. (6) It is likely that an abnormal molecule could compete with another normal factor in the formation of these complexes.

ACKNOWLEDGEMENTS

We are happy to thank D. Benamon-Djiane and C. Regnier, who prepared purified factor VII.

REFERENCES

1. Alexander B., G., Landwher Evolution of a prothrombin conversion accelerator in stored human plasma and prothrombin fractions. *Amer. J. Physiol.*, 159, 322 (1949).
2. Altman R., H. C. Hemker, Contact activation in the extrinsic blood clotting system. *Thromb. Diath. haemorrh.*, 18, 525 (1967).
3. Benamon-Djiane D., F. Josso, J. P. Soulier, Purification de la prothrombine humaine par chromatographie sur DEAE-Sephadex. Propriétés de la prothrombine purifiée. *Coagulation* 1, 259 (1968).
4. Biggs R., H. L. Nossel, Tissue extract and the contact reaction in blood coagulation *Thromb. Diath. haemorrh.*, 6, 1 (1961).
5. Denson K. W. E., R. Biggs, P. M. Mannucci, An investigation of three patiens with Christmas disease due to an abnormal type of factor IX. *J. Clin. Path.*, 21, 160 (1968).
6. Hemker H. C., M. J. P. Kahn, Reaction sequence of blood coagulation. *Nature*, 215, 1201 (1967).
7. Hjort P. F., Intermediate reactions in the coagulation of blood with tissue thromboplastin. *Scand. J. Clin. Lab. Invest.*, 9, suppl. 27 (1957).
8. Hougie C., J. J. Twomey, Haemophilia Bᴍ: a new type of factor IX deficiency. *Lancet*, 1, 698 (1967).
9. Josso F., O. Prou-Wartelle, Interaction of tissue factor and factor VII at the earliest phase of coagulation. *Thromb. Diath. haemorrh.* 17, suppl 17, 35 (1965).
10. Nossel H. L., *The contact phase of blood coagulation*. Blackwell Scientific Publications Ed., Oxford (1964).
11. Nossel H. L., Differential consumption of coagulation factors resulting from activation of the extrinsic (tissue thromboplastin) or the intrinsic (foreign surface contact) pathways. *Blood*, 29, 331 (1967).
12. Rapaport S. I., K. Aas, P. A. Owren, The effect of glass upon the activity of the various plasma clotting factors. *J. Clin. Invest.*, 34, 9 (1955).
13. Rapaport S. I., P. F. Hjort, M. J. Patch, and M. Jeremic, Consumption of serum factors and prothrombin during intravascular clotting in rabbits. *Scand. J. Haemat.*, 3, 59 (1966).
14. Shanberg J. N., T. Matsuoka, Studies regarding the effect of foreign-surface contact on the one-stage prothrombin time determination. *Thromb. Diath. haemorrh.*, 15, 442 (1966).
15. Somer J. B., P. A. Castaldi, Studies on coagulation factor IX in haemophilia B, *Abstracts* of XIIth *Congr. Internat. Soc. Hemat.*, New York, (1968), p. 180.
16. Soulier J. P., C. Blatrix, M. Steinbuch, Fractions 'coagulantes' contenant les facteurs de coagulation adsorbables par le phosphate tricalcique. *Presse Med.*, 72, 1223 (1964).
17. Soulier J. P., O. Prou-Wartelle, New data on Hageman factor and plasma thromboplastin antecedent: the role of 'contact' in the initial phase of blood coagulation. *Brit. J. Haemat.*, 6, 8 (1960).
18. Verstraete M., C. Vermylen, Hemophilia B associated with decreased factor VII activity. *Thromb. Diath. haemorrh.*, 6, 613 (1961).

DISCUSSION

Hemker: When we investigate the shortening of an extrinsic coagulation time under the influence of contact activation in the course of several hours with several deficient plasmas, we see a negligible shortening in factor xii-deficient plasmas, which is only a little more pronounced-in factor xi-deficient plasma; but other deficiencies, and especially factor ix deficiency, all show the same effect as normal plasmas except of course a factor vii deficiency. This indicates an action of factor xii and possibly factor xi on factor vii. These experiments were carried out by Dr. Altman in our laboratory.

We also found a quantitative correlation between the amount of factor vii present and the degree of activation obtained. The same holds for the concentration either of a purified contact product or of factor xii. I am rather in favor of Dr. Josso's explanation. The discrepancies between his experiments and ours may be explained by a difference in the factor ix-deficient plasma we used. I wonder if Dr. Josso could tell us what he thinks are the real differences in these different factor ix-deficient plasmas.

Josso: It seems that patients with hemophilia BM have an abnormal factor ix molecule which may act as an inhibitor of factor vii conversion.

Denson: We had three patients with hemophilia BM and we could demonstrate that their plasma contained a competitive inhibitor in the thromboplastin-factor vii-factor x reaction. There was apparently no abnormality in the factor vii molecule.

Hemker: This indeed would also explain the differences we find in contact activation experiments. I think that we have to consider that activation product acts on factor vii directly and not via factor ix but that in the presence of an abnormal factor ix molecule the reaction may be inhibited.

FACTOR VII AND TISSUE THROMBOPLASTIN

H. PRYDZ

The extrinsic coagulation system is an alternative way for the activation of factor x in blood coagulation. The reactions are triggered by tissue thromboplastin (factor III), and the presence of factor VII and calcium ions is necessary.

Patients lacking factor VII often have a bleeding tendency of varying clinical significance (1, 2), although no definite physiological role has been assigned to this system in current models of normal hemostasis. It may serve as a rapid means of generating the small amounts of thrombin necessary for the subsequent activation of the slower intrinsic coagulation. Due to the intracellular (microsomal) localization of tissue thromboplastin, cell damage is a prerequisite for exposure of this factor to plasma.

There are, on the other hand, reports of thrombo-embolic episodes in patients with a severe congenital factor VII deficiency, and other severe cases without clinical symptoms are discovered (3, 4). The extrinsic system is therefore apparently not indispensable for normal hemostasis and the occurrence of thrombosis.

The reaction initiating this pathway is the activation of factor VII by tissue thromboplastin. Factor VII purified from human serum 8 to 10 thavsanb fold (5) is a glycoprotein homogeneous in starch gel electrophoresis and in analytical disc electrophoresis when 50-60 µg of protein is used. Two bands are observed when 100 µg or more is applied to one gel. In isoelectric focusing, factor VII from serum or plasma gave two bands at pH 5.7 and pH 6.6. The pH 6.6 band disappeared when the preparations were dialysed against EDTA before the isoelectric focusing was carried out. This observation indicates that factor VII will bind a divalent cation, thus giving rise to an extra band, in accordance with the ability of factor VII to bind calcium (6).

Such factor VII preparations were free of detectable activities of the other coagulation factors tested (II, IX, and x). By injection of these preparations into rabbits, antisera were obtained hrat selectively removed factor VII activity completely from plasma or serum while the levels of the other coagulation factors (II, IX, and X) were left essentially unchanged (7). These antisera were also used to demonstrate that neither plasma from Dicumarol-treated normal controls nor that from patients with severe congenital factor VII deficiency contained any cross-reacting antigens (7). These findings have recently been confirmed (8, 9).

Such reasonably pure preparations of factor VII were used to study various physical parameters and the composition of the carbohydrate portion. Gel filtration on calibrated columns and sucrose gradient centrifugation gave molecular weights for factor VII from plasma or serum (table 1) in good accordance with earlier data (5). The un-

Table 1. Molecular parameters of factor VII

	sedimentation coefficient	Stokes' radius	molecular weights
Factor VII from plasma	4.61 ± 0.41	35.3 ± 0.5	$59\,000 \pm 6\,100$
Factor VII from serum	4.11 ± 0.25	30.0 ± 1.1	$44\,700 \pm 4\,300$

activated form of factor VII in plasma has a greater molecular weight than factor VII isolated from serum produced by intrinsic coagulation. Factor VII is activated by the intrinsic system, and factors XII, XI, VIII, and IX are required (10). We are currently studying factor VII activated by tissue thromboplastin to see if it has the same reduced molecular weight or is noticeably different from the intrinsic-activated factor VII. Nothing is known about the nature of this change in molecular weight, but it is reasonable to assume that a peptide or a glycopeptide is split off, in analogy with several other reactions in the blood coagulation mechanism. Such a peptide would be of a neutral character, since no changes were observed in the molecular charge upon activation.

The coagulation activity, the antigenic activity, and the calcium-binding capacity of factor VII preparations were abolished or greatly reduced by relatively brief periodate exposures (7). Although the periodate effect provided only circumstantial evidence for the functional significance of the carbohydrate portion, we felt that the ob-

servations justified a closer look at the composition of these carbohydrates. In a number of analyses we have found glucose and fucose to be
present. Two preparations contained a small amount of hexosamine,
which was absent in four other samples (11). Glucose is an uncommon
but not unknown component of glycoproteins (12). It has been identified by chromatography as well as by glucose oxidase. A tightly bound
macromolecular contaminant containing glucose cannot yet be completely excluded.

   The very small amounts of purified factor VII make the quantitative
estimations somewhat variable (table 2). The total carbohydrate

Table 2. Carbohydrate content in factor VII preparations*

Glucose (%)	Fucose (%)	Total (%)
16.8 ± 7.3	6.7 ± 3.7	23.6 ± 3.6

* Based on analysis of 6 preparations, two of which contained small amounts of hexosamine.

content is on the order of 20 to 25%, the main part of which reacts
like glucose.

   Bovine factor VII is reported to have a molecular weight of about
60,000 (13), and the probably activated form studied by Tishkoff,
Williams and Brown had a molecular weight of 33,900.

   Tissue thromboplastin is a protein-phospholipid complex (14) connected with the endoplasmic reticulum (15, 16). By solubilization with
deoxycholate (DOC), the complex is split into two components, A and
B (17), which can be further purified separately. Each component is
by itself inactive, but the procoagulant activity is regained upon recombination (17) and subsequent removal of DOC. A time-consuming
re-aggregation of fractions A and B into large membranous structures
takes place concomitantly with an increase in the procoagulant
activity (18), which is bound to the membranes. These membrane
structures are obviously of basic importance to the activity of tissue
thromboplastin. A similar splitting of tissue thromboplastin has been
reported by Deutsch, Irsigler and Lomoschitz (19).

   Fraction A consists almost entirely of protein (97-100%) and fraction B of 80-90% phospholipids (17). Nemerson recently described a
similar protein fraction (20). Fraction B alone will give rise to the same

membranous structures as A and B together, but when formed in the absence of fraction A the membranes are inactive in the extrinsic coagulation. A membranous structure is thus in itself not enough. There is, however, also some specificity in the composition of the membranes formed by fraction B, since membranes formed from phospholipids in other fractions of the eluate give no tissue thromboplastin activity when recombined with fraction A, although they appear identical in the electron microscope. Fraction A, the protein part, appears from membrane and gel filtration data to have a molecular weight of about 50,000 or slightly less.

THE INITIAL REACTIONS OF THE EXTRINSIC SYSTEM

Hougie (21), using factor VII- and factor x-deficient plasma, established that factor VII acted in a catalytic way in the production of extrinsic prothrombin converting activity. The level of factor VII influenced the rate of appearance of this activity rather than the yield, while factor x had a substrate role in determining the final yield of converting activity.

Straub and Duckert (22) concluded that tissue factor and factor x in the presence of calcium were substrates in a reaction catalyzed by factor VII and that the product of this reaction interacted with factor v to form the extrinsic activator.

Williams (15) reported that tissue thromboplastin acted like an enzyme in the activation of factor x, but later modified his view (23). Factor VII, calcium, and tissue thromboplastin form a stoichiometric complex and are not in any substrate-enzyme relationship to each other. Factor VII may be activated by its adsorption to tissue thromboplastin to give the complex enzymatic activity towards factor x.

Nemerson and Spaet (24) described a saline extract from butanol-treated rabbit brain activating factor x in the presence of factor VII. In the postulated absence of factor VII, a slow activation took place. Later, Nemerson (25) agreed with Williams and Norris (23) that a factor VII-calcium-tissue thromboplastin complex was formed which had enzymatic activity towards factor x. This complex was inhibited by DFP and by soybean trypsin inhibitor. No activated factor VII could be solubilized from the complex. The reaction between tissue thromboplastin and factor VII is very rapid (25).

We have approached these problems by studying the two partial functions of tissue thromboplastin, the binding of factor VII and x and the activation of these two factors by the two isolated components A and B obtained after DOC splitting (17). This work is still in progress. We have so far demonstrated that fraction B (the phospholipid component) will bind either factor VII or X in a sedimentable form. The active protein(s) in fraction A did not sediment, and their binding capacity is currently being studied by means of gel filtration.

So far, we have purified factors VII and X from serum. They are already activated, and no further activation is obtained with tissue thromboplastin. Such purified factors lose their activity quite rapidly at 37°C. We have therefore studied the ability of fraction A and B to protect the already activated factors against loss of activity at 37°C, which implies that this stabilizing influence is in some way related to activation.

In such studies we found that fraction B (the phospholipid fraction) had a stabilizing effect upon both factor VII and X. Fraction A (the protein fraction) had a marked effect upon factor X and a mixture of VII and X, but no effect on factor VII. It is obviously necessary to repeat these experiments with unactivated, purified factors, and this approach may then be of some help in establishing the molecular events in these initial steps of the extrinsic system.

REFERENCES

1. Voss, D., B. A. Waaler, *Thromb. Diath. haemorrh.* 3 ,375 (1959).
2. Owen, C. A. et al., *Amer. J. Med.* 37, 71 (1964).
3. Hall, C. A. et al., *Amer. J. Med.* 37, 172 (1964).
4. Godal, H. C., K. Madsen, R. Nissen-Meyer, *Acta Med. Scand.* 171, 325 (1962).
5. Prydz, H., *Scand. J. Clin. Lab. Invest.* 17, suppl. 84 p. 78 (1965).
6. Prydz, H., *Abstr. 1st Meeting, Fed. Europ. Biochem. Soc.*, London (1964).
7. Prydz, H., *Scand. J. Clin. Lab. Invest.* 17, 66 (1965).
8. Denson, K. W. E., The use of antibodies in the study of blood coagulation, Blackwell, Oxford (1967).
9. Goldstein, R., G. Schindler, *Abstr.* XII *Congress, Int. Soc. Hematol.*, New York (1968).
10. Johnston, C. L., P. F. Hjort, *J. Clin. Invest.* 40, 743 (1961).
11. Prydz, H., *Abstr. 4th Meeting, Fed. Europ. Biochem. Soc.*, Oslo (1967).
12. Radhakrishnamurthy, B., G. S. Berenson, *J. Biol. Chem.*, 241, 2106 (1966).
13. Deutsch, E., et al., *Abstr.* XI *Congress, Int. Soc. Hematol.* Siydney (1966).
14. Cohen, S. S., E. Chargraff, *J. Biol. Chem.* 136, 243 (1940).
15. Williams, W. J., *J. Biol. Chem.* 239, 933 (1964).
16. Hvatum, M., H. Prydz, *Biochem. Biophys. Acat* 130, 92 (1966).
17. Hvatum, M., H. Prydz, *Abstr. 4th Meeting, Fed. Europ. Biocehm. Soc.*, Oslo (1967).
18. Prydz, H., M. Hvatum, *Abstr. 3rd Meeting, Fed. Europ. Biochem. Soc.*, Warsaw (1966).
19. Deutsch, E., K. Irsigler, H. Lomoschitz, *Thromb. Diath. haemorrh.* 12, 12 (1964).
20. Nemerson, Y., *Abstr.* XII *Congress, Int. Soc. Hematol.*, New York (1968).
21. Hougie, C., *Proc. Soc. Exp. Biol. Med.* 101, 132 (1959).

22. Straub, W., F. Duckert, *Thromb. Diath. haemorrh.* 5, 402 (1961).
23. Williams, W. J., D. G. Norris, *J. Biol. Chem.* 241, 1847 (1966).
24. Nemerson, Y., T. H. Spaet, *Blood* 23, 657 (1964).
25. Nemerson, Y., *Biochemistry* 5, 601 (1966).

DISCUSSION

P. M. van der Plas: The use of filipin as a tool in coagulation research

Lipid clusters (c q. phospholipid clusters) are thought to play a role at different sites in the coagulation procedure:

1. At the formation of a complex between factors v, x, and lipid. This complex converts prothrombin into thrombin.
2. At the formation of a complex between factors viii, ix, and lipid, which activates factor x.

The existence of these two complexes is reasonably certain. Phospholipids are possibly also necessary for the reaction between factor vii and the proteins present in tissue-extract. This is what specifically interests us in the context of Dr. Prydz's work.

We tried to obtain more information about the function of lipids in blood-clotting by the use of some polyene antibiotics, such as nystatin, pimaricin, amphotericin b, and filipin. These antibiotics act by interaction with lipids. Very probably, sterols play an important role in this interaction, although they appear not to be absolutely necessary. In clotting studies the most useful polyene is filipin. The other polyenes give a lower inhibition or are poorly soluble in a suitable medium.

The effect of different amounts of filipin on the clotting time of a modified prothrombin time according to Quick is shown in table 1. The clotting time was measured as follows: 1 part plasma; 1 part

Table 1. Effect of filipin on prothrombin – time. (Clotting times are given in seconds means of 5 experiment)

Filipin conc.(M)	Dilution of Brain thromboplastin		
	Undil.	1 : 3	1 : 10
$7 \cdot 10^{-5}$	38	43	59
$3,5 \cdot 10^{-5}$	32	42	58
$1,75 \cdot 10^{-5}$	21	32	50
	16	21	28

filipin suspension or blank; and 1 part brain extract are mixed at 37°; after 30 seconds, 1 part CaCl$_2$ 25mM is added and the clotting time is recorded. It is clearly seen that the clotting times depend on the filipin concentration: the higher the concentration the longer the clotting times.

To see whether the action of filipin is dependent of the cholesterol content of the lipid in coagulation tests as it is in many other test systems, we mead lipid suspensions differing in cholesterol content. we mixed inosithin and cholesterol, and used these mixtures in a cephalin-kaolin clotting time estimation. The test was carried out as follows: 1 part plasma, 1 part filipin sus pension or blank, and 1 part lipid-kaolin mixture were mixed at 37° and after 5 minutes 1 part CaCl$_2$ (25 M) was added and the clotting time was recorded. Four different inosithin-cholesterol mixtures were used. Mixture A contained only inosithin; mixtures B, C, and D inosithin and 10, 20, and 40 per cent cholesterol by weight, respectively.

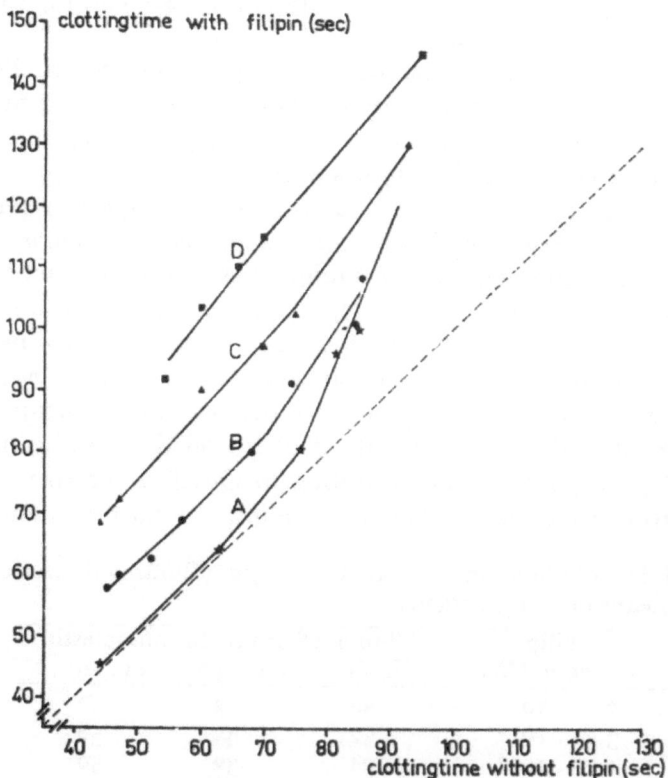

Fig. 1 Influence of filipin on cephalin-kaotin time

In figure 1 the not-inhibited and inhibited clotting times are compared. The variation in clotting time was obtained by the use of different dilutions of the above-mentioned inosithin-cholesterol mixtures. All inhibited clotting times were recorded in the present of a constant filipin concentration (2.10^{-5} M). It is evident that the degree onhibition increases with the cholesterol content.

On the basis of these (and other) experiments, we must conclude that the composition of micelles in clotting is important for the degree of inhibition obtained with filipin.

The question of the exact localization of the inhibition remains to be solved. Since the clotting mechanism initiated by RVV can be inhibited by polyenes, we must conclude that the formation or action of a complex formed by factors v, x, and lipid is inhibited. We attempted to answer the question of whether a complex between factors VIII, IX, and lipid can be inhibited, by means of a two-stage test:

stage one	*stage two*
diluted factor v-deficient plasma	factor x-deficient plasma
lipid suspension (low conc.)	lipid suspension (high conc.)
filipin suspension or blank	filipin suspension or blank
CaCl$_2$	

In this test, a complex may be formed between factors VIII, IX, and lipid in the first stage, and in the second stage a complex between factors v, x_a, and lipid is formed. This makes it possible to differentiate between inhibitory action of filipin in the VIII-IX-lipid complex and in the v-x-lipid complex. In figure 2 the presence of filipin in the first or second stage is indicated by the signs in brackets.

Figure 2 shows that addition of filipin to the first stage only $(+,-)$ causes a much more pronounced inhibition than the same quantity of filipin present in the second stage only $(-, +)$. In the case $(-,-)$, no filipin was used, and in $(+,+)$ filipin was added to both stages. On the basis of these experiments we must assume that a complex is indeed formed between factors VIII, IX, and lipid and that it is sensitive to filipin.

Lastly, a lipid-protein complex may be involved in the reaction between tissue-extract and factor VII. Another possibility is that the lipid present in tissue extract is necessary for the formation of the complex between factors v, x, and lipid only. At the moment we do not have conclusive experimental evidence either to prove or disprove a role of micelles at the level of the activation of factor vii, although preliminary experiments have revealed inhibition of the activation of factor vii by filipin.

Deutsch: For several years we have done experiments on the separation and recombination of tissue thromboplastin. By treatment with pyridine, a protein and a lipid fraction can be obtained, each of which has a negligible activity, but both recover full activity after recombination. I think this proves that tissue thromboplastin contains a protein moiety as well as a lipid moiety.

Esnouf: Dr. Nemerson has shown that the factor x activation by mixtures of factors iii and vii is only inhibited by DFP when factors iii and vii are both present together. Pre-incubation of either reactant with DFP is without effect.

Prydz: I have never tried to inhibit the combination of tissue thromboplastin and factor vii, but I have tried to look into the esterase activity of factor vii that has been activated and separated from the tissue

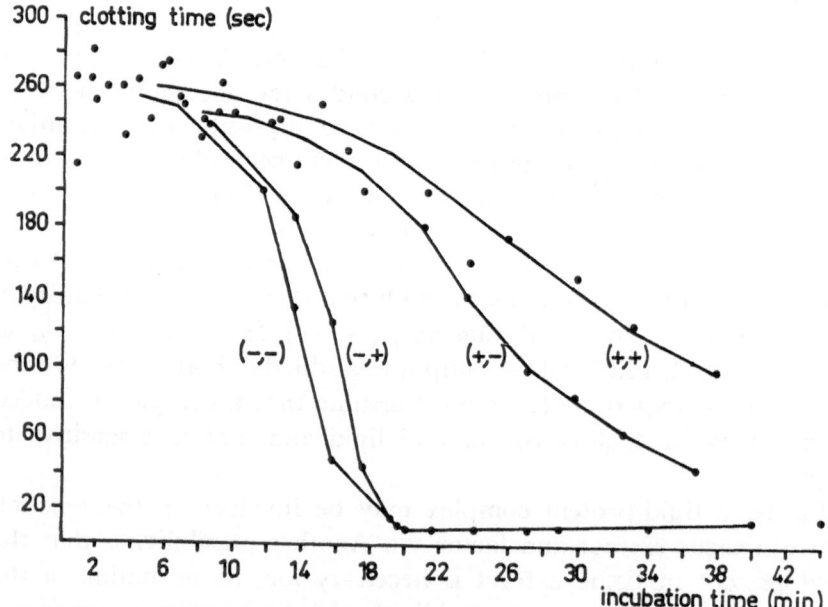

Fig. 2. Influence of filipin on two-stage clotting test incubation mixture: Fv deficient plasma assay mixture: Fx   „   „

thromboplastin-factor VII product. I have never been able to find any esterase activity, but this may have been due to the choice of the wrong substrate and it may be worth-while to re-investigate this problem.

At the moment, I have the following tentative picture of the reaction mechanism that starts the extrinsic clotting: phospholipid serves as a binding template for factors VII and X, possibly factor VII is activated by this binding, whereas factor X is activated by a protein-protein interaction. The phospholipid fraction (fraction B) binds factor VII, whereas fraction A (the protein part) has no such binding capacity. Crude tissue thromboplastin as well as the recombined fractions A and B also bind factor VII.

A disadvantage of our experiments is that they were done with factor VII from serum, which is already activated. We have not been able to demonstrate any further activation of factor VII by the various fractions. What we can demonstrate is a stabilization. Purified factor VII loses its activity quite rapidly when incubated at $37\,°C$ in the presence of, for instance, fraction A or buffer. Fraction B has some stabilizing effect, but incubation with recombined fractions A and B or a crude thromboplastin has a marked stabilizing activity compared to the single fractions.

In the case of factor X we have a different situation. Fraction A has a marked stabilizing effect on activated factor X. Tissue thromboplastin, which here again was reconstituted from purified fractions A and B, had a similar effect. Fraction B has a slight or insignificant stabilizing effect, and a buffer control shows a loss of factor X activity during incubation. It is dangerous to conclude that stabilization has something to do with activation. We hope to repeat these experiments with unactivated factor VII, but it is difficult to go through the purification procedure and still end up with an unactivated factor VII. I think that the DEAE chromatography contributes to part of the activation of factor VII. Yet this approach, if successful, may be able to tell us something more about the details of the triggering of the extrinsic coagulation system.

ENZYME SYSTEMS TRIGGERED BY THE CONTACT FACTORS

C. R. M. PRENTICE

It has been recognized that some of the enzymes concerned with coagulation and fibrinolysis have several substrates of differing specificity. Not least amongst these are the contact factors, Hageman factor (factor XII), and plasma thromboplastin antecedent (factor XI). They appear to form the pathway through which the plasma response to contact with abnormal surfaces is channelled. In addition to coagulation, they play a part in fibrinolysis and in the inflammatory reaction through their role in kinin formation. Some aspects of these reactions will be discussed.

For further information, the comprehensive reviews of Ratnoff (20) and Eisen (5) should be read. Additionally, Sherry et al. (22) have summarized important information relating to the esterolytic properties of these factors and of plasma that has been contacted with glass.

THE CONTACT FACTORS AND FIBRINOLYSIS

Several investigators have suggested that activated Hageman factor is able to activate plasminogen (9, 18). Iatridis and Ferguson (10) found that when the euglobulin fraction prepared from normal plasma was incubated in glass, progressively increasing fibrinolytic activity was noted. In the presence of kaolin the process was accelerated. A similar fraction prepared from Hageman-factor deficient plasma did not show such activity, even in the presence of kaolin. When, however, the contact factors were added to this preparation, normal fibrinolytic activity was restored. Hexadimethrine, an agent which inhibits the activation of Hageman factor, also inhibited the development of fibrinolytic activity under these conditions (4). Thus, the fibrinolytic mechanism appears to be dependent, in some manner, on activated Hageman factor.

Studies on patients with Hageman trait or plasma thromboplastin antecedent (PTA) deficiency have produced conflicting results. Iatridis and Ferguson (10), and Holemans (8) found that, in patients with Hageman trait, fibrinolytic activity was diminished and the normal rise of such activity following exercise and venous occlusion was impaired. Similarly, Ratnoff (20) has demonstrated that a patient with PTA deficiency had defective fibrinolysis. Conversely, Holemans found that one patient with Hageman trait had an exaggerated fibrinolytic response to intravenous nicotinic acid, an agent known to stimulate this process. Nilsson (19) has also found fibrinolytic activity to be normal in these patients.

The basis for these conflicting reports has not yet been resolved, but it seems clear that fibrinolytic activity is not mediated solely through the contact factors.

Purified fractions of bovine or human activated Hageman factor do not induce lysis *in vitro*. Neither can fibrinolysis be induced in dogs by the injection of ellagic acid, a known activator of Hageman factor (2). The reports of some investigators that 'contact factor' stimulates lysis must be viewed with some caution, because in most cases these preparations have been contaminated by other proteins, including plasminogen, as demonstrated by the fact that they generate plasmin when streptokinase is added to them.

CONTACT FACTORS AND THE INFLAMMATORY REACTION
The implication of Hageman factor in the inflammatory reaction was based on the observations of Armstrong, Keele, Jepson and Stewart (1) and Margolis (15) that plasma, following exposure to glass, developed the ability to induce pain and increase vascular permeability in experimental animals. Margolis (16), noting that Hageman factor deficient plasma failed to produce these changes under similar conditions, suggested that they were mediated by activated Hageman factor.

In support of this evidence, Ratnoff and Miles (21) found that purified activated Hageman factor, when added to diluted plasma, stimulated the production of a permeability-producing factor. This may be indentical to PF/dil as described by Miles and Wilhelm (17). Kinetic studies showed that activated Hageman factor acted as an enzyme to produce permeability factor from an inactive substrate. The formation of PF/dil was inhibited by hexadimethrine bromide (Polybrene) (4, 21).

Further studies showed that activated Hageman factor could induce in plasma the formation of agents which contracted smooth muscle (14), produced pain (13), and dilated blood vessels (7). Similarly, when injected into a rabbit ear chamber, it caused the leucocytes to adhere to vascular walls and migrate into extravascular spaces (7).

These experiments suggest that activated Hageman factor has an enzymatic action on the precursor substance kallikreinogen to release kallikrein. This enzyme, in its turn, acts upon the prokinins to form the pharmacologically active kinins. As might be expected, esterolytic activity appears in plasma on exposure to glass, since both PF/dill and plasma kallikrein are esterolytic. The precursors of PF/dil and kalli-krein can be separated chromatographically, thus indicating that Hageman factor acts on at least two different substrates. There are certainly other enzymes in plasma which activate kallikreinogen. One such agent can be distinguished from activated Hageman factor by the fact that is not inhibited by hexadimethrine bromide (3).

Somewhat puzzling in the light of these observations is the fact that people with Hageman trait appear to respond normally to infective or inflammatory disorders. One such patient developed a staphylococ-cal abscess with pus formation, and responded normally to the tuber-culin and Shick tests, indicating that the presence of this factor is not essential for these responses (20). On the other hand, Margolis noted that the inflammatory reaction to an intracutaneous injection of kaolin was defective in one patient with Hageman factor deficiency.

The fact that surface contact causes both increased fibrinolytic activity and kinin formation has led to the suggestion that plasmin, or other products of the fibrinolytic process, might be responsible for kinin formation. Eisen (3) suggested that the two processes occurred mainly independently, since he found that streptokinase produced marked fibrinolysis but poor kinin-forming activity. Also, ε -amino caproïc acid (EACA) in -hibited the fibrinolytic but not the kinin-forming response of plasma to contact with silica surfaces. In contrast, other workers have suggested that plasmin is the main kinin-forming enzyme.

It is possible that plasmin produces kinins indirectly through an ac-tion on kallikreinogen, or that both kallikreinogen and kininogen be-long to the protein substrates of plasmin (5).

CONTACT FACTORS AND GOUT

The possibility that Hageman factor is concerned in the production of acute gouty arthritis was first made by Kellermeyer and Breckenridge (11), who showed that microcrystalline sodium urate, as found in affected joints, activated Hageman factor. Since synovial fluid contains both Hageman factor (12) and the precursor of a permeability producing factor, it is possible that Hageman factor mediates the inflammatory pathways in gouty arthritis. Moreover, kinins can be demonstrated both in inflammatory joint effusions (6) and in synovial fluid incubated with urate crystals.

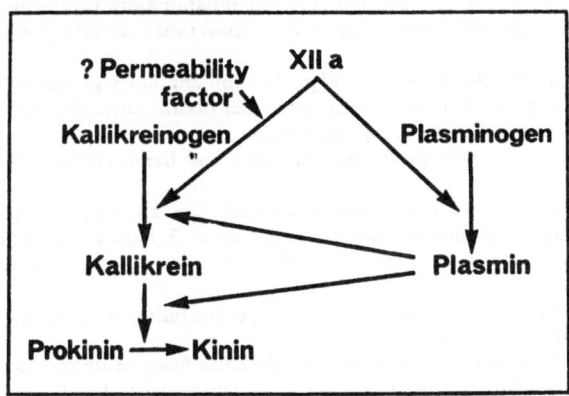

Fig. 1. Tentative mechanism by which activated Hageman factor participates in the kinin-forming and fibrinolytic enzyme systems.

It is evident, therefore, that the role of the contact factors extends widely outside the process of blood coagulation. Although much progress has been made in *in vitro* experiments, more information is required as to the significance of these phenomena in view of the good health of patients with Hageman factor deficiency.

REFERENCES

1. Armstrong, D., C. A. Keele, J. B. Jepson, J. W. Stewart, Development of pain producing substance in human plasma. *Nature*, 174, 791 (1954).
2. Botti, R. E., O. D. Ratnoff, Studies on the pathogenesis of thrombosis: An experimental 'hypercoagulable' state induced by the intravenous injection of ellagic acid. *J. lab. Clin. Med.*, 64, 385 (1964).
3. Eisen, V., Kinin formation and fibrinolysis in human plasma. *J. Physiol.* 166, 514 (1963).
4. Eisen, V., Effects of hexadimethrine bromide on plasma kinin formation, hydrolysis of p-tosyl-l-arginine methyl ester and fibrinolysis. *Brit. J. Pharmacol.*, 22, 87 (1964).

5. Eisen, V., Fibrinolysis and the formation of biologically active polypeptides. *Brit. med. Bull.* 20, 205 (1964).
6. Goldfinger, S., K. L. Melmon, M. E. Webster, A. Sjoerdsma, J. E. Seegmiller, The presence of a kinin-peptide in inflammatory synovial effusions. *Arthritis Rheum.*, 7, 311 (1964).
7. Graham, R. C., Jr., R. H. Ebert, O. D. Ratnoff, J. M. Moses, Pathogenesis of inflammation II. In vivo observations of the inflammatory effects of activated Hageman factor and bradykinin. *J. exp. Med.*, 121, 807 (1965).
8. Holemans, R., H. R. Roberts, Hageman factor and in vivo activation of fibrinolysis. *J. lab. Clin. Med.*, 64, 778 (1964).
9. Iatridis, S. G., J. H. Ferguson, Effect of surface and Hageman factor on the endogenous or spontaneous activation of the fibrinolytic system. *Thromb. Diath. heamorrh.*, 6, 411 (1961)
10. Iatridis, S. G., J. H. Ferguson, Active Hageman factor: A plasma lysokinase of the human fibrinolytic system. *J. clin. Invest.*, 41, 1277 (1962).
11. Kellermeyer, R. W., R. T. Breckenridge, The inflammatory process in acute gouty arthritis. I. Activation of Hageman factor by sodium urate crystals. *J. lab. Clin. Med.*, 65, 307 (1965).
12. Kellermeyer, R. W. ,R. T. Breckenridge, The inflammatory process in acute gouty arthritis. II. The presence of Hageman factor and plasma thromboplastin antecedent in synovial fluid. *J. lab. Clin. Med.* ,67, 455 (1966).
13. Margolis, J., Plasma pain producing substance and blood clotting. *Nature*, 180, 1464 (1957).
14. Margolis, J., Activation of plasma by contact with glass: Evidence for a common reaction which releases plasma kinin and initiates coagulation. *J. Physiol.*, 144, 1 (1958).
15. Margolis, J., Activation of a permeability factor in plasma by contact with glass. *Nature*, 181, 635 (1958).
16. Margolis, J., Hageman factor and capillary permeability. *Aust. J. exp. Biol. Med. Sci.*, 37, 239 (1959).
17. Miles, A. A., D. L. Wilhelm, Enzyme-like globulins from serum producing the vascular phenomena of inflammation: I. An activable permeability factor and its inhibitor in guinea pig serum. *Brit. J. exp. Path.*,, 36, 71 (1955).
18. Niewiarowski, S., O. Prou-Wartelle, Role du facteur contact (Facteur Hageman) dans la fibrinolyse. *Thromb. Diath. haemorrh.*, 3, 593 (1959).
19. Nilsson, I. M., Personal communication.
20. Ratnoff, O. D., The biology and pathology of the initial stages of blood coagulation. *Progress in Hematology*, 5, 204 (1966).
21. Ratnoff, O. D., A. A. Miles, The induction of permeability-increasing activity in human plasma by activated Hageman factor. *Brit. J. exp. Pathh.*, 45, 328 (1964).
22. Sherry, S., N. K. Alkjaersig, A. P. Fletcher, Observations on the spontaneous arginine and lysine esterase activity of human plasma and their relation to Hageman factor. *Thromb. Diath. haemorrh.*, suppl. 20, 243 (1966).

DISCUSSION

K. W. Pondman: The complement system, its relations to other triggered enzyme systems in the blood plasma

In fibrinolysis there is a kinin-like activity that is simultaneously produced. I would like to propose an alternative pathway for the generation of this kind of tissue toxin. This is derived from results obtained in complement studies.

$$E \quad + \quad A \quad \longrightarrow \quad EA$$

$$EA \quad + \quad \boxed{C1} \xrightarrow{\ Ca^{++}\ } EAC\overline{1}$$

$$EAC\overline{1} \quad + \quad C4 \quad \longrightarrow \quad EAC14$$

$$EAC14 \quad + \quad C2 \xrightarrow{\ Mg^{++}\ } EAC142$$

$$EAC142 \quad \longrightarrow \quad EAC\overline{142}$$

$$EAC\overline{142} \quad + \quad \boxed{C3}_{complex} \longrightarrow E^{\bullet} \quad \begin{array}{l}(stroma \\ (hemoglobin\end{array}$$

$$\longrightarrow decay$$

Schematic representation of the complement fixation reaction, with 'sensitized' sheep erythrocytes, used as the target cell for complement action.

E = sheep erythrocyte.

A = specific antibody against sheep cell antigenic determinants.

c1, etc. = first component of complement, etc.

c̄1 = activated first component of complement, etc.

$\boxed{c1}$ = the first component of complement consists of three subcomponents called c1q, c1r, and c1s, which are united by a ca⁺⁺ ligand. c1s is a pro-esterase that activates to esterase during the fixation reaction.

$\boxed{c3}$complex = series of late-acting complement components c3 through c9. c9 is the really lytic component.

E* = the resulting damaged erythrocyte that hemolyses spontaneously in time.

The complement system is as complicated in handling as the clotting system. Immunologically, complement usually acts on immune aggregates, but it can occasionally act in their absence. It consists of nine components, referred to as c1 to c9. Figure 1 supplies information with respect to the reaction sequence of complement components in an immune system. Some of these components have very particular activities, especially in regard to their biological effects. I should like to discuss some of the biological effects of complement components in *in vivo* as well as *in vitro* systems.

The components of complement must act in sequence to allow its biological effects to take place. Complement-fixation reactions are usually studied by close examination of the activity of complement in immune haemolysis and bacteriolysis. Figure 2 shows that there are other

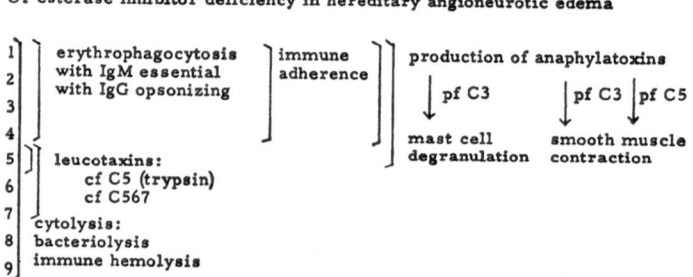

Fig. 1 Complement activity in biological phenomena

biological effects of the complement system. Immune hemolysis and bacteriolysis require all 9 complement components. Other phenomena require only the initially acting components in the series, and these components have to act in the same sequence as in immune hemolysis and bacteriolysis. For example, one phenomenon in which a limited number of complement components participate is the immune phagocytosis reaction. As shown in this figure 2, in phagocytosis only four components have been found to participate and permit the process to reach completion.

Figure 2 also shows which components are active in other biological phenomena. In general, it is found that once c1, c2, c4, and c3 react with each other, biologically active principles are generated. It is likely that the same activities will appear regardless of the principles that initiate the complement component interaction. This is important with respect to our views on the pathways of the simultaneously occurring activities generated by the clotting factors or fibrinolytic factors. The production of anaphylatoxins, as we prefer to call them, is a consequence of the interaction of some of the components of complement. A permeability factor derived from the third component of complement is a very small fragment with a molecular weight of

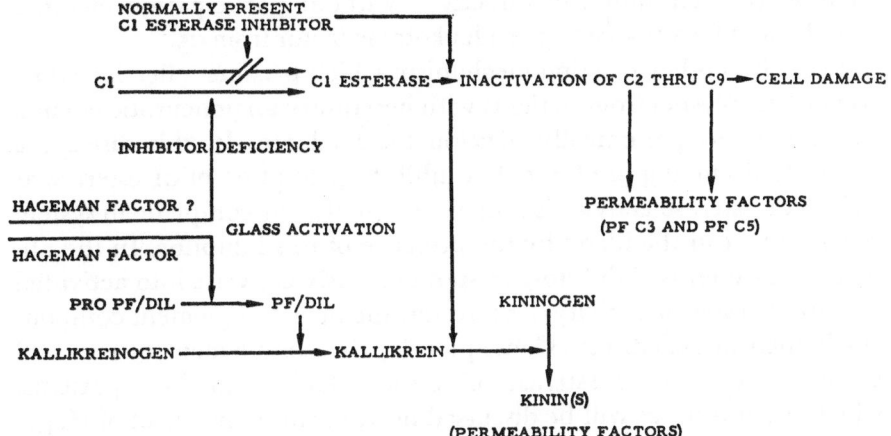

Fig. 3. Alternative pathways for generation of tissue toxinus

8,500 that generates kinin-like activity. This results in increased permeability of vessel walls in small tissue arteries or in arterial cutaneous vessels; smooth muscle contractions occur and can cause visceral pains. Whereas this anaphylatoxin is a factor derived from c3, there is another tissue toxin derived from C5. Both these toxins are generated from complement by the interaction of the first five components. If we can demonstrate that some of the clotting factors can act in generating the activities of these toxins, we may have produced evidence for another pathway in the production of tissue toxins.

It is worthwhile to mention also that the production of leukotaxins, factors that cause polymorphonuclear leucocytes to migrate, is mediated either by activated c5 alone or by the action of trypsin on c5 or by c5 in conjunction with the sixth and seventh components of complement.

It has been demonstrated that plasmin is capable of transforming cr into an 'activated' form in which an esterase is active. cr is a proesterase. Once this component is activated, the other components act in a chain reaction and therefore give rise to the formation of the above-mentioned tissue toxins, including also the principles that promote phagocytosis and leukotaxis.

All this depends on the presence or absence of anticoagulants. If you work in a milieu containing citrate, oxalate, or EDTA, it is quite definite that those factors will not be produced, since the interaction of c_2, c_3, and c_4 requires magnesium ions. It is also of interest here to mention that plasmin will directly – without participation of other complement factors – generate a leukotaxic factor from c_5.

There is another reaction mechanism which becomes effective when you use the plasma from patients with hereditary angioneurotic edema. These patients periodically develop local edema. In this disease, a naturally occurring inhibitor that inhibits generation of c_I esterase as well as c_I esterase activity is absent. Normally, the complement system is kept intact in the blood by the presence of this inhibitor. In the absence of c_I esterase inhibitor, c_I spontaneously converts into activated c_I with c_I esterase activity. As a result, the next complement component is then attacked, etc. Consequently, the complement system will be activated. The c_I esterase inhibitor is lacking in these patients, which permits us, as will be discussed now, to study the effect of Hageman factor on complement activation.

Recent experiments by Donaldson have shown that activated Hageman factor is capable of transforming c_I to c_I esterase in a purified preparation. She has also noted that the Hageman factor preparations used were not free of plasminogen. It is therefore reasonable to assume that activated Hageman factor can transform plasminogen into plasmin, which in turn will activate c_I into c_I esterase. It is possible to propose an alternative pathway for the generation of tissue toxins by saying that in angioneurotic edema plasma, c_I will be activated by activated Hageman factor and produce c_I esterase, a reaction resulting in the concomitant activation of the other components from c_2 through c_9. This will lead to generation of permeability factors and leukotaxins.

To return again for a moment to the inhibitory specificity of the c_I esterase inhibitor of blood, it is of interest that this factor also acts as a kallikrein inhibitor. In angioneurotic edema, the path towards generation of kinin activity seems to be uninhibited as well.

If we accept the idea that Hageman factor is the first step in the initiation of the fibrinolytic mechanism, then it is for the first time acceptable to propose the hypothesis that the four important mechanisms are interrelated by means of the Hageman factor. Activation of Hageman factor by rough surfaces, for instance local areas of vessel wall damage, may lead to clotting, fibrinolysis, activation of the complement system, or the formation of kinins. Which of these reactions will actually take place may be a function of the quantitative aspects of the kinetics of these reactions.

Prentice: It is quite true that there is a connection between the action of complement, activated Hageman factor, kinins, and plasmin. Although in the laboratory one can manipulate these systems, they are probably relatively independent *in vivo*. If you take streptokinase and add it to plasma in various dilutions, you will get fibrinolysis and very little kinin formation. Although one can get those various mechanisms going by adjusting the conditions, it is probable that the lytic system and the kinin-forming system are relatively independent. One wonders, although one knows that plasmin can produce kinin and can activate the complement system, whether this is the prime mechanism by which these systems are triggered or whether it is a secondary and relatively unimportant mechanism.

Vreeken: It is very difficult for me to understand that Mr. Hageman, who must have a severe deficiency in four systems, has no illness at all.

Vroman: Mr. Hageman is not as well as you may have hoped. He died of massive thromboses.

Prentice: After having first fallen off a train.

ENZYME KINETIC EVALUATION OF COAGULATION SYSTEMS

H. C. HEMKER

Enzyme-kinetic evaluation of data obtained in clotting tests suffers from all the drawbacks inherent to enzyme kinetics in general and, on top of that, has some extra difficulties peculiar to the field of blood coagulation. In general, the enzyme-kinetic approach starts by designing a model of the reaction(s) under study and then calculates what the kinetic behaviour of that model would be, compares experimental data with this calculated behaviour, and finally concludes whether or not the model is in agreement with the results of the experiments. A logical consequence of this approach is that the only conclusion that can be drawn with certainty is that a given model does not fit the observed facts. It is impossible to prove that a model in agreement with the observations is a fair representation of reality.

Extra drawbacks, peculiar to the field of blood coagulation, are:

a. An accurate method for the measurement of reaction velocities is lacking. In practice, we have to make do with coagulation-time estimations, which are highly inaccurate. Moreover, there is no clearcut relation between a clotting time and a reaction velocity in the coagulation reaction mechanism.

b. We lack an accurate method for measuring the concentration of reactants. In practice, we express these concentrations as the proportion relative to the activity in normal plasma.

Nevertheless, some of the relations found between clotting time and coagulation-factor concentration are so intriguing that one cannot help trying to find a suitable model for their explanation.

The first finding of this kind was that in prothrombin-time estimations of the 'Thrombotest' type there is a perfectly rectilinear dependency of the coagulation time upon the dilution ratio of a normal plasma sample (figure 1).

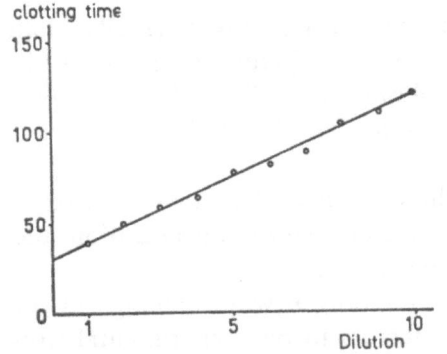

Fig. 1. A clotting time-dilution graph
(t-D graph).
Reaction mixture: 0.25 ml Thrombotest reagent,
0.05 ml sample.
Each point represents the mean of 20 estimations.

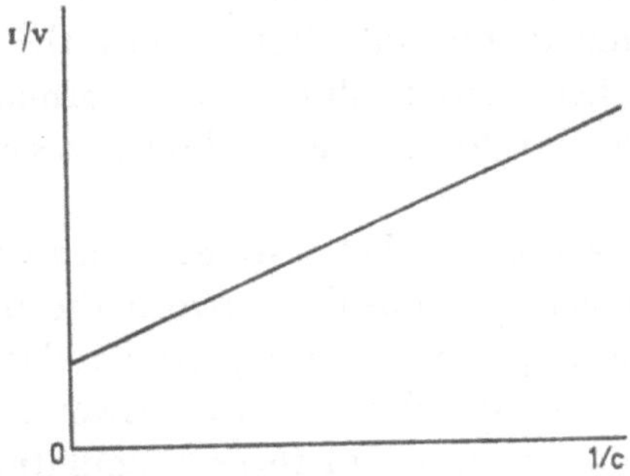

Fig. 2. A Lineweaver-Burk plot.

Prothrombin-time estimations of the *Thrombotest type* are those in which a fixed amount of factors I and V and thromboplastin is always present in the reagent, whereas the concentration of factors II, VII, and X is determined by the sample added. The dilution ratio we define as the ratio between the volumes of the sample before and after dilution. Therefore, a dilution ratio of unity indicates an undiluted sample. Now the analogy between the t-D plot depicted in figure 1 and a classical Lineweaver-Burk plot is immediately obvious (figure 2). In a Lineweaver-Burk plot, there is a rectilinear relationship between the inverse of a reaction velocity and the inverse of a concentration. Recognition of this analogy leaves us with two working hypotheses:

a. The clotting time is directly proportional to the inverse of the reaction velocity in a rate-limiting step of the coagulation reaction sequence.
b. The dilution of the plasma sample is proportional to the inverse of the concentration of *one* rate-limiting substrate.

We shall try to prove the second hypothesis first. Dilution of the plasma sample with buffer, as in the experiment shown in figure 1, affects the concentration of factors II, VII, and X in an analogous way. Dilution with a plasma deficient in one factor only, will affect nothing but the concentration of that factor. With this kind of experimental approach we were able to show that as long as the proportion of the concentration of factor x to that of factors VII and II is equal to or smaller than that in normal plasma, only the amount of factor x is relevant. In other words: dilution of a normal plasma in a 'Thrombotest' experiment is for all practical purposes equal to changing its factor x content (1).

From the above, we must draw the conclusion that there is a rectilinear relationship between the inverse of factor x concentration and clotting time in the experimental system studied.

This conclusion may answer the question of why a change in the concentrations of three coagulation factors in our experimental situation has the same effect as simply changing the concentration of the substrate in a uncomplicated enzymatic reaction; it leaves us with the still greater problem of why factor x should behave like a substrate in the reaction that sets the pace under our experimental conditions.

The solution to this problem is to be found in the fact that the situation in a coagulation test does not satisfy all the conditions for the validity of steady-state kinetics. At least one condition for the assumptions of steady-state kinetics does not hold: we can never assume that substrate is present in excess over the enzyme if we do not know whether factor x is to be regarded as substrate or enzyme in the reaction studied. Omission of the assumption $S \gg E$ from the set of assumptions leading to the standard formula of enzyme kinetics i.e. to:

$$\frac{k_{+2}}{V} = \frac{1}{E} + \frac{K_m}{E.S.}$$

leads to a slightly different formula, viz.:

$$\frac{k_{+2}}{V} = \frac{1}{E} + \frac{1}{S} + \frac{K_m}{E.S.}$$

In this formula, E and S occupy symetrical places, from which it follows that it does not matter whether factor x is to be regarded as a substrate or as an enzyme (2). If we now construct a system consisting of plasma congenitally deficient in factor x, thromboplastin, Ca^{++}ions, and varying concentrations of factor x, we expect to find the same lineair relationship as exists in a thrombotest experiment. This however, proved not to be the case. The coagulation times obtained with decreasing concentrations of factor x approach a limit (figure 3). This limit is the so-called 'buffer time', which is observed when no sample containing factor x is added. Obviously, a factor x activity must be present in the congenitally factor x-deficient plasma used as a reagent. We worked out a graphical method for the estimation of this activity (2, 3), which turned out to be between 1 and 2 per cent of normal plasma activities in various batches of reagent. When the concentration provided by the sample and the concentration present in the

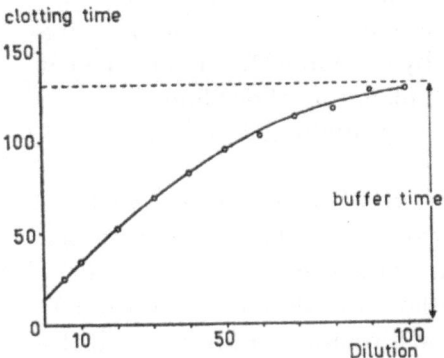

Fig. 3. Uncorrected t-D graph of a factor x test.
Reaction mixture: 0.1 ml. factor xdef. plasma
                              0.1 ml. thromboplastin
                              0.1 ml. sample
                              0.1 ml. CaCl$_2$ 25 mM.
Each point represents het mean of 20 estimations.

Fig. 4. Corrected t-D graph of a factor x test, based on the data in Fig. 3.

reagent were added (the real concentration in the experimental system thus being calculated), a perfectly linear relationship was again found between coagulation time and the inverse of factor x concentration (figure 4). This result was obtained with congenitally-deficient reagent as well as with a reagent made with plasma from a patient with acquired factor x deficiency (amyloidosis) (4).

To tackle the problem of why factor x shows such deceptively simple behaviour in a reaction sequence known to be very intricate, we investigated whether plots analogous to figure 4 could be obtained with other reagents, as a means of studying the behaviour of other factors.

The results indicated that all reagents deficient in one of the three factors II, v, or VII, showed the pattern described above. But a reagent deficient in two factors (factor VII-x reagent according to Bachman) (5) or reagents containing added Russell's viper venom (Borchgrevink's factor v reagent) (6) or the factor x estimation according to

Bachman (7) did not give similar results, and the same holds for estimations in the intrinsic system (factor VIII, IX, XI, and XII).

It thus seemed that in all systems where the extrinsic coagulation system is operative and where only one factor is rate limiting, the coagulation time bears a rectilinear relationship to the inverse of the concentration of the rate limiting factor.

Before trying to explain this behaviour we must first face the criticism that has been given to our approach by, for instance, Dr. Biggs, (8), who says that, essentially, our measurements concern nothing but a fibrinogen-fibrin conversion mediated by thrombin. If this were true it would indeed provide a most elegant explanation of our findings: each linear graph produced would then be essentially a Lineweaver-Burk plot of the action of trombin on fibrinogen.

Major objections can be raised to this view: *In the first place*, we have seen above that systems more complicated than those measuring one factor of the extrinsic system by means of a plasma specifically deficient in only this one factor do not show the simple rectilinear t-D graph. Nevertheless, in such systems the formation of fibrin is still the final step of the reaction process. *Secondly*, we were able to estimate that the activation energy of the reaction that is rate-limiting in a factor II estimation is only half as big as the activation energy of the fibrinogen-fibrin conversion under the same conditions, which indicates that these are different reactions. *In the third place*, the variation of the clotting time with the inverse of the concentration of factors V and X as observed in our one-stage tests is exactly comparable to the variation of the prothrombinase concentration with the inverse of these concentrations in a purified system (9). This last finding also provides indirect support for the hypothesis that clotting times can serve as a direct estimation of the reaction velocity in a rate-limiting step of the clotting system.

The major problem remaining to be solved is then how to find a reaction mechanism of blood coagulation from which the kinetic behaviour we observe can be explained. This cannot be an unmodified enzyme cascade, because a mathematical investigation of kinetic properties of a cascade has shown that such a system always causes an accelerated rise of the final product (10).

We have therefore considered a modified cascade incorporating three peculiarities of the coagulation system:

a. Prothrombinase can be considered to be a stoichiometric product of factors v_a, x_a, and phospholipid (9).

b. Prothrombinase is extremely labile.

c. In the last step of the coagulation reaction sequence, a small amount of enzyme (thrombin) is generated in the presence of a tremendous excess of its substrate (fibrinogen). Under these circumstances, the initial velocity of the formation of fibrinogen can equal the formation velocity of thrombin (transient state kinetics) (4).

These considerations lead to the following reaction scheme:

$$x \xrightarrow{\text{VII}_a} x_a$$

$$x_a + v_a + \text{ph. lip} \xrightleftharpoons{\hspace{1cm}} \text{prothrombinase} \longrightarrow \text{inactive prod.}$$

$$\text{II} \xrightarrow{\text{prothrombinase}} \text{thrombin}$$

$$\text{I} \xrightarrow{\text{thrombin}} \text{fibrin ('transient state kinetics')}$$

Analysis of the kinetic behaviour of this system of reactions has shown that here coagulation time can indeed be a linear function of the concentration of factors II, V, X, and VII (4, 10, 11).

REFERENCES

1. Hemker, H. C., R. Altman. Siepel, E. A. Loeliger, Kinetic aspects of the interaction of bloodclotting enzymes. II The relation between clotting time and plasma concentration in prothrombin time estimations. *Thrombos. Diathes. haemorrh.* 17, 349 (1967).

2. Hemker, H. C., P. W. Hemker, E. A. Loeliger, Kinetic aspects of the interaction of blood clotting enzymes. I Derivation of basic formula's. *Thrombos. Diathes. haemorrh.* 13, 155 (1965).

3. Hemker, H. C., Kwantitering in de bloedstollling. *Maandschr. Kindergeneesk.* 32, 503 (1964).

4. Hemker, H. C., A. D. Muller, Kinetics aspects of the interaction of blood clotting enzymes. V The reaction mechanism of the extrinsic clotting system as revealed by the kinetics of one-stage-estimations of coagulation enzymes. Thrombos. Diathes. haemorrh. 19,368 (1968).

5. Loeliger, E. A., F. Koller, Behaviour of factor VII and prothrombin during late pregnancy and in the newborn. *Acta Haemat.* (Basel) 7, 152 (1952).

6. Borchgrevink, C. F., J. G. Pool, H. Stormorken, A new assay for factor v (Proaccelerin-Accelerin) using Russell's viper venom. *J. Lab. Clin. Med.* 55, 625 (1960).

7. Bachman, F., F. Duckert, F. Koller, The Stuart-Prower factor assay and its clinical significance. *Thrombos. Diathes. haemorrh.* 2, 24 (1958).

8. Biggs, R., In: A discussion on triggered enzyme systems in blood plasma organized by R. G. Macfarlane F. R. S. Proc. Roy. Soc. B 173, 421 (1969).

9. Hemker, H. C., P. W. Esnouf, P. W. Hemker, A. C. W. Swart, R. C. MacFarlane, Formation of prothrombin converting activity. *Nature* 215, 248 (1967).

10. Hemker, H. C., P. W. Hemker, General kinetics of enzyme cascades *Proc. Roy. Soc.* B 173, 411 (1969).

11. Hemker, H. C., J. M. C. Wimmers, On the reaction mechanism of the extrinsic clotting system. *Proc. Europ. Fed. Biochem. Soc.*, Vienna A 120, 82 (1965).

DISCUSSION

Deggeller: I still do not understand why one gets a linear graph when clotting is plotted versus the inverse of concentration. I feel that the complicated reaction mechanism that is behind the coagulation system makes it impossible to develop mathematical equations which predict a velocity-concentration relationship.

I do not think that you can deduce the complex-formation hypothesis from the kinetics of coagulation reactions as Dr. Hemker has done, because there are too many factors and hence too much uncertainty about reaction constants to permit a clearcut conclusion.

This does not mean that I do not believe that the enzyme kinetics are useful in the study of blood coagulation, but I feel that they are more applicable to purified systems in which one can vary one reactant at will. I should like to illustrate this with some of our own experiments (to be found in full detail in K. Deggeller: *The human prothrombin activating enzyme.* Thesis, Amsterdam 1968). Plots of the inverse of the concentration of the factors x_a and v_a against the velocity of prothrombin activation in a mixture of factors II, v, x, phospholipid, and Ca^{++} lead us to assume that factors x_a and v_a adsorb onto phospholipid and that both play an analogous role in the activation of prothrombin.

Hemker has proposed a mechanism in which the adsorption of x_a and v_a onto phospholipid results in the formation of prothrombinase, based on experiments with purified bovine material. Our findings with purified human material support this hypothesis.

Hemker: Everybody – including myself – when confronted with the kinetics of impure systems arrives at the objections expressed by Dr. Deggeller. I think that when one approaches the methodological problems with some care, no doubt can remain concerning the value of the kinetic approach, even in impure systems. First of all, it should be observed that kinetic considerations can *never* prove a certain mechanism to be true. This holds even for the basic scheme of enzyme kinetics: $E + S \xrightleftharpoons{} ES \longrightarrow E + P$. Kinetic experiments can *disprove* a certain postulated mechanism, because from a given mechanism the kinetic behaviour can be calculated unequivocally. By sheer serendipity we found that there is a rectilinear relation between clotting time and the inverse of the concentrations of factors II, V, X, VII, and phospholipid when varied one at the time. The same relation was not found with factors VIII, IX, XI and XII, or when factors VII and X were varied together, thus excluding a trivial cause of these results. When we found this (1964), the only available reaction mechanism for the blood coagulation process was the cascade hypothesis, and it could be easily shown that this mechanism did *not* account for the observations. We thus tried to find a modification of the cascade mechanism that would give the least complicated reaction scheme that was in accordance with the observed facts. In 1965 (F.E.B.S. Congress, Vienna), we postulated that mechanism to be:

$$X_a + V + \text{phospholipid} \longrightarrow \text{prothrombinase} \longrightarrow \text{inactive product.}$$

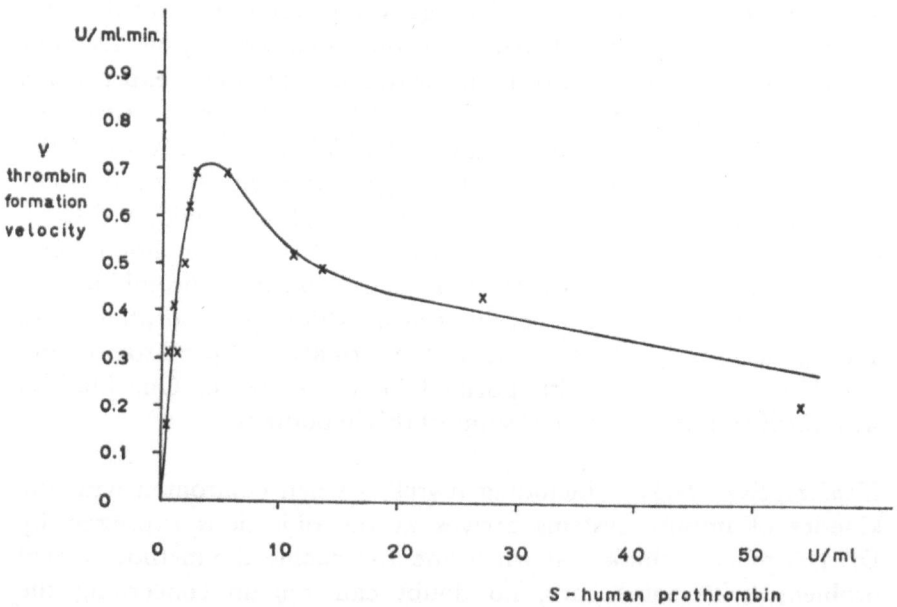

Fig. 1. The dependence of reaction velocity on concentration of substrate (human prothrombin).

Developments since 1965 supported this view remarkably well, which is a piece of sheer luck, because more complex mechanisms might explain just as well the kinetics observed. Once this mechanism has been shown to be acceptable by various independent means, including the kinetics of pure systems, one has obtained an indirect proof of the basic hypothesis in kinetics of impure systems, namely that clotting time in such a system is directly proportional to the inverse of the initial reaction velocity in the rate-limiting step.

Deggeller: I should then like to draw attention to a phenomenon which has thus far not been observed when the prothrombin conversion in purified bovine systems was studied, i.e. in the activation of human prothrombin there is an inhibition by excess substrate (figures 1, 2, and 3). There is a linear relationship between substrate concentrations (S) and the inverse of the reaction velocity (1/v) at high substrate concentrations. This can be explained by the reaction mechanism:

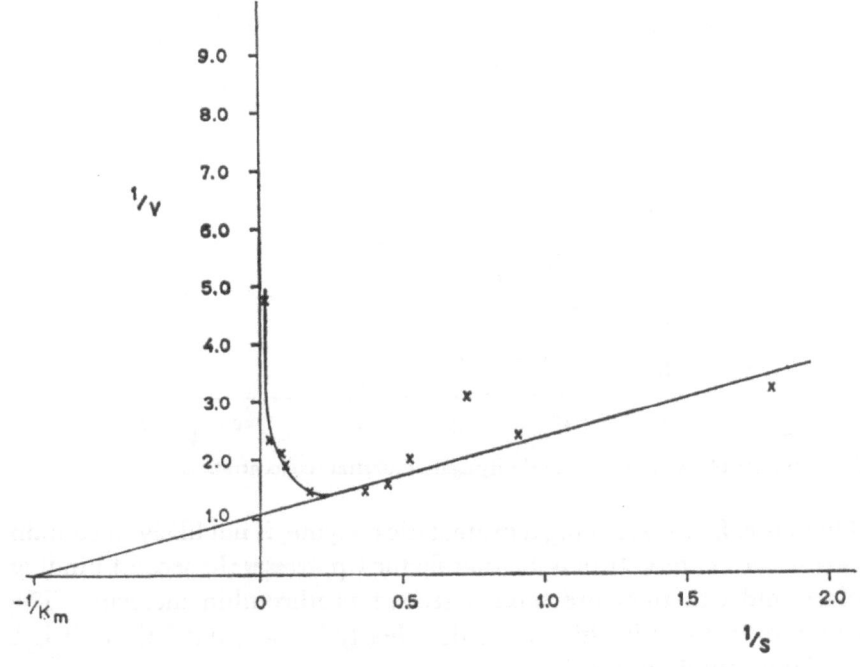

2. Lineweaver-Burk plot of the data in Fig. 3.

$$\text{E} + \text{S} \;\rightleftharpoons\; \text{ES} \;\longrightarrow\; \text{E} + \text{R}$$

$$\text{S} + \text{ES} \;\rightleftharpoons\; \text{ESS}$$

in which ESS is an inactive complex of two substrate molecules (S) plus the enzyme (E). This is the standard mechanism for inhibition by excess substrate; it is a common reaction that occurs when two different binding places meant to bind one molecule of substrate together, bind two molecules instead. When both active binding sites are confronted with another molecule (prothrombin in this case) they cannot form a product. This finding implies that there are two active binding sites on the prothrombin-activating enzyme. This is not known for any of the proteolytic enzymes such as trypsin or chymotrypsin as far as I know.

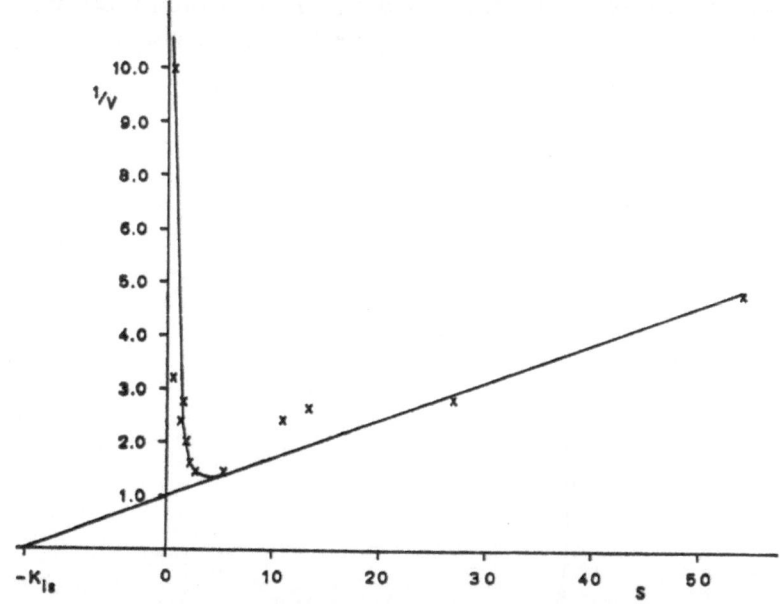

Fig. 3. Inverse plot of the reaction velocity against substrate concentration.

Therefore, factor x_a, being a proteolytic enzyme, is not likely to contain two active centers. It may be that factor v possesses the second binding place and can therefore bind a second prothrombin molecule. The action of factor v in this case is not clearly known, but I think it is a good topic for discussion.

Denson: Could the substrate inhibition with prothrombin not be due to antithrombin III in the prothrombin preparation?

Deggeller: We did experiments with three types of prothrombin preparations having different specific activities, and calculated that the degree of inhibition per unit factor II activity produced by all three was exactly the same. One cannot assume that one has purified an independent inhibitor like antithrombin III together with the prothrombin in exactly the same way in three different preparations.

Esnouf: I would like to ask Dr. Deggeller whether in the scheme that I suggested earlier, i.e., x_a binding v binding prothrombin, prothrombin could prevent the binding of x_a and v and thereby reduce the reaction velocity when present in excess.

Deggeller: I have taken that possibility into serious consideration but we found, as you have, that both factors v and x_a adsorb onto phospholipid independently of each other. The association on the phospholipid and the formation of the enzyme is exactly similar. I do not see how we can postulate an additional force, i.e., chemical binding, between factors v and x_a, and still get the same results. The adsorption onto phospholipid seems sufficient to explain the formation of the enzyme. There is no need to postulate the formation of additional chemical bonds between factors v and x_a.

Esnouf: Factor v stimulated the reaction between x_a and prothrombin. This stimulation occurred in the presence of calcium ions. It is possible that we are looking at two different types of bonds: interprotein and protein-phospholipid. Both of these forces may be acting in slightly opposite directions in the complete system. In your experiments you had a prothrombin concentration greatly above normal. Perhaps that was sufficient to displace some x_a, getting say two molecules of prothrombin around one molecule of factor v rather than one molecule of x_a and one of prothrombin.

Hemker: I think that at the moment the experimental findings are sufficiently explained by the following assumptions (see figure 4):

a. Factor x_a has an active centre that binds factor II and subsequently converts it into thrombin.

b. Factor v_a has a centre that binds the factor II molecule at a place different from that by which factor x_a acts. When factor x_a and factor v_a are adsorbed in a favorable juxtaposition on a phospholipid surface, they offer two different binding sites for one prothrombin molecule. After binding of the prothrombin molecule by these two sites, the active site of factor x_a causes the prothrombin $\longrightarrow$ thrombin conversion. This arrangement creates a much more effective prothrombinase than does *a*.

c. When an excess of prothrombin is present, two molecules bind to each x_a-v-phospholipid complex, one via x_a, the other via v. The activity of the complex is thereby reduced to that of factor x_a alone, (as in *a*).

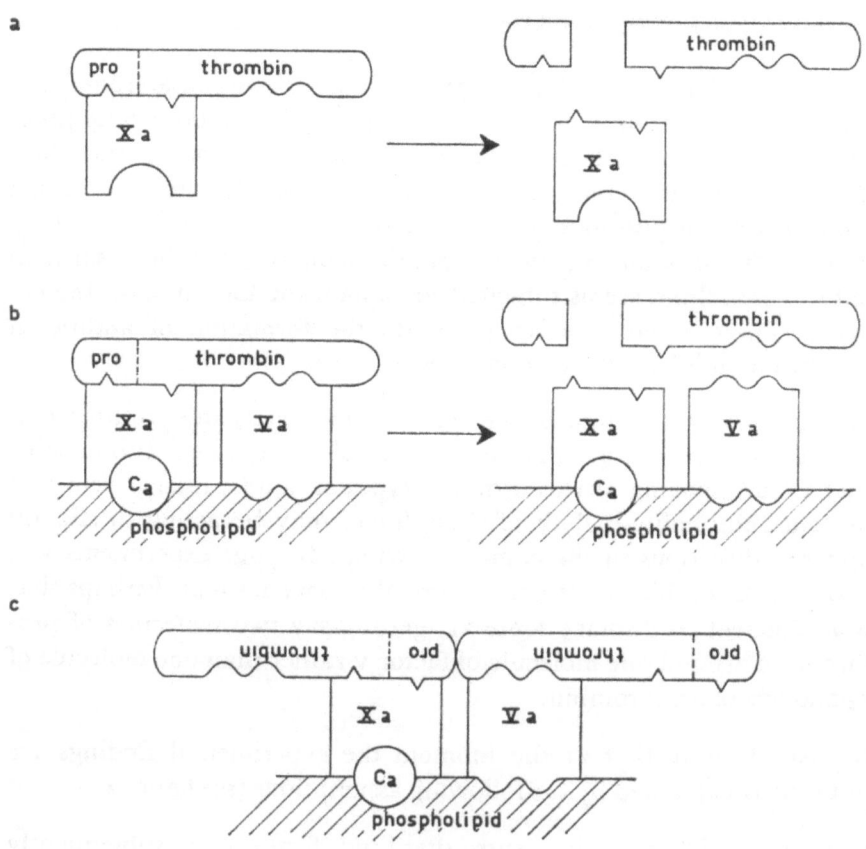

Fig. 4

ROUND TABLE DISCUSSION

CHAIRMAN: E. DEUTSCH

The round table discussion, open to all participants of the conference, was held to select the most fruitful working hypotheses for studying the reaction mechanism of blood clotting. To keep the discussion from becoming bogged down in details, thirteen statements (formulated by Hemker, Swart, and Vroman) each representing one partial coagulation reaction, were taken as guidelines, so that no major aspect of clotting would remain untouched. Some of the statements were formulated to encourage discussion rather than as pronouncements of absolute truths.

The essence of the various discussions is given below, each preceded by the relevant statement and summarized in a conclusion. In editing the tape recordings, we made no essential changes, but did our best to avoid duplication of material already presented in the lectures.

I.   XII ———→ XII$_a$

Upon contact with a surface, factor XII *is activated by an unknown mechanism*

Vroman: I wish to de-emphasize everyone else's knowledge. We should be prepared to reverse our ideas about the whole problem of contact activation and the possible reaction sequences involved. I think that factor XI may be activated and then activate XII, or that they may both be activated together. Moreover, there is the intriguing problem of the possible role of fibrinogen in contact activation, as I have mentioned in my discussion of Dr. Prentice's paper.

Prentice: I would like to comment on Dr. Vroman's very interesting observations on the adsorption of proteins from plasma. Dr. Vroman plated glass with plasma solutions and then, using an anti-fibrinogen antiserum, showed that the main adsorbed protein was fibrinogen. But one cannot exclude the possibility that other proteins, such as Hageman factor, are adsorbed on the surface too. Possibly they are adsorbed in the same proportion as they occur in plasma, i.e. 300 mg of fibrinogen as against 1 μg of factor XII.

Vroman: The adsorbed material doesn't react with anti-human globulin and anti-albumin at all. So it cannot be a mere representation of the protein population in plasma. On the other hand, our anti-fibrinogen is not absolutely specific. If you look at the problem in terms of activity, perhaps one molecule of factor XII for every 5,000 molecules of fibrinogen is enough to explain everything that you find in coagulation.

It may be the same with complement factors. That is why I am a little hesitant about kinetics when you work with surfaces. We have unknown concentrations, unknown orientations, plus the possibility of changing activities, so we really do not know exactly what we are dealing with.

Hemker: This indeed is the reason why in our kinetic calculations on the generation of prothrombinase activity on a phospholipid surface we assume reversible adsorption, in which case these objections do not hold. I agree that at this moment a kinetic treatment of irreversible adsorption – as discussed here – is not feasible.

Deutsch: Have you done any experiments with a purified factor XII solution and have you used it to cover a glass surface?

Vroman: We have used Dr. Ratnoff's factor XII, and under our conditions that went onto every surface; and any other protein that we have tried goes on as well. It seems that any protein will go anywhere as long as there are no other proteins getting there first.

Haanen: The inner surface of a glass tube that has contained normal plasma for some minutes, and that afterwards has been rinsed 10 times and dried, can correct thromboplastin generation of a factor XII-deficient plasma. This proves, I think, that factor XII indeed is adsorbed.

When normal plasma is kept in a tube for three hours, this tube, after rinsing and drying, no longer corrects factor XII-deficient plasma. The plasma that has been stored in this way is still able to coat a new tube so as to activate Hageman-deficient plasma. I think this can be explained by assuming that the adsorbed and hence activated factor XII combines with factor XI, and that this complex is inactivated because factor XI is labile. The quantity of factor XII in normal plasma seems to be greater than the amount necessary to coat a glass tube.

This theory sheds no light on the mechanism of factor XII activation, but it does suggest a role of factor XII as the prime factor involved in contact activation.

Hanahan: When I hear of activated factors I think that proteolytic enzymes, like the Hageman factor, should be activated from pro-enzymes. Has anyone shown that such an activation occurs?

Haanen: The activation of our highly purified factor XII preparations proved to be reversible. Therefore, I think that a change in tertiary structure upon adsorption is more probably the cause of the activation than cleavage of a covalent bond, which is known to be the mechanism in pro-enzyme $\longrightarrow$ enzyme transitions.

Prentice: That view is shared by Margolis. It is also supported by observations of the activation of factor XII by urate crystals. Physical properties of these crystals, such as crystal size and possibly charge, appear to be very important for the degree of activation obtained. This suggests the action of a physical process such as adsorption rather than a chemical process.

CONCLUSION
Adsorption of factor xii onto a surface possibly initiates the clotting process by bringing about a reversible change in the tertiary structure of the factor xii molecule.

II.   xii$_a$ + xi ⟶ contact product
Activated factor xii and factor xi interact to form a stoichiometric product (contact product) that may act both while adsorbed and when released.

Deutsch: I propose that this proposition be discussed in two parts; first, the evidence that factors xii and xi interact stoichiometrically.

Haanen: I can only give the suggestive evidence discussed in my paper. More evidence for our proposed mechanism will have to wait until a purified factor xi preparation is available.

Deutsch: If nobody thinks there is evidence against this proposition, we can discuss the question of whether factors xii and xi act both while adsorbed and when released?

Vroman: If you pour plasma out of plastic into glass and back again you get a shorter clotting-time, so you have transferred some activated yet soluble moiety.

Deutsch: It seems that the molecule has undergone a physical transformation that persists after factor xii is released from the surface.

Haanen: For a surface, two different roles are feasible; first, it can serve to increase the local concentration of factors xii and xi and thus the chance for both to interact; second, it can change the conformation of factor xii so as to make it reactive towards factor xi.

CONCLUSION
Although conclusive evidence is still lacking, it seems an attractive hypothesis that factors xii and xi react at a surface and form an active contact product that can be released from the surface.

III.

$$CP$$
$$IX \longrightarrow IX_a$$
$$CP$$
$$VII \longrightarrow VII_a$$

Factors VII and IX can be activated by the contact product (CP).
Alternative pathways exist for the activation of both factors.

Hemker: This proposition brings us directly to the question, why does plasma clot at all via the intrinsic mechanism? Rapaport has given us good evidence that factor VIII needs activation by thrombin before it can take part in the formation of the intrinsic factor x activating enzyme. We must then ask: Where does this thrombin come from? I think that the activated contact product can activate factor VII. This factor VII$_a$ then activates a slight amount of factor x, which with factor v produces the initial amount of prothrombinase necessary for the formation of thrombin, which then activates factor VIII. By this activation of factor VIII the intrinsic pathway can become operative.

Denson: We found recently that after incubation of platelets in plasma they produced a type of extrinsic thromboplastin, but this was never developed in the absence of Hageman factor. This could be a mechanism by means of which the first traces of thrombin are formed for the initiation of the intrinsic clotting mechanism.

Hemker: This is an interesting possibility, but I am convinced that platelets are not essential, because all of our experiments were done with plasma that was virtually platelet-free.

Duckert: We did some experiments with concentrates of prothrombin, factors VII and x, etc. We apparently had no contact factor in the mixture, and still we found activation of factor VII to about three times its original activity; after that it decreased to the starting activity.

In this system, prothrombin underwent the same type of variation but not as pronounced as that of factor VII, and it returned to its original level after a certain period of incubation. At that time we had thrombin, but I do not know the exact nature of this activation. During the first phases of the experiment it was impossible to demonstrate the existence of thrombin and there was no contact factor present. So I wonder if we may have another way of activating factor VII.

Hemker: In our laboratory Swart did some experiments that indicated that factor VII may possibly be activated in a non-enzymatic way when you adsorb it onto a surface and elute it again.

On the other hand, Bruning has proved that in the presence of Hageman factor and factor XI the activation of factor VII occurs very much faster than in their absence during a purification procedure by means of adsorption.

CONCLUSION

Factor VII may be activated in various ways, among others by contact product. Contact product probably activates factor IX in presence of calcium ions.

IV.   Thrombin

$$\text{VIII} \longrightarrow \text{VIII}_a$$

Factor VIII *must be activated by thrombin before it can participate in the coagulation reaction.*

The discussion on the activation of factor VIII was opened by a general discussi on onthe increase of factor VIII activity *in vivo* during exercise. Some speakers (Magnusson, Blombäck, Prentice, Manucci) thought that this increase does not reflect the presence of more normal factor VIII in the blood stream because:

1. the *in vivo* recovery of factor VIII preparations of post-exercise blood was the same as from normal blood;
2. it had no increased capability to neutralize factor VIII inhibitors; and
3. it had a short *in vivo* half-life time.

Others (Denson, Stibbe) had had exactly the opposite experience. Manucci reported a rise of factor VIII in heparinized patients after stress, which seems to exclude thrombin as the cause of the *in vivo* increase. However, none of the speakers had reason to doubt the validity of the evidence produced by Rapaport for the activation of factor VIII by thrombin.

CONCLUSION

The mechanism of *in vivo* increase of plasmatic factor VIII activity with exercise, etc., is still unclear. It is probably unrelated to the coagulation process *per se*. The coagulation process probably requires activation of factor VIII by thrombin.

V. $$x \xrightarrow{E} 2\,X_a$$

Factor x can be activated in at least three ways: by the extrinsic factor x activator, by the intrinsic factor x activator, and by Russell's viper venom. Activation results in the acquisition of esterolytic properties and is accompanied by a reduction of the molecular size to about half the original.

Deggeller: Factor x is activated by Russell's viper venom through an enzymatic mechanism, and normal enzymatic kinetics are found.

In the intrinsic mechanism you find a stoichiometric relationship between the amount of factor VIII present and the amount of factor x_a formed. This is contradictory to normal enzymatic activation. It could be due to the lability of factor VIII after it has been converted to the factor x activating enzyme, but I do not think that this is the case.

If you omit factor x from the incubation mixture and add it after ten minutes, you will still observe a rise in prothrombin-activating enzyme after this addition. The lability of the enzyme should be the same when the substrate is absent. So the question of the mechanism of factor x activation in the intrinsic coagulation pathway seems still open.

Hemker: I should like to know how you excluded the possibility that the lability of factor VIII is brought about by the presence of the factor x preparation in some way or other?

Deggeller: That is perhaps an answer to the problem. You could perhaps look at it this way, that factor VIII is an acceptor of a part of factor x that is removed from the molecule. This is in agreement with the theory of Seegers, who proposed an inhibitor to be bound by factor VIII.

Hemker: I do not want to try and propose a detailed mechanism, but something of the sort is certainly a possibility. Another possibility is that addition of factor x causes the generation of minute amounts of thrombin which activate and subsequently inactivate factor VIII.

Hanahan: It seems to me that there is a bit of a dilemma posed by what you mean by activated factor x. During the activation with Russell's viper venom you get an electrophoretically and chromatographically single species of protein. Still, there could be more than one type of activated factor x; for instance, one generated via the intrinsic system and another via the extrinsic system. There is no doubt that the intact or original system may be much more complex than our *in vitro* systems. Dr. Deggeller referred to the fact that factor x_a and phospholipid interact. We have never been able to interact factor x with phospholipid under any conditions short of degradation of the molecule. However, if you activate it with Russell's viper venom or trypsin, it will then react, but only in the presence of calcium ions.

This might indicate that there are two different systems, and certainly this presents a problem in trying to come to an unique hypothesis.

You can separate prothrombinase activity by Sephadex chromatography into v, phospholipid complex, x_a, and calcium ions. When you reconstitute them, you have an active preparation again. The components are not active individually unless they are used in very high concentrations. This is true at least for factor x_a. In our experience, factor v has never been active on prothrombin. So in our experience, unactivated x does not react with phospholipid.

CONCLUSION
The mechanism of factor x activation by Russell's viper venom seems to be a straightforward enzymatic reaction. The other ways of activation – via the intrinsic and extrinsic system – are much less clear. Factor x must be activated to be adsorbed by phospholipids; calcium ions are necessary for this adsorption.

VI. $VIII_a + IX_a + Ca^{++} +$ phospholipid $\longrightarrow$ factor x activator

The intrinsic factor x activator consists of factors VIII_a and IX_a adsorbed in a favourable way onto a phospholipid micelle.

The meaning of the word 'activated' when used to describe a more reactive form of a coagulation factor was discussed first. All the speakers agreed that two essentially different forms of activation probably exist.

First, there is the pro-enzyme → enzyme transition, well known for many proteolytic enzymes, which occurs in the activation of factor II and probably in that of factors IX and x. This activation is irreversible;

the product is a proteolytic and/or esterolytic enzyme. Another type of activation is seen with factors v and vIII. This type appears to differ from the former, because in the first place it is not proven that activation of factor v is essential. Rapaport defends the point of view that activation of factor vIII by thrombin is necessary, but Denson holds the opposite view. The result of the activation of factors v and vIII is not a clearcut enzymatic activity, but rather opens the possibility of a potentiation of the activities of factors x_a and IX_a respectively. The activation of factor v is reversible (Esnouf, Kahn); that of factor vIII also appears to be reversible under certain circumstances (Stibbe). The activation of factor v is probably accompanied by a dimer $\longleftrightarrow$ monomer transition for the bovine species and with a tetramer $\longleftrightarrow$ monomer transition in human blood (Kahn, Hemker).

Although there seems to be sufficient reason for differentiation in the activation reactions of blood-clotting factors, there does not seem to be enough substantial evidence at the moment to define two different mechanisms. Hence, the terminology v_r and $vIII_r$ (indicating *re*active) should not be used, and the suffix *a* added to the roman numeral should merely indicate a form of coagulation factor more active than the plasma precursor (Haanen, Deggeller, Denson).

No one on the panel defended the cascade mechanism against the complex formation given in proposition vi. The experiments of Hemker and Kahn and of Hougie, Denson and Biggs seem to provide enough preliminary evidence to maintain the complex-formation theory as the most favourable working hypothesis.

CONCLUSION
The proposition is sustained.

VII.   vii + tissue lipoproteins → extrinsic factor x activator
The extrinsic factor x activator is formed by tissue lipoproteins and factor vii.

In answer to a question posed by Hanahan, Prydz described his experiments on the separation of tissue thromboplastin:

Prydz: We make a deoxycholate (DOC) extract of a saline extract of homogenized human brain and ultracentrifuge it for 2 to 3 hours at 100,000 g. The supernatant is submitted to gel filtration on Sephadex G-100.

If we remove the deoxycholate by dialysis or gel filtration, we will recover tissue thromboplastin activity. Immediately after the removal of DOC this activity is very low, but if we leave the solution at 4° for 24 to 48 hrs the activity increases. This coincides with the appearance of the large membrane aggregates seen on electron-micrographs. So it appears that these membrane structures are in some way of importance to the activity. When the supernatant is submitted to gel filtration in the presence of DOC, we find three fractions: a front-fraction and fractions A and B. The front-fraction contains phospholipid and forms membranes when we remove DOC. These membranes, though identical in electron-microscopical appearance, have no activity, not even when the protein fraction A is added to them. There must thus be a chemical specificity in the membrane structure which is not detectable by electron micrography.

Hanahan: As I understand it, in your chromatographic elution pattern on Sephadex after DOC treatment, fraction A was protein and fraction B contained 80 to 90% phospholipids besides protein. It seems very strange that a lipoprotein or lipid-like fraction B would elute after a protein (fraction A) from a Sephadex colum; this seems to be the reverse of what one would expect. Anything that has 80 to 90% lipoprotein in it will tend to come out in the void-volume on G-100 Sephadex.

Prydz: Not in the presence of DOC. If you remove the DOC before you submit the preparation to gel filtration, all lipoproteins will come out in the void-volume. Fraction A, the protein fraction, is not completely free of phospholipid when you obtain it from the first column chromatography. You have to rechromatograph it to remove the last few per cents of phospholipid. Fraction A has a tendency to stabilize factor x; there seems to be some specific interaction between these proteins, but I hesitate to call it an activation. Fraction A appears to be similar to the protein described by Nemerson and Spaet. It does not induce coagulation in the absence of phospholipid.

Deutsch: The procedure of Nemerson and Spaet does not completely separate the protein and phospholipid parts. The only methods I know by which it is possible to separate the protein and lipid parts and to recombine them again into an active thromboplastin are the DOC

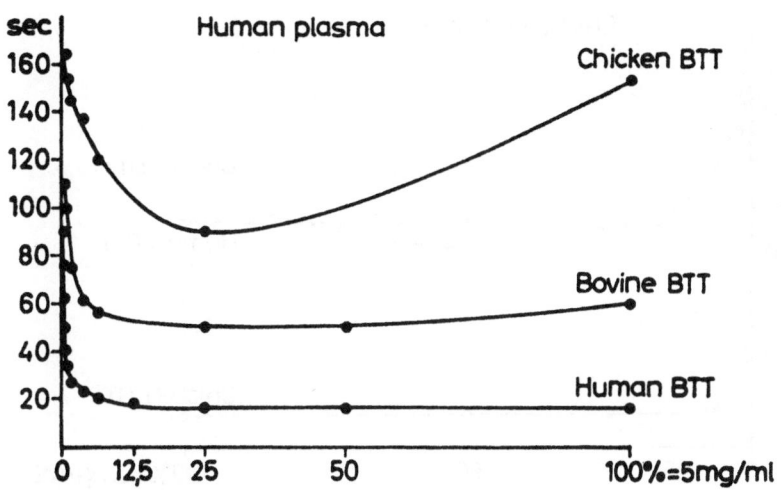

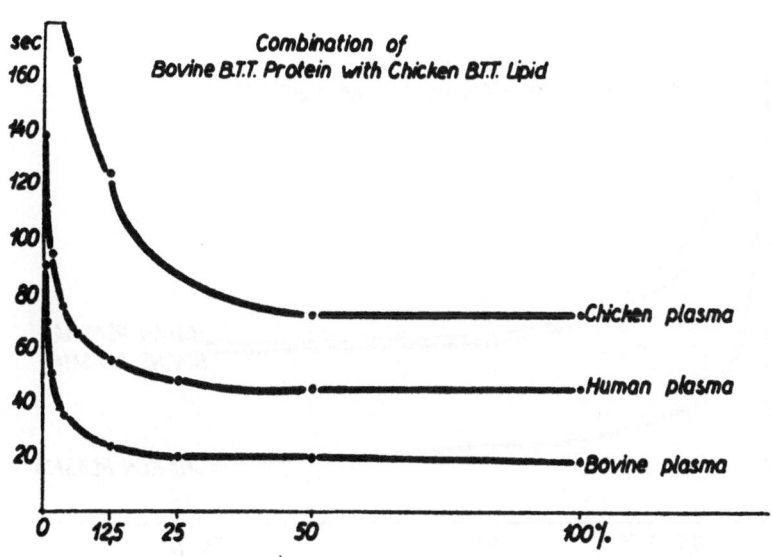

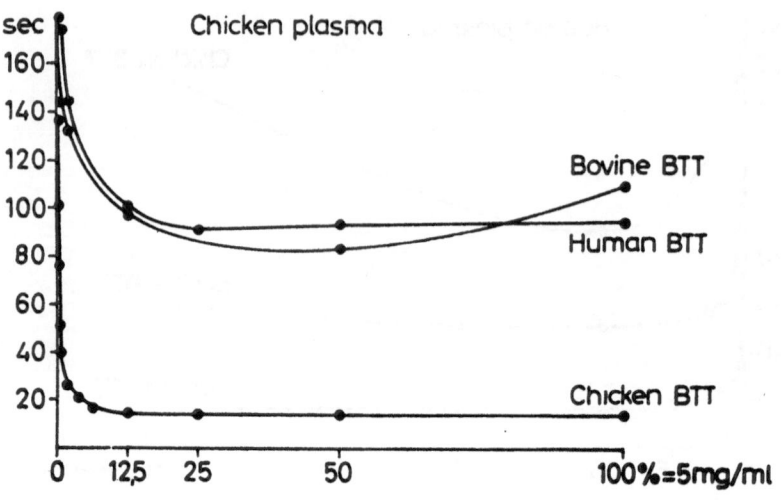

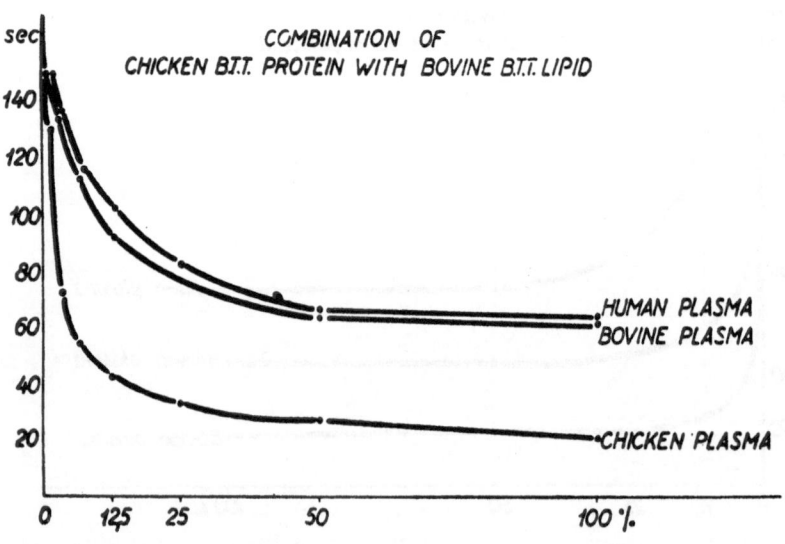

procedure of Prydz and our own procedure using pyridine. The protein we obtained gave an active thromboplastin when combined with purified phosphatidyl ethanolamine or phosphatidyl serine. We have not been able to find any other protein which was able to form an active thromboplastin when it was combined with either synthetic phosphatide or with the original phospholipid of the thromboplastin. If you recombine human thromboplastin protein with bovine thromboplastin lipid and test it against human, bovine, or chicken plasma, you find the highest activity with the human plasma. If you do the same experiment using chicken thromboplastin protein and human brain thromboplastin lipid, you see the highest activity with chicken plasma. So the species specificity is linked to the protein preparation. We were not able to find significant differences in the lipid composition of the different thromboplastins by means of thin layer chromatography.

We also did a few experiments with thromboplastin and purified fractions VII and X, and tested the esterase activity which developed. If the tissue thromboplastin acted directly on factor X, we did not get esterase activity. We got it only if we added factor VII. I therefore do not think that tissue thromboplastin will act directly on factor X in the absence of factor VII despite the interaction between factor X and the fraction A protein in Prydz's experiments.

Denson: I did experiments in a system in which the factor VII activity was completely blocked by the use of a specific antibody. Factor X seemed to be activated directly by tissue thromboplastin there.

Duckert: Sometimes an antigen retains its activity when part of an antibody-antigen complex; or did you remove factor VII by a precipitating antibody?

Denson: No, but the antibody completely blocked the factor VII activity in a factor VII assay.

Hemker: Thromboplastin when used in e.g. a prothrombin-time estimation has at least two actions: we know that a protein is necessary to activate factor VII and we know that phospholipids are necessary at the level of factors V and X_a. But is phospholipid also necessary somewhere in the course of the activation of factor X, either for the activation of factor VII or the activation of factor X by factor VII?

Van der Plas: Filipin, which is a substance known to interact with phospholipid micelles, does under certain conditions probably inhibit the activation of factor VII by thromboplastin, so I believe that a protein is necessary for the activation of factor VII as well as a phospholipid. I do not know what is necessary for the activation of factor x by factor VII. Our data, however, are only preliminary.

Prydz: As far as I know, the polyene antibiotics such as filipin would interact only with phospholipid micelles containing sterols. We have done some preliminary experiments on the phospholipid component of tissue thromboplastin, and we do not find any sterols.

Van der Plas: Recently, it has been demonstrated that sterols are not essential for the action of filipin on phospholipids.

CONCLUSION
The exact nature of the extrinsic factor x activator is still unknown.

VIII. $V \longrightarrow 4 V_a$
Factor v can be activated by thrombin or Russell's viper venom, but also in a non-enzymatic way. Activation is accompanied by reduction to one half (bovine) or one quarter (human) of its original molecular weight.

Hemker: Dr. Kahn and I have been able to demonstrate that factor v is activated by the procoagulant protein from Russell's viper venom (RVV). The purified fraction that we used was supplied by Dr. Esnouf.
    I think that it has been unequivocably shown by MacFarlane that factor x is activated by RVV, but it seems that factor v is activated by a protein contained in the same, highly purified fraction. Human factor v activated by Russell's viper venom is much more stable than human factor v activated by thrombin or by non-enzymatic means. This made it possible for us to estimate its molecular weight. Human factor v activated by Russell's viper venom appears to have about one fourth of the molecular weight of unactivated factor v. Activated factor v had a molecular weight of about 130,000 as compared to approximately 510,000 in the unactivated factor v.

Prentice: I agree with Hemker that a partially purified factor v preparation can be 'activated' or made more reactive by Russell's viper venom. This activated factor v appears to be considerably more stable than thrombin-treated factor v. This suggests that activation by Russell's viper venom is different from that by thrombin. I think that Rapaport has suggested that the interaction between the venom and factor v is stoichiometric.

Hemker: We have never obtained the impression, though, that factor v activated by Russell's viper venom is more stable than plasma factor v. In view of the experiments which show that factor v activated by Russell's viper venom has a molecular weight of only 130,000 as compared to 510,000 for the unactivated factor, a stoichiometric mode of activation appears very unlikely.

Prentice: Dr. Denson suggested that factor VIII has some intrinsic activity before it is treated with thrombin. We sought for similar activity in factor v. However, when native factor v was included in the prothrombin converting principle, immediate generation of thrombin did not occur following addition of prothrombin. One possible conclusion is that factor v is inactive in the circulation and must first react with some circulating enzyme before it can participate in the coagulation process.

Hemker: Dr. Deggeller, too, found a definite lag period in the generation of prothrombinase activity with human factor v when no thrombin was added.

Deggeller: We estimated the prothrombinase formation upon incubation of factors x_a and v, phospholipid, and calcium ions. We had to add some thrombin to the system in order to get immediate full activity of the prothrombin-activating enzyme. When we omitted thrombin from the mixture we definitely had a lag period of some minutes. Probably, there is some thrombin formed during this lag period with the not entirely pure reagents we used. We were unable, though, to make exact measurements in the systems with very low thrombin concentrations. I think that factor v is inactive as it circulates in the blood and that it must react with thrombin or via another mechanism. We must still explain how the first molecules of thrombin are formed before the activated form of factor v is available.

Hemker: In our chromatographic experiments it was difficult to keep factor v in its inactive, high molecular weight form. We did not require enzymes in order to get it into its activated low molecular weight form. The conditions that were most successful for maintaining factor v intact were 50% glycerol and high concentrations of magnesium ions. I think that it may be possible that factor v is converted into an active form non-enzymatically. This agrees with the findings of Jobin and Esnouf, who obtained yields clearly above 100 per cent during their purification procedures for bovine factor v. Gel filtration on polyacrylamide 300 columns shows that after activation with Russell's viper venom there is a clear shift of the factor v activity to a greater elution volume. In the absence of magnesium ions there is much more denaturation of factor v activity but also a shift to the lower molecular weight region.

Denson: I just want to ask Dr. Deggeller again if he thinks that factor v circulates in an inactive form? This would support the experimental finding that factor x_a converts prothrombin directly to produce the first trace of thrombin.

Deggeller: I have no experimental evidence to support that.

CONCLUSION
Factor v can be converted into a more active form, by thrombin, by an enzyme from Russell's viper venom, and non-enzymatically. The physiological way(s) of factor v activation and its nature are not known.

IX. $v_a + x_a + c_a^{++}$ + Phospholipid $\longrightarrow$ Prothrombinase
Prothrombinase consists of factors v_a and x_a adsorbed in a favourable juxta-position onto a phospholipid micelle.

Josso: I would like to present some data from experiments done on the activation of human prothrombin. We labelled purified prothrombin with radioactive iodine. Then the prothrombin was activated by complete prothrombinase – namely, in a mixture of phospholipid, calcium ions, and factors v and x_a prepared according to Esnouf and Williams. We found a partial conversion of prothrombin into thrombin after one minute. More radioactive thrombin was formed after three minutes, and after five minutes all the radioactivity was in the thrombin.

We then activated prothrombin with only factor x_a in a high concentration. Only after two hours was all of the radioactivity found in the thrombin.

I think these findings support the hypothesis that factor x_a carries the enzymatically active site of prothrombinase, and that it may have a slight activity in the absence of factor v and phospholipid.

Prentice: I think that most people who have worked with factor x_a and prothrombin have seen thrombin formation over a long period of time with large amounts of these factors.

Deutsch: I too think that for slow activation, factor x_a alone is enough.

Duckert: I would like to ask Dr. Esnouf about the adsorption of factors x_a and v_a onto phospholipid. What is the rate of formation of these complexes? We did some experiments showing that we had an adsorption of factor x_a onto lipid in the presence of calcium and we were able to centrifuge the complex. By removal of the calcium ions by dilution, EDTA, or oxalate, we were able to split the complex and to recover the original factor x activity in the supernatant and the lipid part in the sediment.

Esnouf: Factor x_a is bound to the phospholipid surface in the presence of divalent metal ions almost as soon as the different components are mixed together. There is an equilibrium here between the concentration of x_a, phospholipid, and metal ions; the concentration of each affecting the amount of factor x_a that can be recovered in the phospholipid pellet. The amount of factor x_a that is bound depends not only on the surface charge but also, we think, on the way in which the phosphate groups are arranged on the surface. If you use pure phosphatidic acid, the apparent amount of the factor x_a that is adsorbed is less than that obtained with mixed micelles of lecithin and phosphatidic acid. If you take phospholipid which has had x_a adsorbed onto it in the presence of calcium, then on dilution, some x_a dissociates off the surface. This process can be hastened very quickly by adding a small amount of Mg-ions, which leads to a complete elution of the x_a from the surface.

With purified reagents (x_a, v, II) one does not require phospholipid to get thrombin generation; however, one does require divalent metal ions, not necessarily calcium ions. On the other hand, in plasma there is an absolute requirement for phospholipid.

Hemker: Dr. Kahn and I did similar experiments with factor ix, and we found this factor to be adsorbed exactly as Dr. Esnouf described for factor x. Another point is that we never succeeded in obtaining prothrombinase activity without the presence of phospholipid, and neither has Dr. Deggeller, I think.

CONCLUSION

The proposition is sustained as far as the generation of a complete prothrombinase is concerned. It is stressed that factor x_a alone has slight prothrombinase activity.

X. *To be active in the coagulation process, a phospholipid micelle needs a mosaic surface structure formed jointly by hydrophobic and hydrophilic loci and/or a mosaic charge surface pattern.*

Hanahan: Normally, in the dispersions of phospholipid used, you are always beyond the critical micellar concentration, and so they will exist as very high molecular weight complexes. The question that really has to be defined is whether there is an active component in these micelles or there is a smaller molecular weight unit that is the active moiety.

When there is a small molecular weight unit, it will be in an equilibrium situation with the larger micelles, and the equilibrium is certainly toward the formation of the high molecular weight components.

We usually consider the phospholipid micelle with its hydrophobic groups oriented inward and its charged groups on the outer surface. However, given the importance of hydrophobic groupings in protein interactions, it would be interesting to know how the phospholipid really interacts with, for instance factor v; whether charged groups are important or whether the hydrophobic portion of the molecule is involved.

I think that with factors ix_a and x_a you have charged group interactions, and that they would occur on the surface, but you might find a different type of association with factor v.

Esnouf: Dr. Papahadjopoulos, when he was in Cambridge, carried out some preliminary studies on the binding of clotting factors onto monolayers made with mixed lipids which were active in clotting.

The particular mixture he took was phosphatidic acid and phosphatydyl choline. He found that in order to stop x_a binding onto the phospholipid surface, only a relatively low film pressure was required. In one experiment with factor v, considerably higher pressures were required to reduce the amount of factor v bound. This would suggest that factor v was penetrating into the phospholipid film. This implies a hydrophobic interaction for this factor and a weaker ionic equilibrium reaction with x_a. It would appear that these results support Dr. Hanahan's concept of this mechanism.

Hemker: We used barium stearate as a model for a system that was just hydrophobic and nothing else. We observed the adsorption of factors v and x onto the barium stearate and the elution from the barium stearate. We observed, as Vroman did earlier, that factor v is readily adsorbed onto barium stearate and then retains some of its activity, but it proved impossible to elute the factor v from the barium salt. We found that factor x adsorbed onto barium stearate also; however, it shows no activity in the adsorbed state. But it can be partially eluted from the barium stearate, and then shows activity again.

This suggests that, while factor v is bound via hydrophobic bonds to barium stearate, it leaves its active center free. Factor x, on the other hand, has a more or less hydrophobic active center which is buried in the barium stearate upon adsorption. No factor x activity is observed on the resuspended barium stearate powder after contact with normal citrated plasma, whereas the activity can be eluted. It is just the other way round with factor v. This also supports the idea that factor v is bound to the phospholipid via a hydrophobic bond, whereas the binding of factor x_a to phospholipid must be essentially different from that to barium stearate, i.e. presumably polar.

Esnouf: Another interesting thing about factor v is that on amino acid analysis it shows a high number of hydrophilic residues. In fact, factor v is readily soluble in distilled water and then remains very stable. It remained quite stable for at least two months at room temperature in Oxford. Dr. Hemker has shown that factor v will adsorb onto any hydrophobic surface, such as polystyrene latex particles, barium stearate, and phospholipid. Presumably, factor v is capable of undergoing conformational changes in the presence of a hydrophobic surface. This may account, in part, for its apparent accelerating effect in clotting.

CONCLUSION

The proposition is sustained; the importance of the existence of hydro-philic and hydrophobic loci is stressed.

XI. *Prothrombin (factor* II*) should be considered an entity that is independent of factors* VII, IX, *and* X. *No covalent bonds exist between factors* II, VII, IX *and* X *in plasma.*

Magnusson: I think that it is really too early to comment on this ques-tion. One has to wait for evidence in the way of amino acid sequence determinations before one can say whether the factors are genetically related to one another.

Considering their remarkably similar chemical properties (evi-denced by the great difficulties encountered in attempts to separate the factors by various purification procedures), and their common and apparently unique dependence on vitamin K for their biosynthesis, I believe it may well turn out that they have genetically related struct-ures which have evolved from a common ancestor, probably through gene doubling and separate evolution of the resulting genes.

It is quite obvious, for example, that trypsinogen, chymotryp-sinogen, elastase, and prothrombin have all evolved from the same common ancestral gene. We know this because of our recently acquired knowledge of the amino acid sequence of thrombin, which is in large part homologous to those of the other enzymes mentioned. It may very well be that proconvertin, Stuart factor, prothrombin, and anti-haemophilic factor B are all related to prothrombin in an analogous way.

There is also the other question of whether or not some of them are actually formed as chemical derivates from prothrombin in plasma or even in the hepatic cells before secretion into the bloodstream. This would mean, of course, that they are synthesized by the same gene. If one were to find amino acid sequence evidence that, for example, proconvertin is an entirely different protein from prothrombin, then one could exclude this possibility immediately. If, on the other hand, one found that two or more of the factors have a long string of amino acid sequence in common, then one could still maintain the 'derivative hypothesis'.

Esnouf: This proposition covers a problem that has bothered a lot of people. I wonder whether prothrombin might be one large piece of something which seems to dissociate into lots of other little bits of other things recognized by other people under different names.

Swart: I would argue in favour of the existence of four separate factors, on the basis of evidence coming both from adsorption experiments and from salting-out experiments. Perhaps the adsorption evidence is not new, because factors VII, IX, and X have been removed from plasma by selective adsorption onto Bentonite, but in that case their activity has been destroyed. When adsorbed onto aluminium hydroxide, the factors can be eluted virtually quantitatively. When the concentration of aluminium hydroxide is 1%, all four factors are adsorbed from the plasma. When the concentration of $Al(OH)_3$ is reduced to a very low level, factors VII and X are adsorbed quite preferentially. I think that this indicates the existence of separate factors. In salting-out experiments at high pH, all factors precipitate really together, while at pH 5.5 factors II and VII and X precipitate separately at about 7% saturation of ammonium sulphate apart. As far as I know, no breaking of covalent bonds between proteins can be brought about by ammonium sulphate. These experiments may thus indicate the existence of separate factors.

Deutsch: If you apply human plasma to a DEAE-cellulose column, factor VII will pass through the column, whereas the other factors are adsorbed. This argues for the fact that factor VII is a separate factor.

Swart: If you are referring to experiments with ion-exchangers, the objection has been raised that occasionally other N-terminal and C-terminal amino acids are found after chromatography than were seen before chromatography. This is an argument from the Seegers group. My arguments are based on salt fractionation and adsorption onto aluminium hydroxide, and are therefore based on the same techniques that Seegers uses to make his prothrombin consisting of four factors tightly linked together. He has never reported differences between these factors when working with this technique. Perhaps the pH in his salting-out experiments was too high. In that case he would find the four factors together. He also used a very high concentration of adsorbent, which does not favour differential adsorption either.

Denson: The development of highly specific antibodies to the individual purified clotting factors, prothrombin, factor VII, factor IX, and factor X, also suggests that these four factors exist as separate entities in plasma.

CONCLUSION
No conclusive evidence can be given to support this proposition, yet suggestive new evidence for its correctness can be presented.

XII. *Prothrombinase converts prothrombin (mol. wt.* ∽ *68,000) into thrombin (mol.wt.* ∽ *32,000). Thrombin converts fibrinogen into fibrin monomers.*

Magnusson: Let us look at a model of the tertiary structure of bovine α-chymotrypsin based on the x-ray diffraction analysis by Blow, Sigler, and Matthew in Cambridge. We see that it consists of three polypeptide chains, A, B, and C.

The N-terminal isoleucine of the B-chain starts a bit of amino acid sequence that is highly homologous in chymotrypsin, trypsin, elastase, and thrombin. In the tertiary structure the isoleucine-16 is hydrogen or ion-pair bonded to aspartic acid-194, which lies in the C-chain and immediately precedes the active serine-195. The imidazole group of histidine-57 forms one hydrogen bond with serine-195 and another with aspartic acid-102. This set of interactions is considered by Blow, Birktoft and Hartley to be the essential feature of the active centre of the pancreatic serine-proteinases.

The activation of chymotrypsinogen to chymotrypsin occurs when the peptide bond from arginine-15 to isoleucine-16 is split, so that the isoleucine is free to form the previously mentioned bond to aspartic acid-194. This new bond probably alters slightly the tertiary structure around aspartic acid-194, so that the hydrogen bond from serine-195 to histidine-57 can be formed, giving the active enzyme. As long as isoleucine-16 is not N-terminal, we still have the zymogen. As soon as it becomes N-terminal, the zymogen becomes active enzyme. We know that this is also true for prothrombin activation to thrombin.

Furthermore, we know now from our amino acid sequence studies on thrombin that the B-chain of thrombin also has all the other sequence features that were mentioned above and that have been involved in the mechanism of activation and activity of chymotrypsin and the

other pancreatic serine proteinases. Any system that activates prothrombin to thrombin, whether it be called prothrombinase or something else, must therefore directly or indirectly cause the proteolytic
cleavage of this particular peptide bond which, in prothrombin, blocks
that isoleucine which on activation to thrombin is to become the N-
terminal of the B-chain.

Haanen: What can be thought to be a likely explanation for the occurrence of residual prothrombin left in the serum in cases where there is a
deficiency in the first steps of the clotting system – in haemophilia for
example? Why, in these case, is prothrombinase unable to convert all
prothrombin to thrombin?

Hemker: Prothrombinase in plasma is an extremely labile substance.
If you cannot form it with a velocity that is high enough or in an
amount that is high enough to ensure the persistence of a certain concentration of prothrombinase for a certain length of time, it simply will
not be there long enough to convert all the prothrombin present into
thrombin. You therefore have prothrombin left at the end of your
reaction.

Haanen: Perhaps that is true, but I find it hard to believe since the
whole reaction occurs within a few seconds. I think that prothrombinase is not so labile that it is broken down within so few seconds.

Hemker: Residual prothrombin is found in serum especially in those
cases where coagulation is slowed down.

Deggeller: We have only a part of the picture of the total mechanism
at this moment. There must be a mechanism to destroy prothrombinase, and there must be inhibitors in the plasma to prevent clotting of
all the blood when there has been some local stasis and clotting. There
must be other mechanisms besides antithrombin and antithrombo-
plastins which regulate this process.

Haanen: I agree with Dr. Deggeller that there is no doubt a very
potent anti-factor x_a and that traces of x_a will be inactivated immediately in plasma. You must have an explosive generation of factor x_a and
thrombin in order to clot plasma, and you must certainly have a lot of

factor x_a to convert the prothrombin. If you have small amounts, these will be neutralized quickly by the anti-factor x_a, which has an almost infinite capacity to inhibit x_a.

CONCLUSION

The proposition is sustained. Our knowledge of the equilibrium between activators and inactivators that governs the efficiency of the coagulation process still is inadequate.

XIII. *Fibrin-stabilizing factor (factor* XIII*) catalyses the formation of covalent bonds connecting adjacent fibrin molecules.*

Referring to the discussion after Blombäck's paper, *Duckert* stated that the number of covalent bonds formed between fibrin monomers by factor XIII_a is 1-2 per monomer according to one method and 2-3 according to another method, so that the most likely number is 2. There may be other linkages between monomers in the final fibrin structure, but these are not known.

CONCLUSION

The proposition is sustained.

CHAPTER II

PHYSIOPATHOLOGY

THE MECHANISM OF HAEMOSTASIS

E. A. LOELIGER

The Dutch proverb 'The best is the enemy of the good' sounds like one of Parkinson's laws but only means that the search for an ideal solution often implies the neglect of an available satisfactory solution. I am always reminded of this proverb when I encounter the almost palpable distaste, if not total resistance, shown by students, physicians, and biochemists at the mention of haemostasis. I hope nonetheless that you will bear with me. Since, as a process, haemostasis is so complex and is still so poorly understood that any attempt to discuss it briefly is doomed to failure, and since there are simply too many new concepts and complicated reactions to commit to memory at one sitting, I shall attempt to convey as much basic material and as few details as possible.

By way of introduction, let me begin with a few remarks concerning terminology. The literal definition of haemostasis is the arrestation of blood, in other words the stopping of bleeding, sometimes also called haemostypsis. Haemostasis or the stopping of bleeding must be sharply distinguished from the blood clot formation, which is simply the gelification of liquid blood *in vitro* as a consequence of fibrin formation. Spontaneous haemostasis and blood clot formation are preceded by reactions referred to collectively as the haemostasis mechanism and the coagulation mechanism, respectively. I shall discuss the former; the latter has been extensively dealt with in Chapter I.

The mechanism of primary haemostasis is represented in figure 1; the Arabic numbers (1, 2, 3, 4) show the sequence of events that commences when a small cut is made in skin by a standard lancet. During the first 15 to 30 seconds after the injury, the axon reflex leads to an *initial vasoconstriction* (1) and in this period only a very small amount of blood emerges from the wound. After this, blood flows out of the opened vessels, i.e. capillaries, venules, and arterioles. As the blood flows from the opened vessels, the platelets become attached to the

damaged basal membrane of the vessel wall and to the collagenous
fibres in the perivascular connective tissue. This is called *platelet adhesion* (2); it is dependent not only on platelet factors but also on a
protein present in the blood (Von Willebrand factor). The thrombocytes clinging to the injured vascular structures attract other
platelets from the passing stream; this phenomenon is called *platelet
aggregation* (3). Within a short time, the opening in the vessel is filled
and the blood-flow is blocked. The bleeding has been arrested without involvement of the coagulation mechanism or coagulation of
the blood. Concurrently with the aggregation of the thrombocytes,
vasoactive amines liberated from them cause a powerful and prolonged
second vasoconstriction at the arteriolar level (4). The interval between
the occurrence of the injury and the arrestation of the bleeding is called
the bleeding time; this interval usually lasts 1 to 2 minutes, even in
patients whose blood has little or no capacity to coagulate. For a
small skin wound, the platelet aggregations possess just enough resistance to withstand the blood pressure, even when the second vasoconstriction has been abolished, probably because in the skin they receive
support from the resistance offered by the firm connective tissue.

It follows from reactions 2 and 3 that the arrestation of the flow of
blood at the site of a microtrauma would be abnormal if there were a
shortage or inadequate functioning of the thrombocytes (i.e. thrombocytopenia or thrombocytopathy). In Von Willebrand's disease, also
called vascular haemophilia and angiohaemophilia, the lack of the so-
called bleeding factor, a plasma protein closely related to coagulation
factor VIII, causes pathologically prolonged bleeding. The marked
prolongation of the bleeding time often seen when the thrombocyte
count lies above 2 million per cubic millimetre may be related to an
ineffective aggregation in which the platelet plug breaks up repeatedly
before the opening in the vessel can be completely filled up (snowstorm
phenomenon). Another cause of the prolonged bleeding time could
be a relative shortage of vaso-active amines in the platelets, resulting
in an insufficient vasoconstriction. The prolonged bleeding time seen in
uraemia and after the administration of certain medicaments (particularly acetosal, to which there can be a hereditary sensitivity) is due
to a thrombocytopathy, since after transfusion of normal platelets the
bleeding time becomes normal. The explanation of the prolonged
bleeding time seen in paraproteinaemia is a different one: in this

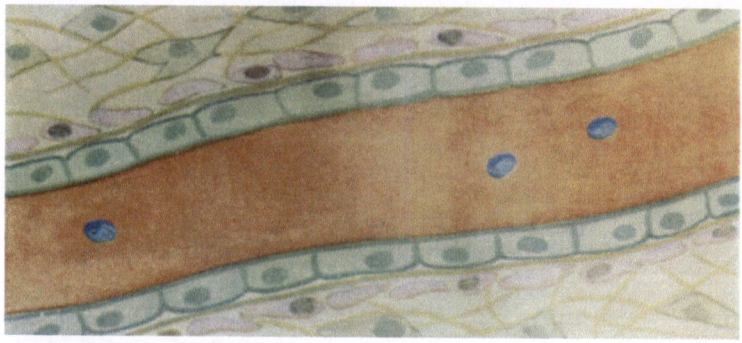

Fig. 1. Normal vessel.

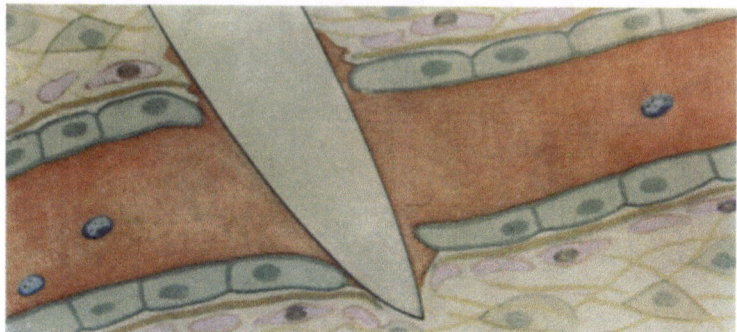

Fig. 2. Lesion.

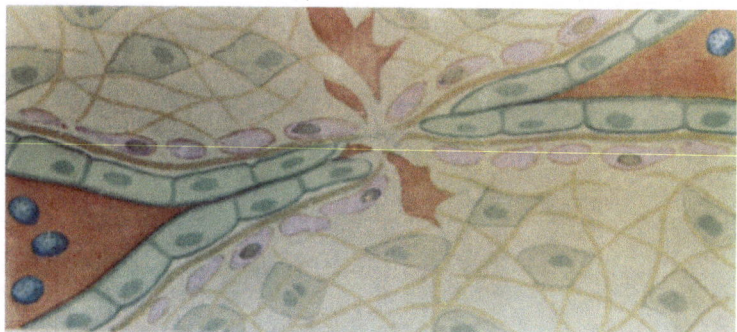

Fig. 3. Contraction by axone reflex.

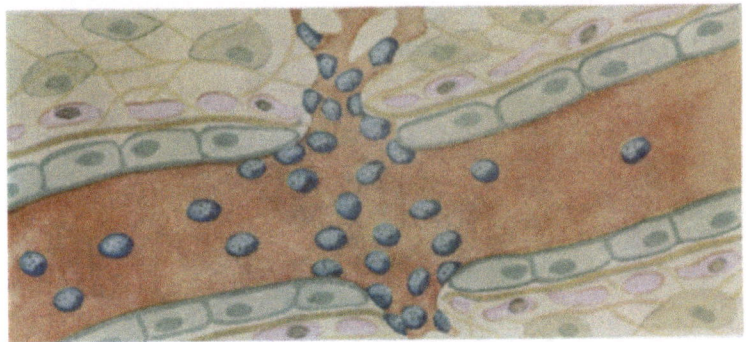

Fig. 4. Bleeding, adhaesion of platelets.

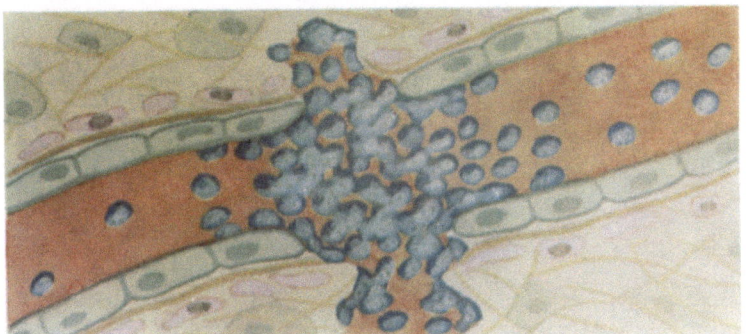

Fig. 5. Platelet aggregation, plug formation.

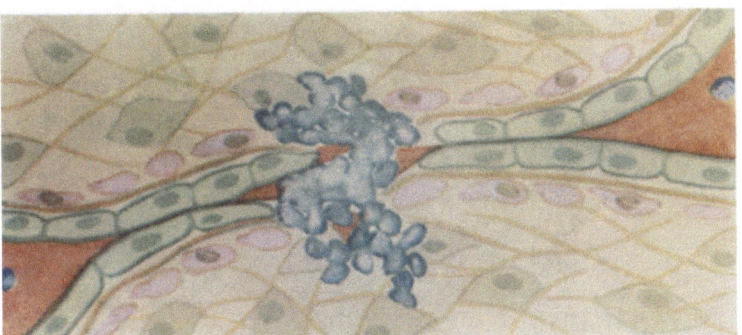

Fig. 6. Viscous metamorphosis, second retraction.

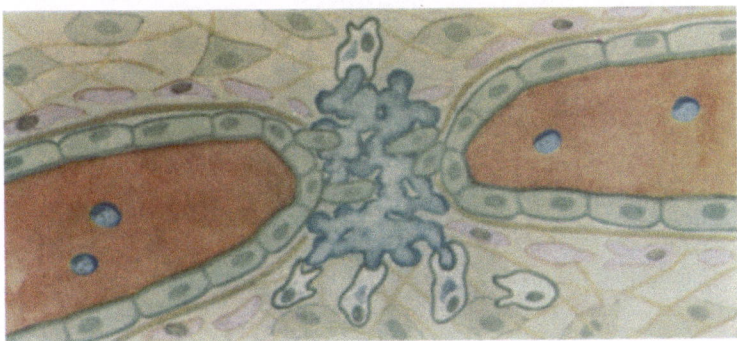

Fig. 7. Reparation.

case the pathological protein probably interferes with the reaction between the platelets and the basal membrane and collagen fibres.

The understanding of reaction 4, the vasoconstriction induced by biologically active amines, is far from complete, primarily because of the lack of experimentation on functions specific to the vascular wall. The Rumpel Leede test for the determination of capillary fragility is in no sense specific for the vascular component in haemostasis: a severe capillaropathy with a strongly positive Rumpel Leede phenomenon has no haemostatic significance whatsoever if the thrombocyte function is adequate. This does not hold, of course, for the general occurence of anatomical vascular pathology in which, as for instance in pan-vasculitis (sepsis, auto-immune diseases), fibroelastosis (Ehler-Danlos syndrome), and angiomatosis (including Osler's disease), very severe haemorrhagic phenomena often occur.

But to turn to normal haemostasis: in wounds caused by injury to somewhat larger arteries located in regions with less elastic and less firm perivascular connective tissue than is found in the small skin lesion demonstrated in figure 1 – whether this concerns the extraction of a tooth, a tonsillectomy, an accidental injury, or a cut made with a surgical knife – primary haemostasis is not completed after 1-2 minutes. This becomes clear from observations in persons with a disturbed coagulation mechanism, in whom such wounds, after an interval of a few hours, frequently lead to severe haemorrhage; this postoperative haemorrhage is greatly feared in the practice of surgery. Here after cessation of the second vasoconstriction, the arterial plugs have apparently been unable to offer sufficient resistance to the arterial pressure; an adequate consolidation of the thrombocyte plug, called *viscous metamorphosis*, has not taken place. Viscous metamorphosis is very distinctly dependent on normal functioning of an important part of the coagulation mechanism, i.e. the part that is responsible for the formation of thrombin. Thrombin induces (in addition to fibrin formation) the amalgamation of thrombocytes (by activation of the contractile substance thrombosthenin and possibly the action of coagulation factor XIII, etc.). Thus, individuals suffering from a significient absolute or relative vitamin K deficiency (shortage of factors II, VII, IX, and X), haemophiliacs (shortage of factors VIII or IX), patients with circulating anticoagulants, etc., all belong to the group of patients in whom haemostasis seems normal initially (normal bleeding time, no abnormally high loss of blood during operation) but in whom an increased loss of blood occurs several hours after the trauma. An exception to this is formed by patients whose blood coagulation is clearly retarded *in vitro* by the presence of *moderate* quantities of heparin (iatrogenic) or antiphospholipoprotein (auto-immune anticoagulant). In these cases the thrombin formation *in vivo*, and with it the viscous metamorphosis of the platelets, appears hardly or not at all disturbed, probably due to the strong heparin-neutralizing properties of the thrombocyte (platelet factor iv) and a high phospholipid content of the platelet (platelet factor iii).

It is an extremely interesting point that the last step of the blood-coagulation mechanism, the formation of fibrin, or in other words the actual coagulation, has almost no importance for haemostasis itself. This fact is demonstrated by the many patients in whose blood the precursor of fibrin, fibrinogen (factor i), is largely missing (afibrinogenaemia) or occurs in such a pathological state that there is grossly pathologic formation of fibrin (dysfibrinogenaemia). Such patients show no or only limited haemorrhagic manifestations.

A final remark on haemostasis in the uterus: here, both the special anatomy of the arteries and the local perivascular structures contribute to the limited consequences of coagulation disturbances with respect to menstruation and to the fact that even severe thrombocytopenia and thrombocytopathy are rarely accompanied by dangerous meno- or metrorrhagias. This does not hold, however, for the defibrination syndrome, in which both platelet functions and coagulation factors are severely disturbed or reduced. When this syndrome is accompanied by accelerated fibrinolysis, as in the obstetrical amnionic-fluid embolism, it is almost or entirely impossible to stop the bleeding.

Put even more briefly, the haemostasis mechanism has three important phases: phase 1, thrombocyte adhesion and aggregation; phase 2, vasoconstriction; and phase 3, firm platelet plug formation under the influence of thrombin. In the operation of this mechanism a role is played by the perivascular anatomical structures (skin, uterus).

MORPHOLOGY OF THE PROCESS OF HAEMOSTASIS

J. J. SIXMA

This discussion concerns several morphological aspects of the process of haemostasis and is based on a number of electronmicroscopical photographs.

Figure 1 shows an ellipsoidal cross-section of a normal thrombocyte present in the circulation as a small disk. This blood platelet has a membrane resembling the normal cell membrane but arising as an intracellular membrane of the megakaryocyte. An expression of this origin may lie in the presence of a layer (protein?) seen on the outer surface of the platelet membrane, whereas the erythrocyte membrane, for instance, is smooth. The most striking organelles in the blood platelet are the alpha granules, whose function is unknown; and there is also a system of tubules some of which are connected with the surface. At the extremities of the oval cross-section there are a number of small tubules running as a ring along the periphery of the disk-shaped platelet. In a cross-section taken more parallel to the flat surface of the disk, these microtubules are seen longitudinally. The platelet also contains mitochondria, remarkable for their relatively simple structure, and glycogen particles. Here and there, very dark granules thought to contain serotonin are also seen. In pseudopodia there are microfibrils lying parallel to the cell membrane. These fibrils are also present in the circulating platelet, but are seen there much less distinctly since they form a criss-cross pattern under the membrane (figure 2). On the structural basis of the fibrils and the microtubules, we have formulated a hypothesis in which the disk shape of the thrombocyte is explained as the result of the contactile fibrils, which give the platelet the smallest possible circumference, and of the ring of microtubules, whose rigidity opposes the contraction of the fibrils in one direction. Some support for this hypothesis is provided by the finding that thrombosthenin, the contractile protein of the blood platelet, apparently has a structure similar to that of the fibrils.

The haemostatic plug (*'clou hémostatique'*) is built up of blood platelets attached to collagen, to which new platelets continue to attach themselves until the picture of a viscous metamorphosis develops, i.e. the platelets have lost their granules and are packed together so tightly that the results appear to be a viscous mass when seen with the light microscope. Electron-microscopical investigation, however, shows that each platelet retains its identity, i.e. possesses an intact cell membrane.

With respect to the diverse aspects of this process, the following may be said:

1. *Adhesion:* Blood platelets attach themselves to collagen fibrillae as well as to collagen in the form of a basal membrane. The mechanism of this adhesion is unknown, although it is known to be independent of the presence of calcium. The platelet membrane lies closely adjacent to the collagen fibrils, at a distance of 20 to 30A.; the membrane is interrupted at various places, making contact where the collagen shows dark bands. The adherent platelets have lost their cellular organelles. Adhesion to the collagen is accompanied by a release reaction in which adenosine diphosphate (ADP) is one of the substances liberated. This ADP triggers the next phase, i.e. aggregation of the platelets.

2. *Aggregation* (figures 3, 4, and 5): Under the influence of ADP (as well as adrenalin and serotonin), the platelets become attached to each other. This reaction requires calcium and a small amount of fibrinogen, and a role is possibly played by another plasma factor which is thermostable. Aggregation is preceded by a change of shape in which the platelets become spherical and their volume increases by about 30 per cent. It is assumed that no degranulation of the platelets takes place during aggregation.

In recent years it has become clear that ADP, when present in more than a given concentration at 37°C, intitiates a release reaction in which ADP is liberated as well as other substances. This explains why a small amount of ADP released by collagen can result in a large platelet aggregate. The small amount of ADP in turn triggers further release of ADP, so that a kind of autocatalytic process leads to the formation of a

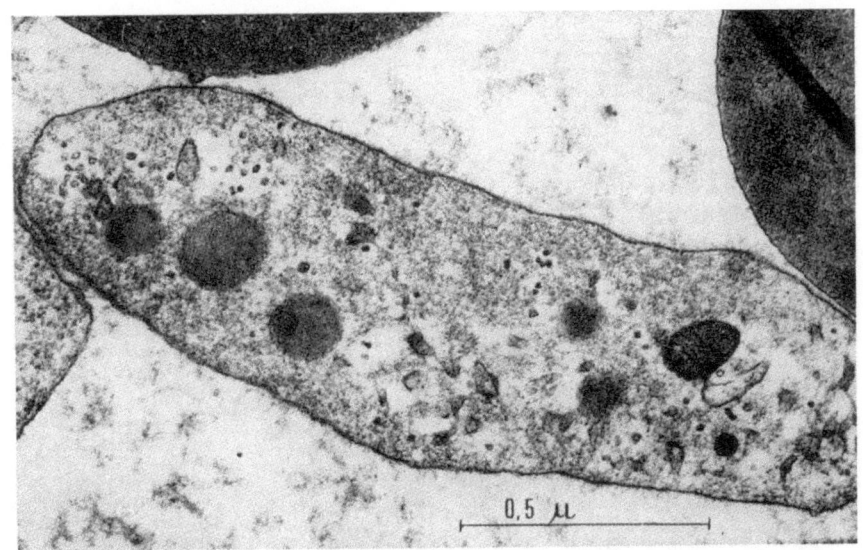

Fig. 1. Cross-section of a normal blood platelet. Glutaraldehyde fixation. Top and top right: parts of red blood cells. Top left: a number of microtubules in cross-section with, below, three α-granules. Left: a mitochondrion, recognizable by its double membrane. Tubules and glycogen particles are scattered throughout. *Folia Med. Neerl.*, 10, 1967.

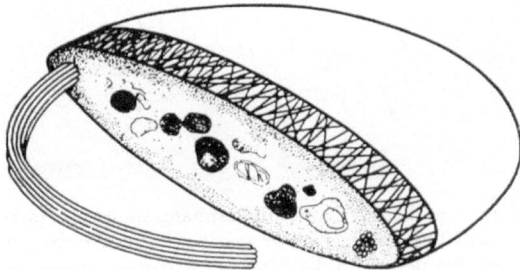

Fig. 2. Diagram of a blood platelet showing the bundle of microtubules at the periphery and the microfibrils localized in a submembranous layer.

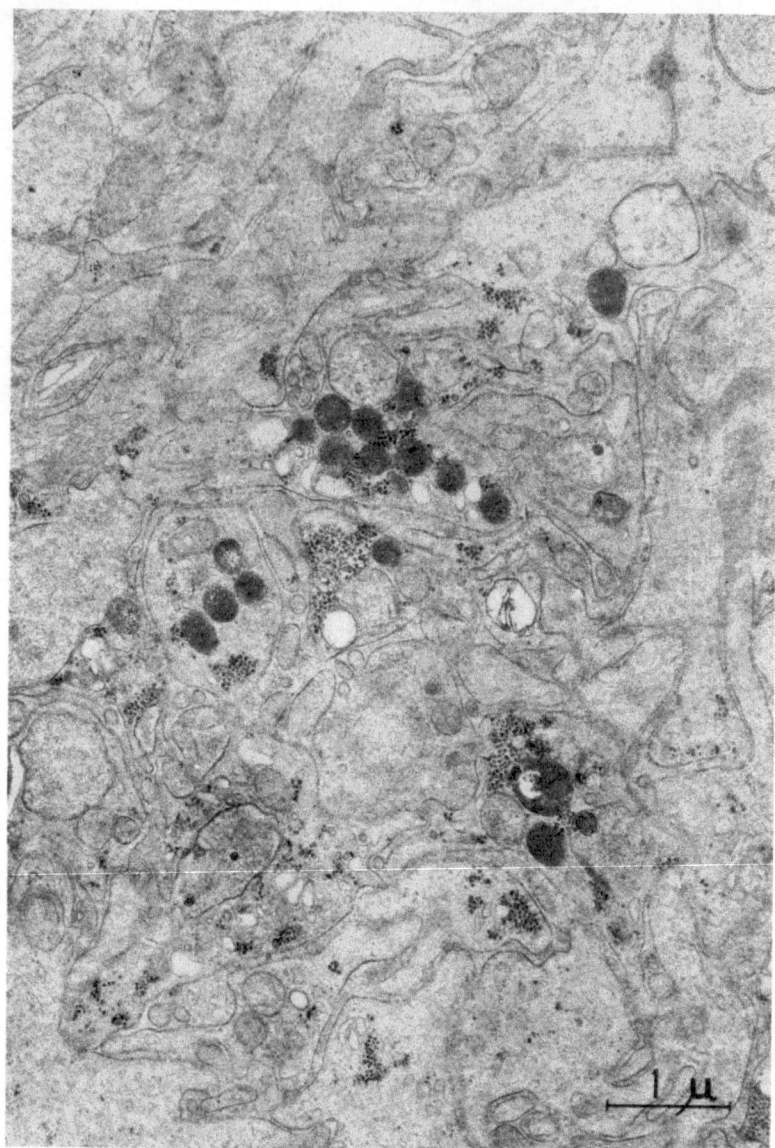

Fig. 3. An aggregate induced by adenosine diphosphate, showing a picture similar to that of viscous metamorphosis. The platelets are densely packed and degranulated. Those in the upper right corner show the peripheral balloon-type extrusions present in these aggregates. Some dense granules are still present. Glycogen is conspicious in a field in the upper right corner.

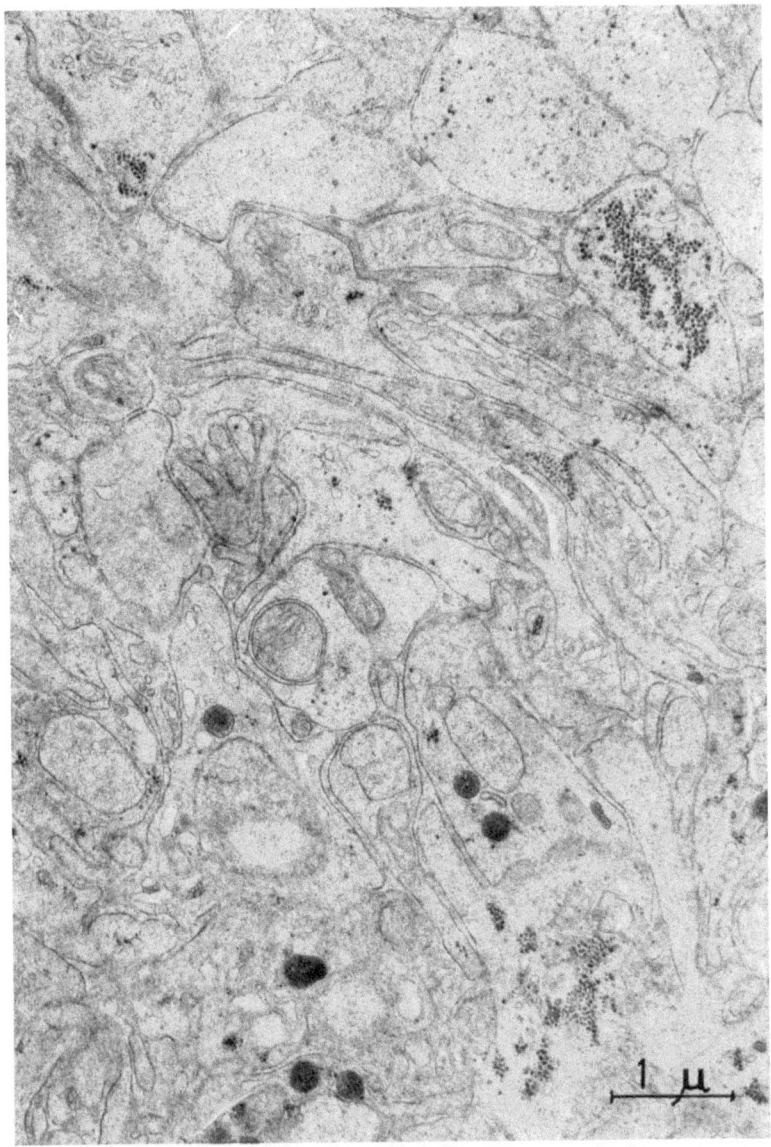

Fig. 4. Detail of the same aggregates as those shown in figure 3, demonstrating that granules are sometimes retained in a platelet.

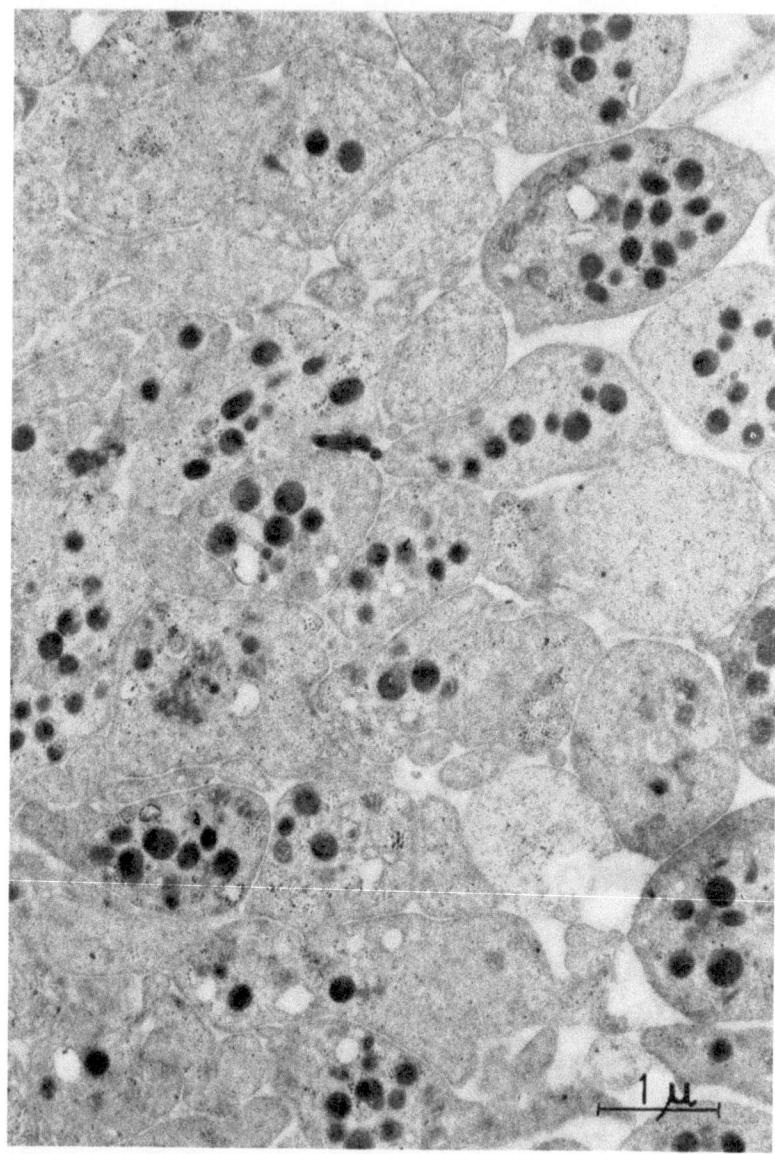

Fig. 5. Part of an aggregate induced at a lower concentration of adenosine diphosphate, showing that most of the granules are retained. The platelets are less densely packed and there are fewer pseudopods.

plug of platelets that fills up the lesion in the vascular wall, after which no new platelets arrive at the site of the lesion.

3. *Viscous metamorphosis:* After a platelet plug has formed, degranulation of the platelets occurs, accompanied by an increase in the density of the packed platelets as the result of a kind of retraction. It is assumed that this so-called viscous metamorphosis is initiated by thrombin formed during the preceding process. How this is thrombin formed *in vivo* is not known, but that its formation is triggered by the presence of thromboplastin seems an obvious assumption. The latter is known to activate factor VII, which then – via factor X and factor V – provides for the conversion of prothrombin into thrombin. A deficiency of factor VII would therefore be expected to disrupt the viscous metamorphosis, but observations in factor-VII-deficient dogs have demonstrated the formation of a normal plug under these circumstances.

In the past year not only we (1) but also Mills, Robb and Roberts (2) have demonstrated that when a release occurs during ADP aggregation there is also a degranulation showing a picture similar to that of viscous metamorphosis (figures 4 and 5). It may therefore be concluded that ADP itself causes a viscous metamorphosis and that the latter occurs when a release reaction takes place. In our opinion, it seems both more reasonable and more probable that during the release reaction ADP is responsible for creating a situation in which thrombin can be easily formed, e.g. in the spaces between the platelets on the surface of the plasma membrane.

REFERENCES

1. Sixma, J. J., J. J. Geuze, Degranulation during ADP induced aggregation. *Vox. Sang.* 15, 309 (1968).
2. Mills, D. C. B., I. A. Robb, G. C. K. Roberts, The release of nucleotides, 5-hydroxytryptamine and enzymes from human blood platelets during aggregation. *J. Physiol.* (Lond.) 195, 715 (1968).

An excellent review on 'The ultrastructure of blood platelets in normal and abnormal states' by Hovig appeared recently in *Series Haematologica.* Volume 1. 2 (1968).

LABORATORY INVESTIGATION

INDICATION, ASSAY PROCEDURES, DIAGNOSIS, AND ADVICE

J. J. VELTKAMP, ANNEMARIE D. MULLER AND
E. A. LOELIGER

I. INDICATION

Laboratory investigation of anomalies in the haemostasis mechanism are requested on the basis of four fundamentally different considerations:

- To exclude haemorrhagic diathesis prior to the performance of a blind biopsy (kidney, spleen, liver).
- To determine the cause of a manifest haemorrhagic diathesis for therapeutic purposes.
- To obtain supplementary evidence with respect to diagnosis and therapy, e.g. in auto-immune and liver diseases, malignant neoplasms, disturbances of intestinal resorption, rejection of (kidney) transplants, etc.
- For the determinations related to overshooting of the haemostasis mechanism, resulting in thrombosis (states with increased tendency toward thrombosis, also called thrombophilia).

An isolated haemorrhage in the respiratory tract (haemoptoea, nosebleeds), urogenital tract (menorrhagia, haematuria), or gastro-intestinal tract (haematemesis, melaena) only constitutes an indication when no pathological substrate is found and *a fortiori* when there are also signs that the local bleeding is part of a haemorrhagic diathesis, i.e. of a general tendency to bleed. The same holds *mutatis mutandis* for thrombosis. In the present state of our knowledge, laboratory investigation can be of use only in exceptional cases (e.g. marked familial predisposition).

2. THE INVESTIGATION

2.1. ANAMNESIS

When a clotting defect is suspected, conclusive evidence can usually be found in the patient's history. In this sense hypermenorrhoea, bleeding gums, and easy bruisability (especially in women) are less important than persisting haemorrhages after surgical treatment or extensive traumata. The patient must always be questioned about any history of tooth extractions, tonsillectomy, hernia operation, and the healing of wounds in general. The duration of the phenomena is very important for the determination of the aetiology and pathogenesis of a haemorrhagic diathesis. The character of a hereditary anomaly can sometimes be determined by drawing up the patient's pedigree. It must not be forgotten, however, that in one-third of all the cases haemophilia has a *de novo* genesis. Women can also have a congenital deficiency of coagulation factors in the absence of parental consanguinity. The nutritional data provided by the anamnesis and the description of the defaecation pattern may convey information concerning possible deficiencies of vitamin C, vitamin K, folic acid or vitamin B_{12}, and iron, all of which may accompany a haemorrhagic diathesis. Often, an exact inventarization of drugs used will clarify the situation (oral anticoagulants, aspirin, PAS, antibiotics, laxatives as (contributory) cause of vitamin K deficiency; certain soporifics and hypertensive drugs known to give vascular purpura as side-effect; quinidine, quinine, Sedormid®, digitalis, known as haptenes in accute immune thrombocytopenia; dilution effect of Macrodex®; etc.). Lastly, in any rather sudden severe haemorrhagic diathesis, all possible intoxications must be kept in mind, and investigation must be directed to the identification of a metastasizing neoplasm or an auto-immune disease.

Note: It need hardly be said that a history concentrating specifically on haemorrhagic diathesis is only an indispensable part of a general history to be evaluated in combination with the results of physical, radiological, and laboratory investigations.

2.2. THE LABORATORY INVESTIGATION

The investigation of the various components of the haemostasis mechanism under indications 1 and 2 is based on the interaction between the vascular wall, platelets (see Mechanism of haemostasis, page 143), and coagulation factors.

The first three steps of the investigation of the patient are:

2.2.1. Determination of the bleeding time.

2.2.2. Performance of a flawless venapuncture and the proper collection of a blood sample.

2.2.3. Preparation of a smear from a puncture of the finger.

Two other investigations, i.e. measurement of the capillary resistance (according to Rumpel and Leede) and capillary microscopy, do not provide relevant information for the evaluation of the haemostasis mechanism. We therefore generally omit both, especially since they are time-consuming and the former is also often very unpleasant for the patient.

In the laboratory, the following procedures are carried out:

2.2.4.   Thrombelastography (TEG).

2.2.5.   Platelet count.

2.2.6.   Measurement of the haematocrit.

2.2.7.a. Measurement of the recalcification time in blood or plasma.

2.2.7.b. Measurement of the concentration of factors VIII, IX, XI, and XII, based on a one-stage recalcification technique.

2.2.8.   Measurement of the thromboplastin time (Quick's prothrombin time), Thrombotest, Normotest, and factor v determination.

2.2.9.   Measurement of the fibrinogen content.

2.2.10. Measurement of the thrombin time.

2.2.11. Urea solubility test.

2.2.12. Determination of the clot retraction (and consequently the whole blood clot lysis time).

2.2.13. Determination of fibrin (fibrinogen) degradation products.

The erythrocyte sedimentation rate (ESR) is estimated from the level of the plasma layer in the TEG cuvette; the colour of the serum is noted (icterus, haemolysis); a qualitative investigation is made with respect to a pathological protein composition of the serum (Sia test) and the presence of cryoglobulin (after holding the plasma and serum for 24 hours under refrigeration).

These laboratory investigations (2.2.1-2.2.13) are described in detail in the following sections.

PROCEDURES PERFORMED AT THE BEDSIDE

2.2.1. THE DETERMINATION OF THE BLEEDING TIME ACCORDING TO IVY

A prolonged bleeding time can result from the use of salicylic acid.

Materials

- blood pressure manometer
- lancet (manufacturer: Becton Dickinson & Co., Blood Lancet no. 433; obtainable in The Netherlands from AVAC, Naarden)
- filter paper (obtainable in The Netherlands from Schut en Zonen, Heelsum; no. V 255-90 mm)
- 3 stop-watches

Method

The blood-pressure cuff is applied to one of the upper arms; the inside of that fore-arm is desinfected with ether (stroking with wad of cotton wool from distal to proximal); the lancet is placed in readiness and the pressure in the cuff is brought to 40 mm of mercury. With the lancet, three linear cuts are made (with a firm stroke, avoiding superficial veins). As a rule, bleeding starts only 15 to 30 seconds after the cut has been made. The stop-watches are started at the moment at wich a distinct drop of blood appears (a separate stop-watch is used for each of the three cuts). If no blood appears within 30 seconds, the cuts are spread briefly and firmly by placing a finger on either side of the wound and pressing outward in opposite directions, which is almost always followed by bleeding (the normal values are not affected). At intervals of at least 15 seconds the drops are taken up with filter paper, the wound being touched as little as possible. As soon as the flow ceases, which can be judged from the staining of the papers, the stop-watch is stopped and read. The wound is then covered, especially in cases of prolonged bleeding time. When prolongation is extreme, a pressure bandage is sometimes required.

Normal values:

95% of the normal values lie below 4 minutes; mean and standard deviation:

men   = 50 ± 35 sec
women   = 90 ± 40 sec

Note: Marked hyperaemia (for instance, after exposure of the arm to hot water) does not result in a prolongation of the normal values of more than 30 seconds.

Interpretation of prolonged bleeding time
- Frequency: this is the most frequent of the anomalies found in the laboratory.
- Severity:

$$\left.\begin{array}{l} 4 - \ 8 \ \text{min: mild} \\ 8 - 15 \ \text{min: moderate} \\ > \quad 15 \ \text{min: severe} \end{array}\right\} \quad \text{prolongation}$$

- *Pathogenesis in cases in which prolonged bleeding time is accompanied by a normal platelet count:*
Congenital:
a. thrombocytopathy (three types: Glanzmann-Naegeli, Soulier-Bernard, Hardisty-Caen)
b. deficiency of coagulation factor (Von Willebrand-Jürgens' disease, Rita's disease, etc.)
c. total absence of fibrinogen in blood
d. pathological vascular or connective tissue (?)

Acquired:
a. thrombocytopathy
intrinsic: medicamentous (usually salicylic acid, phenylbutazon), endotoxic (uraemia), neoplastic (myeloproliferative affections)
extrinsic: medicamentous (thrombolytic therapy), paraproteinaemic (coating, possibly also of collagen)

Note: An acquired total afibrinogenaemia or bleeding factor deficiency or an acquired vascular or collagen pathology is not known.

Pathogenesis in cases in which prolonged bleeding time is associated with thrombocytopenia.
In diminished production there is a certain correlation between the severity of the thrombocytopenia and the degree of prolongation:

$$< 50,000/\mu l \ \rightarrow \ > 4 \text{min}$$
$$< \ 5,000/\mu l \ \rightarrow \ > 15 \text{min}$$

but this correlation holds exclusively for normally functioning platelets, as found in cases of diminished production, trapping in the
spleen, or after transfusion of normal platelets.

The same holds to a lesser extent for immune-thrombocytopenia
and especially for cases treated with corticosteroids, which may result
in inhibition of the RES function such that pathological platelets are
not removed and continue to circulate. Such platelets are often functionally inadequate. But in diffuse intravascular coagulation, overloading of the RES also leads to the persistence of functionally inferior
platelets in the circulation; these are thrombocytes that are recircul-
ated when the microthrombi into which they have been incorporated
disintegrate (the so-called serum platelets). Under these circumstances,
even at platelet counts between 50,000 and 150,000 / µl the bleeding
time is often prolonged. No distinct correlation between the platelet
count and the severity of the prolongation of the bleeding time is
found in myeloproliferative affections, but in these cases the platelets
often show pronounced morphological abnormalities.

*Pathogenesis in cases in which prolonged bleeding time is associated with
thrombocythaemia*
Here, too, there is no distinct correlation between prolongation of the
bleeding time and the platelet count. However, cases with severe
bleeding phenomena usually show platelet counts of > 2 million/ µl
and bleeding times of > 15 min. These anomalies disappear together
with normalization of the thrombocyte count, e.g. due to treatment
with cytostatics.

Remarks
- The measurement of the bleeding time according to Ivy is a minor
  procedure and can be repeated many times in succession because of
  the large surface offered by the forearms.
- The procedure leaves no objectionable scars.
- The procedure never results in dangerous haematomas or bleeding
  such as can occur in the measurement of bleeding time according to
  Duke on the ear-lobe (in cases of severe haemophilia and defibrination syndrome).
- In our experience there is no need for modification of the Ivy
  method (which would usually involve larger wounds) or for
  estimation of the so-called 'secondary' bleeding time (Borchgrevink).

2.2.2. COLLECTION OF BLOOD FROM THE PATIENT

> Flawless collection of blood is imperative for relia-
> ble results.

Tubes:

– plastic (polystyrol crystal) tubes: 50 × 15 mm with red cap (Emnosa,
  Rue de Bourgemeestre, Zuun, Belgium)
– conical centrifuge tubes (glass): 100 × 15 mm.

Have ready for venapuncture

1 plastic tube, empty
1 plastic tube containing a pinch of EDTA
1 plastic tube containing 0.1 ml 0.55 M (20%) Na citrate (check to be
sure that no evaporation of the Na citrate solution has occurred)
1 conical centrifuge tube containing 0.1 ml fibrinolysis inhibitors (25 U
trasylol and 25 mg EACA/ml 1 : 100 diluted human brain thromboplastin).
1 19-gauge disposable needle (1.05 mm)

Venapuncture

Stasis must be minimal, and the puncture clean and flawless. When
completed, the arm should be kept stretched and raised for 3 minutes to
prevent formation of a haematoma. Always cover the wound with a
piece of cotton wool and adhesive plaster.

Procedure for collecting blood

Take up first 2 to 3 ml with a piece of cotton wool.

– in an empty plastic tube, collect about 2 ml blood (TEG)
– in a plastic tube containing EDTA, collect about 1 ml blood (haematocrit + platelet count)
– in a plastic tube containing citrate, collect as close as possible to 4.9
  blood; the 5 ml level can easily be marked on the tube (coagulation
  measurements)
– in a conical centrifuge tube containing an antifibrinolytic mixture,
  allow about 5 ml blood to collect (clot retraction, degradation
  products, etc.).

2.2.3. PREPARATION OF A SMEAR FROM A FINGER PUNCTURE

In an ordinary haematomorphological smear stained according to
May-Gruenwald-Giemsa, platelet aggregation and platelet morphology
can be studied.

HANDLING OF BLOOD SAMPLES IN THE LABORATORY

Rapid and accurate work increases the reliability
of the results.

Blood for thrombelastography should not be allowed to cool unnecessarily.
For out-patients seen in the laboratory, the time up to loading of the
apparatus should not exceed 3 minutes. Blood collected at the bedside
is transported in a thermostatically controlled container; nevertheless,
the procedure should whenever possible be completed within 6 to 8
minutes after sampling.

EDTA *blood:* as rapidly as possible, the haematocrit is determined, the
platelets counted, and, when necessary, a micro–ESR started. EDTA
blood is not suitable for the evaluation of platelet aggregation, since
complete binding of Ca to EDTA makes it impossible for the platelets to
aggregate. EDTA blood is also unsuitable for investigation of the
coagulation (factors I, V and VIII rapidly lose almost all activity under
Ca-free conditions).

Whole blood (without anticoagulant): place in a thermostat at 37°C
without delay and examine for clot formation at regular intervals (e.g.
every half hour).

Citrated blood: after determination of recalcification time, centrifuge at
3,000 r.p.m. for 10 minutes. The resulting lowspun plasma is pipetted
into a plastic tube. In this material, determine the thromboplastin
time, the thrombin time, the fibrinogen content, and, when necessary,
a Thrombotest curve, the Normotest value, and the factor V activity.
Titration of heparin can also be done in this lowspun plasma. For
determination of factors VIII, IX, XI, and XII, and also for holding for
longer periods under deep-freezing (preferably at —70°C), the plasma
is freed of platelets by centrifugation at 20,000 g for 30 minutes.
Preferably, this should be done within 4 hours after venapuncture.

Clotted whole blood (containing fibrinolysis inhibitors)

after allowing to stand for 3 hours at 37°C:
- Measure retraction of the clot.
- Centrifuge at 3,000 r.p.m. for 10 minutes.
- Fill in Ouchterlony plate (see page 194).

– Place remainder in refrigerator ($4\,^{\circ}$C) for 24 hours, for sedimentation
of cryoglobulin (plasma for cryofibrinogen).

2.2.4. THROMBELASTOGRAPHY

> Thrombelastograpy reduces the work load, parti-
> cularly in the precise supervision of anticoagulant
> treatment with heparin.

Materials
– Thrombelastograph 'Hellige' (Manufacturer: Hellige, Postfach 728,
Freiburg im Breisgau, Germany; representative in The Netherlands:
DEPEX, de Bilt) on a vibration-free table.
– Plastic cuvettes (Manufactured and supplied by: EMERGO, Lands-
meer, The Netherlands).

Principle
Optical registration of clot formation on the basis of the developing
elastic properties. In other words, the dynamics of the coagulation
process are measured, as is indicated by the French term *thrombodyna-
mographie*.

Technique
In a slowly oscillating plastic cuvette (period $3\frac{1}{2}$ seconds) containing
the blood sample, a small stainless steel cylinder is hung. This cylinder
begins to turn with the cuvette as soon as the surface of the cylinder
becomes connected with the wall of the cuvette by a sufficient number
of fibrin threads having elastic properties. The cylinder in each sample
is suspended by a thin wire; on this torsion wire is mounted a small
mirror which catches a beam of light. The movements of the cylinder
and with it the torsion wire, mirror, and light beam are directly
visible and are also recorded on a moving film (speed 2 mm per
minute). The exposure time (1 sec.) of the terminal positions are represented on the film. Before the cylinder begins to move, the light
beam is of course stationary, thus giving a single line on the film. The
time elapsing between the venapuncture and the splitting of the line
(start of cylinder movement) is called the reaction time (r value). This
time may be considered to represent the coagulation time. The rate at
which the elasticity of the clot increases is measured as the time required to reach a distance of 20 mm between the two lines on the film
(k value).

The maximal distance reached between the two lines is called the maximal amplitude (*ma* value). After the maximal amplitude has been reached, a relaxation occurs in the internal structure of the clot, probably as the result of fibrinolysis.

The resulting configuration is called a thrombelastogram.

Method for native blood (i.e. without anticoagulant)
Flawless venapuncture is imperative. As soon as the blood begins to flow, the stop-watch is started. About 2 ml is taken up in a wad of cotton wool and the next 2 to 3 ml in a plastic tube. Within 1 to 2 minutes, the cuvettes are filled about two-thirds full directly from the tube (each cuvette takes about 0.6 to 0.7 ml blood). As soon as the cuvettes have been placed in the apparatus, the cylinders are lowered into the blood. Any superfluous blood is removed with a syringe provided with a clean (disposable) needle, after which a thin layer of liquid paraffin is applied to the blood (to prevent evaporation). The position of the light beam is then adjusted and the film started. The time between the venapuncture and the starting of the film, the so-called preparatory interval, is noted. For out-patients this time should be less than 4 minutes and for hospitalized patients not more than 8 minutes. Fifteen and 25 minutes after the venapuncture, the light beam is checked visually and the movements are noted. The film is usually stopped after one to two hours, and is then developed without delay. Before removing the cuvette from the thrombelastograph, notes are again made of the time and amplitude as well as the level and thickness of the plasma layer above the erythrocytes (important for the interpretation of the film).

Analysis of the film obtained with native blood
- Measurement of the *r* value, the so-called reaction time. This is the time elapsing between the moment of venapuncture and the moment that the amplitude measures 2 mm. The interval between venapuncture and starting of the film (preparatory interval) is added to the time calculated from the distance in mm (speed of the film 2 mm/min.) between the beginning of the thrombelastogram and the reaching of the 2 mm result (amplitude).
- Measurement of the *k* value. This is the time elapsing between the moments at which the curve becomes 2 and 20 mm wide. The time in minutes is obtained by dividing the distance in mm by 2.

– Measurement of the *ma* value. This is the greatest distance between the two extremes of the curve. The rate at which the thrombelastogram becomes narrower is estimated, and when appropriate the time required for the two lines to become one is measured (lysis time).

Normal values

The means of threefold determinations, (i.e. three thrombelastograms made simultaneously) obtained in native blood in plastic cuvettes, range between:

r: 15 and 23 min
k: 7 and 13 min
ma: 41 and 53 min

Interpretation of the thrombelastogram obtained with normal blood

General remarks

It will be evident that the *r* value (the clotting time) is highly dependent on the function of the coagulation mechanism, whereas the shape of the thrombelastogram (the *k* and *ma* values) is determined by the quantity and function of the fibrinogen and platelets, both of which must be related to the haematocrit and the sedimentation rate of the erythrocytes, since the measurements are made in whole blood. With very rapid sedimentation the picture resembles that of a plasma thrombelastogram (relatively much fibrin is present between the cylinder and the wall of the cuvette, because erythrocytes accumulate between the bottom of the cuvette and the lower surface of the cylinder). Moreover, fibrinolysis can be so intensive that after some time the two lines again become one (clot lysis time); and furthermore, if the clot becomes detached from the wall of the cuvette (breaking-off phenomenon), movement may cease (pseudolysis).

The r and k values can be too short due to:

1. Improper venapuncture
2. Increase of factor VIII under all forms of stress, including those induced by injection of adrenalin, acute anaemia, or shock.
3. Intravascular haemolysis, in which there is liberation of erythrocytic phospholipid (the so-called erythrocytin), which acts as an accelerator on the coagulation process.
4. Thrombocytosis, in which there is usually no true hypercoagul-

ability but which is accompanied by an accelerated intensification of the viscosity; this of course reduces the *r* time (the onset of fibrin formation occurring about 5 to 8 minutes prior to registration on the thrombelastogram).

Remarks

Uncomplicated thrombocytopenia gives no significant prolongation of the *r* value but only a reduction of the *ma* value; in combination with hypercoagulability, however, a reduction of the *r* value is often found as the sole abnormality.

The r and k values can be prolonged due to:

- Absence or partial deficiency of one or more of the coagulation factors with exception of factors VII and XIII.
- Absence of factor VIII, as seen in severe haemophilia A, gives an *r* value between 60 and 180 minutes; absence of factor IX as seen in severe haemophilia B usually gives an *r* value between 40 and 90 minutes. The *k* value is greatly prolonged in severe deficiencies of both factor VIII and factor IX. A reduction of the antihaemophilic factors to 5 to 25% often gives normal *r* and *k* values.
- Severe factor XII deficiency gives *r* values of 30 to 45 minutes and only slightly prolonged *k* values.
- Serious anomalies in the synthesis of the factors of the prothrombin complex in vitamin K deficiency (also in anticoagulant treatment with coumarin) give pictures indistinguishable from those seen in severe haemophilia.
- Presence of a pathological circulating anticoagulant. Both heparin (exogenous) and auto-immune (endogenous) anticoagulants can result in pictures resembling those seen in haemophilia.
- Excessive cooling of the blood sample (delay in placing cuvettes in the apparatus) causes a spurious prolongation.

In hypocoagulability combined with factors increasing the *ma* value (see below), an increase of the *r* values can coincide with a normal *k* value.

The ma values can be aberrant to different degrees
Less than 40 mm:

Thrombocytopenia, thrombocytopathy, fibrinogenopenia, elevated haematocrit, worn apparatus (fibrinogenopathia? factor XIII-deficiency?).

More than 55 mm:

hyperfibrinogenaemia, low haematocrit, high sedimentation rate (paraproteinaemia; after Macrodex® infusion, etc.).

Shape of the configuration

- Angular irregularities (Stufen Phenomen) may be due to leucocytosis, uraemia, severe hypercoagulability, or can be caused by vibration of the apparatus.
- Gradual narrowing of the configuration occurs in fibrinolysis.
- The severity of the fibrinolysis can be judged from the thrombelastogram:

lysis time of: 5–10 hr = barely increased fibrinolysis
2–5 hr = slightly increased fibrinolysis
1–2 hr = moderately increased fibrinolysis
$\frac{1}{2}$–1 hr = strongly increased fibrinolysis
$< \frac{1}{2}$ hr = very strongly increased fibrinolysis

When strongly increased fibrinolysis is suspected and only a straight line is obtained, a thrombelastogram of a mixed sample should be made immediately (see recalcification thrombelastogram).

A wavy configuration is caused by a defective thermostat, as a result of which the blood periodically becomes too warm, leading to a periodic reduction of the viscosity during the coagulation process.

Procedure for citrated blood or plasma (recalcification thrombelastogram) :
Blood that has been rendered incoagulable by admixture of sodium citrate can in principle also be used for thrombelastography, but due to plasma dilution (addition of the sodium citrate and calcium chloride solutions) and contact activity (even in plastic), the shape and normal values of the configuration differ from those obtained with native blood: the *r* and *k* values are lower, the *ma* value somewhat higher. The normal values of citrated blood are dependent not only on the dilution and the material in which the blood is stored but also on the 'age' and temperature of the blood. In other words, recalcification thrombelastography is only to be applied for the purposes mentioned above when precisely standardized conditions are maintained.

Thrombelastogram of a mixed sample

In principle, this test determines whether normal blood is capable of correcting the defective blood of a patient. The indications for its use are: *demonstration of circulating anticoagulants, circulating antithrombocyte antibodies*, and of *very severe fibrinolysis*.

Because of the possibility of ABO incompatibility and the chance of haemolysis, for which the effect on the shape of the TEG is unknown, use is made of plasma obtained by brief centrifugation (5 minutes) at about 600 r.p.m.; under these conditions the loss of thrombocytes is negligible. Plasma from the patient is prepared at the same time as plasma from a normal subject, to achieve standardization *ad hoc*.

For the mixture, 0.5 ml normal plasma and 0.5 ml patient plasma are combined.

Technique:

For each of the 3 plasmas (normal, mixed, and patient) 0.9 ml is pipetted into separate siliconized test tubes and heated for 3 minutes at 37°C. Recalcification is then performed with a pre-heated calcium chloride solution (0.1 ml 0.2 M). Successively, each of the three tubes is thoroughly shaken, and for each tube a stop-watch is started. The cuvettes are then placed in the thrombelastograph according to the above-described procedure. In immunothrombocytopenia due to sensitization by a medicament, the suspected medicament must be added (in a quantity approximating the level in the plasma of patients treated with this drug).

Interpretation:

If the thrombelastogram of a mixed sample does not diverge clearly from the normal thrombelastogram, a dangerous level of circulating anticoagulants, antithrombocyte antibodies, or severe fibrinolysis is excluded.

2.2.5. PLATELET COUNTING
(Feissly-Lüdin, modified according to Lüdin)

> When the serum shows an unexplained, high potassium- or acid-phosphatase content, thrombocytosis must be considered.

> Thrombocytopenia not only does not exclude thrombosis but may even be a symptom of it.

Solutions and reagents
Cocaine solution according to Feissly:
cocaine HCl   3.0 g
NaCl   0.2 g
Na-azide   0.1 g
Made up to 100 ml with distilled water.

Materials
— erythrocyte pipette
— Thoma counting chamber
— phase-contrast microscope
— blood-pipette shaker

Technique
Venous blood collected on EDTA is drawn into an erythrocyte pipette to the 1.0 mark and then cocaine solution is drawn up until the level reaches the 101.0 mark. The pipette is briefly shaken and then placed in the refrigerator for at least 20 minutes (to obtain haemolysis of the erythrocytes), after which it is placed in the shaker for 3 minutes. The first 2 or 3 drops are then discarded before a counting chamber is filled. Another pipette with cocaine solution is used to fill a second counting chamber serving as a blank. The first counting chamber is then placed in a petri dish provided with a piece of moist filter paper. Sedimentation of the platelets takes 30 minutes. If sedimentation is completed, the platelets all lie in the same plane and the phase-contrast microscope requires only minimal adjustment. The number of platelets in half of the chamber is determined. In moderately severe thrombocytopenia, the entire chamber should be counted; in severe thrombocytopenia, reasonably reliable results can only be obtained by several counts in 10 times less diluted blood prepared with use of a leucocyte pipette.

Calculation

When half a chamber is counted, the number obtained is multiplied by 2,000, since the blood is diluted 100 times and the counted area of the chamber is 20 times smaller than 1 µl. When a larger surface is counted (or a lower dilution is used), the multiplication factor is varied accordingly.

Normal values

1.5 to 3.5 $\times$ 10^5/ µl blood

Sources of error

The counting of thrombocytes, both with the light microscope and the electronic counter, is incomparably more difficult than leucocyte counting. Erroneous counts are therefore not exceptional. Consequently, the result obtained must be checked to see whether it is constistent with the other findings, i.e. the 24-hour value of the ESR, the blood smear, the bleeding time, the clot retraction, and the thrombelastographic results.

Three known sources of error are:

- Faulty technique in the collection of capillary blood: when the blood from the skin puncture does not flow freely and the first few drops are not collected, a false low value is often found because the thrombocyte content of the blood decreases rather rapidly (*in vivo* adhesion and aggregation).
- Faulty evaluation of nuclear remnants from the haemolysed erythrocytes (Howell-Jolly bodies, which in patients without the spleen often reach numbers of 100,000 to 200,000/ µl).
- Contaminations or infections (e.g. with fungi) in the stock solution used for dilution can lead to false high values; this can only be avoided by counting of the blank.

Interpretation

a. Thrombocytopenia:

- Degree:
  mild   – 50,000 to   150,000/ µl
  moderate – 10,000 to   50,000/ µl
  severe   – < 10,000/ µl

– Cause:

increased degradation: toxic, immunological, intravascular coagulation, etc.

simple loss: appreciable bleeding, especially when followed by transfusion of stored blood and plasma expanders.

continuous trapping: in the spleen (the normal spleen contains 30 per cent of the thrombocyte pool); in splenomegaly this value increases considerably.

transient trapping: e.g. after injection of animal proteins, including factor VIII preparations of animal origin.

b. Thrombocytosis and thrombocythaemia:

Under thrombocytosis is usually understood a reactive increase in the number of thrombocytes. Six to 10 days after an operation, childbirth, trauma, etc., the number often rises to 500,000, probably at least partially as a reaction to acute loss of blood, although chronic bleeding also leads to a similar increase, sometimes even to counts of more than 1 million. In many chronic infectious diseases, auto-immune diseases, and malignant neoplasms, numbers up to 1 million can be found. Another well-known form is the (sometimes permanent) thrombocytosis occurring after splenectomy.

Under thrombocythaemia is usually understood a myeloproliferative increase in the number of thrombocytes such as is seen idiopathically or as symptom in leucaemia, myelofibrosis, etc. The possibility of pathological forms must be kept in mind.

Remarks

Counting of thrombocytes in plasma after sedimentation of red cells gives excessively high values, even after correction for the haematocrit, because the thrombocytes from the plasma present between erythrocytes are 'pushed' upward into the supernatant plasma; the plasma between the erythrocytes is thus cleared of thrombocytes.

LITERATURE

1. Feissly, R., H. Lüdin, Microscopie par contraste de phases; applications a l'hématologie. Rev. d'Hémat. 4, 481 (1949).
2. Lüdin, H., Das Phasenkontrastverfahren in der Hämatologie. Acta Haemat. 7, 342 (1952).

2.2.6. HAEMATOCRIT MEASUREMENT

Materials
- Hawksley haematocrit centrifuge.
- Hawksley's plain tubes (without heparin Cat. no A804; manufacturer: Hawksley & Sons Ltd, Peter Road, Lancing, Sussex, Great-Britain).

Technique
The tubes are filled with EDTA blood, heat-sealed without overheating, which would cause haemolysis, and centrifuged for 5 minutes. The height of the red-cell column is read in relation to the total column.

Warning
For coagulation analysis, when haematocrit values of > 65 are obtained the test should be repeated in a fresh sample of citrated blood taken as 0.1 ml citrate 0.55 M + 9.9 ml fresh blood.

2.2.7.*a*. RECALCIFICATION-TIME

> Observation of the behaviour of the blood clot one and three hours after recalcification gives additional information about platelet function, fibrinolytic activity, haematocrit, and the colour and protein composition of the serum.

Principle
Determination of the intrinsic coagulability of decalcified blood or plasma kept under contact-free conditions, is made by measuring the coagulation time of the blood after recalcification.

Materials
- $CaCl_2$ solution: 0.033 M and 0.2 M.
- test tubes: round-bottom glass tubes of 54×11 mm (supplied by Depex, de Bilt, The Netherlands).
- mixing apparatus (Fa. Dijkstra, Geldersekade 20, Amsterdam).

Procedure
The determination is done at 37°C in two glass round-bottom tubes (clean as delivered by manufacturer), one to be provided with 0.05 ml 0.2 M $CaCl_2$ and 1.0 ml citrate blood sample, the other with 0.2 ml

0.033 M CaCl$_2$ and 0.2 ml citrated blood sample, according to the following procedure: The CaCl$_2$ is pipetted into the tubes which are then placed in a water-bath and warmed for a few minutes; the blood is then added without preheating, and the contents of the tube are mixed mechanically. After standing for 2 minutes, the tubes are tilted at 15-second intervals until the blood no longer flows when the tube is held in the horizontal position. The coagulation time is given in seconds. The use of two widely differing strengths of CaCl$_2$ also differing in their final concentration with respect to plasma, has a very definite purpose. The 0.2 M solution gives a much lower dilution effect than the 0.033 M solution, so that pathological circulating anticoagulants are detected more easily; the higher final concentration give greater sensitivity for the detection of clotting defects, and, in addition, the higher final concentration of Ca-ions is advantageous in the exceptional case of sampling irregularities (disproportionally large quantity of citrate solution).

Normal values

For tubes with 0.05 ml 0.2 M CaCl$_2$: 250 seconds (95% confidence limits (c.l.) : 200-300)
For tubes with 0.2 ml 0.33 M CaCl$_2$: 180 seconds (95% cl.: 135-225). These values are dependent not only on the storage time and kind of containers but also on the kind of glass; however, differences in the manner in which the tubes are tilted also effect the readings (due to differences in glass activation).

    Correction for haematocrit: a low haematocrit value gives a shorter coagulation time. This correlation is further strengthened by the frequently high factor VIII level in anaemia, which in itself causes a distinct reduction of the coagulation time.

Pathology

The coagulation time in glass tubes, which in principle should agree with the $r + k$ time in the thrombelastography, is actually about 5 to 7 times shorter. See, therefore, under Thrombelastography. The prolongation of the coagulation time accompanying a rising haematocrit value (pseudo-hypocoagulability) is seen particularly in the measurement with concentrated CaCl$_2$ (the erythrocyte mass being considered as a mechanical anticoagulant).

Remarks

The calcium chloride is placed in the glass tubes first, and only then the blood, in order to standardize contact activation of the blood-coagulation mechanism. The tubes are not cleaned prior to use, because the material used for this purpose (detergents, alkali, or acid) affects the degree of glass-activation. New tubes (as delivered by the manufacturer) give reasonably constant normal values. The coagulation times obtained in severe thrombocytopenia are sometimes appreciably prolonged, especially when there is a high fibrinogen content, because, as already discussed in connection with thrombelastography, the viscosity of the coagulating blood increases more slowly than usual (this corresponds to the high k value of the thrombelastogram).

Interpretation

With respect to the findings one and three hours after recalcification:

- The degree of retraction of the clot is dependent not only on the number and functioning of the thrombocytes but also on the haematocrit value and the fibrinogen content. (See under Clot Retraction.)
- The quantity of erythrocytes pressed out of the retracting clot is determined by the degree of retractibility, the fibrin content, and the fibrinolytic activity. A small amount of sediment indicates a high fibrinogen content and/or low fibrinolytic activity.
- Complete sedimentation of the pressed-out erythrocytes within three hours is an indication of an anomalous protein spectrum.
- The colour of the clear serum has indicative value (and can also, for instance, serve as a check that the plasma derives from a given patient, i.e. by comparison with the colour of the EDTA plasma, the serum from clotted whole blood, etc.).

Recalcification time determined in plasma

The recalcification time can be determined in plasma. Numerous modifications of the basic technique are available; e.g., the partial thromboplastin time (PTT) and the kaolin or celite activated partial thromboplastine time. The capacity for discrimination of the non-activated PTT with respect to a mild hypocoagulability (e.g. mild haemophilia) is less satisfactory than the results obtained when good contact activation is insured by the use of kaolin or celite. It has been found, however, that the kaolin-activated plasma recalcification time (i.e.

the recalcification time obtained without use of a phospholipid preparation) gives still better discrimination, but not better than the recalcification time of citrated blood with 0.033 M CaCl$_2$ (see table 1).

Table 1. Comparison of results obtained with various recalcification methods*

Recalcification methods:	normal clotting time (sec)			Discrimination**
	—2S.D.	mean	+2S.D.	
blood (1/30 M CaCl$_2$)	142	167	192	12/20
blood (1/5 M CaCl$_2$)	176	240	304	5/20
plasma + Inosithin	28	101	174	9/20
plasma + Platelin	24	74	124	9/20
plasma + Thrombofax	11	88	165	7/20
plasma + Tachostyptan	27	87	147	7/20
plasma + Inosithin + kaolin	33	66	99	11/20
plasma + Platelin + kaolin	22	47	72	8/20
plasma + Thrombofax + kaolin	32	49	66	9/20
plasma + Tachostyptan + kaolin	21	52	83	9/20
plasma + kaolin	47	72	97	12/20

* These methods were applied in 20 patients with mild coagulation defects (oral anticoagulant therapy, mild haemophilia A and B), and 20 normals. The combined results of all the techniques demonstrated 15 of the 20 patients to be anomalous (clotting time > mean normal clotting time +2S.D.).
** 12/20, for example, means that the defect could be demonstrated in 12 out of the total of 20 patients.

The advantages of partial thromboplastin times over determination of the recalcification time in blood are:
a. No correction for the erythrocyte mass is required; this advantage is only relative, however, because the citrate concentration in the plasma at higher haematocrit values can become so high that recalcification with the CaCl$_2$ solution used will no longer lead to coagulation.
The disadvantages of the determination in plasma are:
a. An additional procedure is required (centrifugation).
b. Greater expense is involved in the use of commercial phospholipid preparations.

Technique for kaolin-activated plasma recalcification time
Intact citrated blood is centrifuged for 10 minutes at 3,000 r.p.m. The supernatant plasma is then pipetted off, 0.1 ml being brought into a glass tube and 0.1 ml of the kaolin suspension (5 mg/ml Michaelis buffer) added to it. After thorough mixing, incubation is carried out in a waterbath for 10 minutes at 37°C. Recalcification with 0.1 ml CaCl$_2$ 0.02 M is followed by thorough mixing, and after 30 seconds tilting is begun.

2.2.7.*b*. RECALCIFICATION TECHNIQUES FOR THE DETERMINA-
TION OF FACTORS VIII, IX, XI, AND XII

Principle
The corrective capacity of the patient's plasma is tested with respect to the prolonged recalcification time of a plasma deficient in factor VIII, IX, XI, or XII.

Apparatus
- coagulometers (according to Schnittger) (3) with fitting glass tubes (Depex, Steenstraat 85, De Bilt, The Netherlands)
- mixer (Dijkstra, Geldersekade 20, Amsterdam)
- twelve-unit gas-burner for cleaning the electrodes
- toothbrush

Reagents
- platelet-free plasma deficient in the factor to be determined (for factors VIII, IX, and XII congenitally deficient and for XI artificially deficient plasma (according to Horowitz) is used.
- normal platelet-free plasma
- patient's plasma, also free of platelets
- phospholipid (prepared according to Milstone)
- kaolin, light (BDH, Poole, Great Britain)
- CaCl$_2$ 0.033 M

Preparation of reagents
Congenitally deficient plasma (VIII, IX, or XII) blood from a patient with a severe deficiency of the relevant coagulation factor (level < 1% of normal) is collected in a siliconized glass bottle containing 60 ml 3.3% acid citrate dextrose (ACD) under continuous mixing. The blood is then

centrifuged for 30 minutes at 750 g, after which the plasma is pipetted off and centrifugation is repeated for 30 minutes at 20,000 g to free the plasma of platelets (if this were not done, the deepfreezing of plasma containing platelets would result in an indeterminable contamination with phospholipid produced by the break-up of thrombocobytes). The thrombocyte-free plasma is stored in small portions in stoppered plastic tubes at—25°C (not longer than one year).

*Artificially deficient plasma (*xi*) :* Plasma from a normal donor is collected and freed of platelets as described above. After 15 mg celite (Hyflo-Supercel, supplied by Profilta, Amsterdam) has been added per ml platelet-free plasma, the contents are shaken for 5 minutes. The celite is then removed by centrifugation (30 minutes at 20,000 g). The pH is adjusted to 7.0 with 0.1 N HCl or NaOH. The plasma is then divided over a series of 10 ml tubes and held in the water-bath at 37°C for 6 hours, after which it is ready for testing. In the test system (see below) Michaelis buffer is added instead of the plasma dilution to be tested. This buffer time must amount to at least 150 seconds. The reagent is stored in small quantities in stoppered tubes at —25°C (not longer than one year). (See: Horowitz, H. I., Assay of plasma thromboplastin antecedent (PTA) with artificially depleted normal plasma. *Blood*, 22, 35 (1963)).

N.B. Lipaemic plasma is not suitable for use in the preparation of this reagent.

Normal plasma: For the determination of the stable factors IX, XI, and XII, we use a normal plasma pool (30 donors, sex ratio 1:1, mean age 30 years), prepared within 6 hours after the first venapuncture. From each donor, 50 ml citrated blood is collected. This blood is centrifuged for 15 minutes at 1,250 g, after which supernatant plasma is pooled and again centrifuged for 30 minutes at 20,000 g, divided into small portions (e.g. 1 ml), and stored at —25°C in stoppered tubes (for not more than one year). For the factor VIII determinations, we collect 100 ml blood from 4 known donors. In the manner just described, within 2 hours of collection, a platelet-free plasma is prepared and stored in small portions at —70°C. As determined individually against

30 random donors, the 4 donors consistently used show on the average approximately 100% factor VIII activity.

Phospholipid according to Milstone:

Principle
This cephalin suspension represents the portion of human brain tissue that is insoluble in acetone and soluble in ether.

Technique
A 400 g sample of human brain is carefully freed of membranes, washed, and mixed well with 300 ml acetone. After centrifugation the acetone is removed. This procedure is repeated 6 times, always with fresh acetone. The residue is then extracted in 1.8 litres ether overnight at room temperature. The ether is poured off and evaporated over a water-bath at 35 °C. The resulting residue is washed twice, each time for 15 minutes in 900 ml acetone, and spun off, after which the residue is brought into 200 ml ether. After evaporation, any remaining ether is removed under vacuum (75 minutes). About 9.3 g of the waxy cream-coloured to brown residue is suspended in 200 ml Michaelis buffer (Potter). This suspension is then centrifuged for 20 minutes at 1,700 r.p.m. and again for 10 minutes at 2,500 r.p.m. The sediment is discarded. The supernatant fluid, which contains about 2.8 g/100 ml raw cephalin as a milk-white suspension, is distributed in small quantities over rubber-stoppered tubes and stored at —20°C. Before use, this suspension is diluted with Michaelis buffer to a final concentration of 90 mg/100 ml (i.e. about 1:30). (See: Milstone, J. H., The problem of the lipoid thromboplastins. Yale J. Biol & Med. 22, 675 (1950).

Technique
The coagulometers should be allowed to warm up for at least 15 minutes. Use siliconized glass tubes for the dilution of the plasma with Michaelis buffer, and place them on ice. The pipettes belonging to the various dilutions are placed in separate tubes behind the solutions. Take the 1:10 and 1:20 dilutions of the patient sample. Choose the dilutions of the normal plasma such that the expected times of the sample to be determined will lie within those of the normal curve. For this purpose, use the following table:

For suspected haemophilia, according to type:

severe   = 0–1% dilutions normal plasma 1:200, 1:500, 1:1000 buffer time

moderate = 1–5% dilutions normal plasma 1:100, 1:200, 1:500, 1:1000 buffer time

mild   = 5–25% dilutions normal plasma 1:20, 1:50, 1:100, 1:200 buffer time

between 25–100% dilutions normal plasma 1:10, 1:20, 1:40 buffer time

Example of dilution-sequence for test:

Normal plasma 1:20, 1:50, 1:200, buffertime	1st sample 1:10, 1:20, buffertime	2nd sample 1:10, 1:20, buffertime	normal plasma 1:20, 1:50, 1:200, buffertime

Pipette in to the 1st series:
0.1 ml reagent deficient in the factor to be determined
0.1 ml plasma dilution (in indicated sequence)

> Take phospholipid out of deep-freezer, thaw rapidly, and add immediately to the kaolin in the proper concentration (5mg/ml). Mix *very* thoroughly and add

0.1 ml phospholipid/kaolin suspension to the mixture (5 mg/ml).
Mix well and start first stop-watch. When this stop-watch reaches the 2-minute mark, the 2nd series is begun in the same way with freshly prepared phospholipid/kaolin. Two minutes after the second stop-watch has been started, commence the 3rd series.

When the stop-watch reaches 30 minutes, recalcify the 1st series with 0.1 $CaCl_2$ 0.033 M.

Immediately after the addition of calcium, mix the contents of each tube very thoroughly (avoid air-bubbles) and treat each tube separately. Start the corresponding clock on the coagulometer.

The entire 1st series is completed in this way. The electrodes must be placed in the tubes promptly. When the clocks have stopped, note the time, and after brushing the clot off with a toothbrush, burn off the electrodes. The 2nd and 3rd series are also recalcified after 30 minutes of incubation.

Calculation of the results
Make a reference curve by plotting the mean clotting times for each dilution of normal plasma on double-logarithm paper against the concentrations present in the various dilutions ($1:10 = 100\%$, $1:20 = 50\%$, $1:40 = 25\%$, etc.).

Convert the mean clotting time of the test-plasma dilutions into percentages of normal via this curve. N.B. Never extrapolate outside the experimentally determined reference curve.

Screening of one sample for the various factors
When for each coagulation factor, one coagulometer is used, the method can be used to screen for an unknown deficiency in the following way:

Substrate plasma deficient in:	factor VIII	factor IX	factor XI	factor XII
dilutions of plasma to be tested				
normal:	1:10, 1:100	1:10, 1:100	1:10, 1:100	1:40, 1:400
patient:	1:10, 1:20	1:10, 1:20	1:10, 1:20	1:40, 1:80

The lowest plasma dilution is usually $1:10$, but for factor XII it is $1:40$. This exception is made because the reference curve for factor XII only becomes rectilinear on double-log paper at dilutions below $1:40$.

Further details on these methods are to be found in: Veltkamp, J. J., E. F. Drion, E. A. Loeliger, Detection of the carrier state in hereditary coagulation disorders. I *Thrombos. Diathes. haemorrh.*: 19, 279 (1968), II *Thrombos. Diathes. haemorrh.*: 19,403 (1968).

2.2.8. THROMBOPLASTIN TIME (USUALLY CALLED PROTHROMBIN TIME)

The explanation of prolonged prothrombin times is
often provided by the Thrombotest, Normotest, and
factor v assay results.

Principle

The clotting time of plasma is determined under the influence of
tissue thromboplastin. This time is a measure of the rate at which
thrombin is formed via the extrinsic pathway of the reaction mechanism of coagulation.

Reagents

Low-spun citrated plasma.   *Note*: If the haematocrit value is strongly
elevated (70 to 80%), the concentration of the citrate in the plasma
will be so high that there will be no coagulation or only severely
retarded coagulation after recalcification with 0.033 M calcium.
Rather than using a stronger calcium solution (e.g. 0.05 M), it is
better to collect the blood sample in a smaller amount of anticoagulant
(e.g. half the quantity).

Tissue thromboplastin. Human brain thromboplastin can be easily
prepared in the laboratory as follows. An adult human brain is carefully stripped under tepid running tap water and then cut up and
blended in portions in a mixer for about 2 minutes with 1,500 ml
saline solution which has been preheated to 45°C to facilitate extraction and emulsification. The portions are recombined in a glass container. This procedure is carried out at room temperature, the temperature in the mixture being allowed to decrease slowly from 37°C to
20°C. After one hour, the mixture is centrifuged for 30 minutes at
1000 g, and the supernatant fluid (which is usually slightly reddish) is
collected. The reagent is neutralized to pH 7.35 with 0.5 N NaOH, after
which one-tenth volume of buffer is added before it is diluted to optimal strength with buffer/saline (one volume buffer to nine volumes
0.9 g per cent sodium chloride). The optimal strength is determined in
a Quick system with normal human plasma. Usually, 250 to 500 ml
buffered saline can be added to 1,000 ml of the reagent. With this
reagent, the prothrombin time of normal human plasma is 13 to 16
seconds. The reagent is stored in stoppered glass tubes at —20°C in
small amounts. During storage at —20°C, the activity remains rather

constant despite a slight change in physical characteristics: the colour
becomes greyish and small aggregates are formed.

The principle on which this method is based was first described by
P. A. Owren (A quantitative one-stage method for the assay of prothrombin. *Scand. J. clin. Lab. Invest.* 1, 81 (1949)).

Instead of human brain thromboplastin, commercial preparations
are sometimes used, but their sensitivity to disturbances of the extrinsic
system is generally distinctly lower than that of human brain thromboplastin and some of them have a pronounced insensitivity to factor VII.

Buffer: Veronal acetate buffer according to Michaelis (pH 7.4).

Sodium acetate (3H$_2$O)	11.66
Veronal sodium	17.66
Sodium chloride	20.40

made up with distilled (CO$_2$-free) water to 2,400 ml
and hydrochloric acid 0.1 N   600 ml
Check and, if necessary, adjust the pH with a few drops of 0.1 N
HCl or NaOH.

Calcium chloride: 0.033 M solution (keep in mind that some commercial
thromboplastins contain calcium).

Technique
The reaction should take place at a temperature of 37°C. A 0.1 ml
sample of the plasma to be tested is mixed with 0.1 ml pre-heated
thromboplastin and incubated for 30 seconds.

After the addition of 0.1 ml CaCl$_2$ and mechanical mixing, the
clotting time is measured either with a Kolle hook (stainless steel) or,
especially in cases of long prothrombin times, by tilting as for the
measurement of the recalcification time of citrate blood.

Remarks
Both the CaCl$_2$ solution and the thromboplastin solution are brought
into conical glass tubes and held in a water-bath at 37°C. It is imperative that the thromboplastin solution be preheated for a minimal
period of 20 minutes; it may then be used for maximally 2 hours,
after which it must be discarded.

Normal variation and accuracy of the determination
The coefficient of variation of the prothrombin time found in normals

amounts, under favourable circumstances, to about 6.5%, the experimental error to about 4%.

Test with diluted thromboplastin
In addition to the measurement of the prothrombin time with undiluted thromboplastin, prothrombin times are determined with 1:10 and 1:100 dilutions of tissue thromboplastin in buffer to exclude or demonstrate an antithromboplastin. The times for thromboplastin diluted 1:10 are 1.5 to 2 times higher than the normal value, and for the 1:100 dilution about 2 to 3 times normal. Because the characteristics of tissue thromboplastin are not very constant, however, these prolongation factors must be checked against 20 normals. When commercial preparations are used, furthermore, the correct calcium concentration must be taken into account.

Interpretation
Shortening of the prothrombin time is seen frequently during the last trimester of pregnancy, and to a lesser degree also in elderly persons. *Prolongation* of the prothrombin time may be due to a deficiency of one or more of the factors II, V, VII, and X or to a pathologically circulating anticoagulant (immune-anti-thromboplastin, PIVKA, etc.). It need hardly be said that a severe deficiency of fibrinogen (factor I) will also lead to a longer or unmeasurable prothrombin time. Pure factor II deficiency can only be measured by means of the prothrombin time when the level of factor II is < 20% of normal. For factors V, VII, and X it holds that the relation of the prothrombin time to the inverse of the coagulation-factor concentration is linear when the tissue thromboplastins used lack factor VII - and factor X like activity, but only when the (albeit limited) concentration in the substrate plasma of the factor to be determined is subtracted from all the concentrations measured.
Geigy Thrombokinase® shows an activity strongly resembling that of factor VII, and consequently the deficiency of factor VII cannot be adequately demonstrated with this commercial thromboplastin.

Interpretation of the test with diluted thromboplastin
Times more than twice normal for human brain thromboplastin in a 1:10 dilution and more than four times normal for thromboplastin in a 1:100 dilution, indicate the presence of a circulating anticoagulant (usually immune-antithromboplastin).

Determination of the activity of Factors II, VII, *and* X

> Factor VII activation *in vitro* can have serious consequences. Its cause is still unknown.

General remarks

Thrombotest and Normotest are two reagents with which the complex formed by factors II, VII, and X, can be determined. Thrombotest is especially sensitive for inhibitors, Normotest for factor VII. For the theory, findings, and interpretations relevant to this subject, the reader is referred to pages 281-389. The procedure indicated by the manufacturer must be followed.

It must be stressed that the activity of factor IX cannot be measured directly with either of these reagents. It can, however, be estimated on the basis of what is known about the turnover of the clotting factors: in cases of sudden disturbances of production, factor IX drops at a rate lying between those of factor VII and factor X ($t\frac{1}{2}$ factor VII = 6 hr; $t\frac{1}{2}$ factor IX = 20 hr; $t\frac{1}{2}$ factor X = 40 hr). In chronically depressed levels of the prothrombin complex, the activity of factor IX generally does not differ essentially from the activity found with Normotest.

Lastly, it must be kept in mind that the results of the investigation of transported blood or stored blood that has been kept for some time can be erroneously high, even when the blood has been kept under contact-free conditions, (i.e. in plastic or siliconized material). The reason for this is activation of factor VII. This holds particularly for blood that derives from women using oral contraceptives and has been held at a low temperature (e.g. 4°C).

Thrombotest dilution curve

> Thrombotest is indispensable for the rapid diagnosis of vitamin K deficiency.

Materials

- Thrombotest: 1 ampoule of 2.2 ml (for 8 determinations) $CaCl_2$: 3.2 mM.
- pooled normal plasma (see p 174)
- disposable glass test tubes: 54 × 11 mm (see page 169).

Principle

The correlation curve of clotting times found with Thrombotest (linear on the Y axis) and the respective dilutions of the plasma (linear on the X axis; $D = 1/C$; C = concentration in per cent) is a straight line.

Technique

Into each of 8 tubes, 0.25 ml Thrombotest (prepared according to manufacturer's directions) is pipetted and then preheated at 37°C for 3 minutes. The determination is started by adding to the reagent 0.05 ml of the plasma dilution to be tested. Three of the tubes are intended for the determination of dilutions of normal plasma and 5 tubes for the dilutions of the plasma to be tested. The clotting times are determined by the tilting technique.

The dilutions used for the normal plasma are 1:2, 1:6 and 1:10, to be determined simultaneously in that order.

The dilutions of the plasma to be tested (5 in all) are chosen in relation to the prolongation of the thromboplastin time (determined with human brain thromboplastin, which gives a normal time of 13 to 16 seconds) as follows:

Thromboplastin times

$\quad$ < 20 sec $\quad$: $\quad$ 1:2, 1:4, 1:6, 1:8, 1:10

$\quad$ 20–40 sec $\quad$: $\quad$ 1:2, 1:3, 1:4, 1:5, 1:6

$\quad$ > 40 sec $\quad$: mix 4 volumes of the test plasma with one volume normal plasma and determine in:

$\qquad$ 1:2, 1:3, 1:4, 1:5, 1:6 (after subtracting 20%, multiply the result by 5/4).

These dilutions are determined in the same way except that the three most diluted samples are first processed simultaneously and then the two least diluted samples.

Remarks

When the dilution curve of the normal plasma has been determined for a given batch of Thrombotest ten times, the mean of these ten values may be used as reference curve for all further work with the same batch.

Interpretation

The slope of the curve reflects the concentration of factor x in the plasma sample (Hemker, H. C., J. J. Veltkamp, E. A. Loeliger: Kinetic aspects of the interaction of blood clotting enzymes. III. Demonstration of an inhibitor of prothrombin conversion in vitamin K deficiency. *Thrombos. Diathes. haemorrh.* 19, 346 (1968)) provided the activity of the four factors of the prothrombin complex shows approximately the same decrease, as is the case in chronic hepatitis, vitamin K

deficiency, and stable oral anticoagulant treatment. So the result is
also an approximation of the activity of the other three factors of the
complex. In other words: the average activity of the factors of the
prothrombin complex can be obtained indirectly from the slope of the

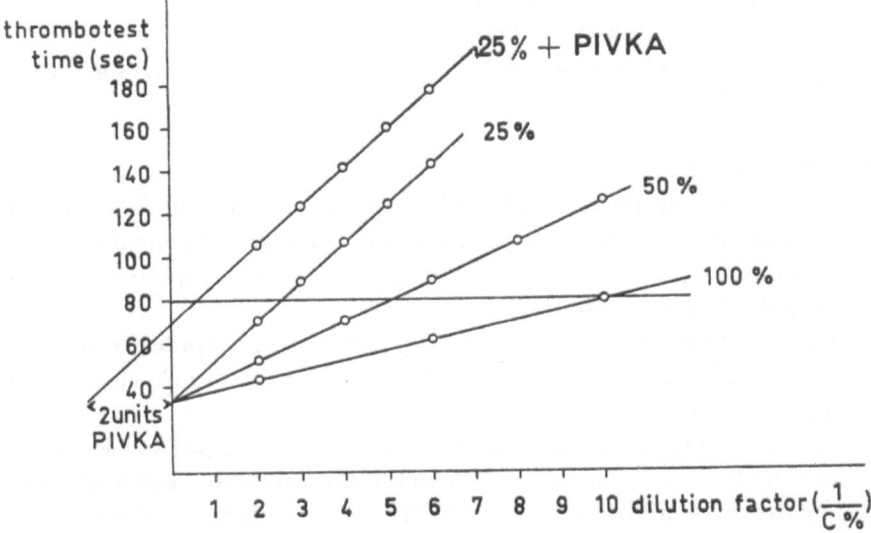

Fig. 1. Thrombotest dilution curves. To read the activity of the prothrombin complex
from the slope of a curve, a line is drawn parallel to the x-axis from the clotting time obtained with 1:10 diluted normal plasma (100 mm from the y-axis). The number of milli-
metres on this line between the y-axis and the sample-line reflects the activity (%) in the
sample, provided the sample-line cuts the y-axis at the same point as the normal-line does.
Otherwise, the procedure must be carried out after parallel displacement of the sample-line.

curve (see figure 1). This does not hold when factor (II or) VII is present
in a much lower concentration than factor X, however, because under
these circumstances the factor present in the lowest concentration is
rate-limiting in the clotting reaction.

The amount of PIVKA present in plasma can be estimated by
measuring the parallel displacement of a sample line when the level of
the factors of the prothrombin complex is below 50 per cent and when
it may reasonably be assumed that the four factors have decreased by
roughly the same amount (chronic hepatitis, prolonged vitamin K
deficiency).

Determination of Factor V

> The severity of an acute hepatitis can be determined
> with the greatest certainty from the activity of fac-
> tor v.

Reagents
- Thromboplastin (pre-heated at 37°C for at least 20 min).
- CaCl$_2$ 0.033 M (pre-heated to 37°C).
- Factor v reagent (human plasma artificially deficient in factor v).
- Normal plasma (stored at —70° or —20°C).

Preparation of factor v-deficient reagent
a. 225 ml human blood is collected in a sterile bottle containing 25 ml
   sodium citrate. After thorough mixing, the blood is centrifuged for
   1 hour at 750 g. The supernatant plasma is then pipetted off and
   centrifuged for 30 minutes at 20,000 g.
b. 1 mg of partly purified Russell's viper venom (2 ampules Stypven®)
   are mixed with 100 ml diluted phospholipid (stock suspension
   diluted 1:10; see page 175).

Equal volumes of plasma and the mixture of phospholipid and Russell's
viper venom are combined, and the pH of this mixture is brought up to
8.5 by dropwise addition of 1 N NaOH. The resulting fluid is divided
over a number of glass tubes (about 10 ml per tube) and sealed off with
Parafilm® before being incubated for about 2 hours at 37°C. After 2
hours, the thromboplastin time of the mixture is determined to see
whether it is already longer than 60 seconds. If not, incubation is
continued until this time has been reached. The pH is then adjusted to
7.3 with 1 N HCl. After rechecking the buffer time, the reagent is
divided over a set of glass or plastic tubes in volumes of slightly more
than 1 ml and the reagent is stored at —20°C. (See: Borchgrevink,
C. F., J. G. Pool, H. Stormorken, A new assay for factor v (proaccelerin-
accelerin) using Russell's viper venom. *J. Lab. clin. Med.* 55, 625 (1960)).

Principle
Measurement of the capacity of a test plasma to correct the prolonged
thromboplastin time of a plasma deficient in factor v. For this purpose,
the test plasma is mixed with the factor V-deficient plasma and the
thromboplastin time of the mixture is determined and compared with
the clotting times obtained by the addition of a known amount of
factor v (dilutions of normal plasma).

Technique

In preparation for the determinations and for purposes of quantification, the following dilutions of the test and normal plasma are made:

test plasma – 1:10 and 1:20
normal plasma – 1:10, 1:20, 1:40, and 1:80.

With each of these dilutions, the following determinations are done:
Bring successively into glass tubes placed in a water-bath at 37°C:

0.1 ml factor v-poor reagent (room temperature)
0.1 ml diluted test plasma (room temperature)
0.1 ml thromboplastin (37°C)

Incubate this mixture for 30 seconds at 37°C.
Start the reaction with:

0.1 ml $CaCl_2$

The measurement of the clotting time is done as described for the thromboplastin time (page 178).

Calculation

The four times obtained with normal plasma are plotted (double – logarithmic paper) on the y axis against 100% (1:10), 50% (1:20), 25% (1:40), and 12.5% (1:80) on the x axis. The best-fitting line is drawn through the four points, and the times obtained for the test plasma can now be converted, on the basis of this standard correlation curve, into percentage factor v activity (percentages > 100% and < 12.5% may be read from the extrapolated part of the line provided the deviations are small, otherwise the 1:5 and 1:160 dilutions of normal plasma must also be tested).

Accuracy of the results

The accuracy is estimated at about 20 per cent (expressed as coefficient of variation).

Remarks

The factor v activity of normal pooled plasma must be corrected with respect to that of normal individuals. At —70°C, factor v remains stable for some months; at —20°C there may be a gradual decrease of activity. Factor v is labile, and must therefore be determined within

6 hours after venapuncture. Degradation is more rapid in oxalate plasma than in citrate plasma, and in EDTA plasma it is so rapid that this plasma is unsuitable for factor v determinations. In hepatitis a factor v content of less than 10 per cent is a very bad sign; an increase of factor v amounting to more that 150 per cent indicates that the hepatitis is cholostatic.

2.2.9. FIBRINOGEN DETERMINATION (ACCORDING TO CLAUSS)

> Fibrinogen has little importance for haemostasis but is probably important as an antithrombotic.

> Rapid determination of the biological activity of fibrinogen is much more useful to the clinician than exact information about the quantity of circulating fibrinogen.

Principle

Measurement of the rate of fibrinogen → fibrin conversion under the influence of an excess of thrombin. Since under these conditions the fibrinogen content is rate-limiting, the clotting time can be used as a measure of the quantity of fibrinogen.

Reagents

Thrombin solution of 60 N.I.H. Units (National Institute of Health) per ml buffer (e.g. Thrombin Roche, Basel, Switzerland). The solution is held at —25 °C in small portions (glass tubes with rubber stoppers), but stocks must not be held for more than 3 months.

For use at 37 °C, thaw until the contents are almost melted and then hold at room temperature. Unused thawed solution must be discarded after 20 minutes. To test the activity of the thrombin solution, it is sufficient to add 0.2 ml of a tenfold dilution (1 volume thrombin solution and 9 volumes buffer) to 0.2 ml undiluted normal plasma, the clotting time should be 10 to 14 seconds.

Technique

The plasma to be tested is diluted 1:10 with buffer. The determination is made at 37 °C.

Into 0.1 ml plasma dilution (pre-heated for 1 minute at 37 °C) blow 0.1 ml thrombin solution and then mix in a mechanical shaker. The moment of coagulation is measured with the Kolle hook. To facilitate calculation of the fibrinogen content, the coagulation time should lie between 10 and 40 seconds. If the coagulation time is shorter than 10 seconds, the plasma is diluted further, in exceptional cases to 1:50. If the coagulation time is longer than 40 seconds, less diluted samples or undiluted plasma is used. The times are converted into mg% on the basis of a standard curve or a Table (see below). Dilutions

Conversion table for expressing clotting time as mg% fibrinogen, based on a plasma dilution of 1:10 in buffer.

Clotting time (sec)	Fibrinogen (mg%)	Clotting time (sec)	Fibrinogen (mg%)
10	500	22	225
11	450	24	208
12	410	26	190
13	380	28	178
14	352	30	165
15	330	32	155
16	310	34	146
17	290	36	140
18	275	38	132
19	260	40	125
20	250		

other than 1:10 must of course be correspondingly corrected (values expressed in mg are based on gravimetric and chemical measurements in a fibrin clot obtained from a given standard plasma). The method has been described by Clauss (Clauss, A., Gerinnungsphysiologische Schnellmethode zur Bestimmung des Fibrinogens. *Acta Haemat.* 17, 237 (1957)).

Accuracy of the method
For precise determinations, the accuracy of the method lies within about 10 per cent of the measured fibrinogen value. It must be stressed once again that fibrinogen is appreciably less stable in oxalated plasma than in citrated plasma, and in EDTA plasma the coagulability of fibrinogen disappears so rapidly that it must not be used for this determination.

Normal values
Between 200 and 400 mg%. The fibrinogen content of blood increases with advancing age (pathophysiological significance?).

Influence of circulating anticoagulants
- *Heparin* (antithrombin) in therapeutic quantities has little or no disturbing effect.
- *Polymerization inhibitors* (in paraproteinaemia) and competitive inhibitors (fibrin or fibrinogen degradation products) may accompany a pronounced pseudohypofibrinogenaemia. The most extreme example of this we have seen was a case of a postpartum defibrination syndrome without bleeding complications in which the biologically determined fibrinogen was about 20 mg%, whereas the gravimetrically determined fibrinogen content was about 400 mg%. In this case the thrombelastogram and the routine clotting tests – neither of which deviated from normal – clearly demonstrated that the cause of the pseudohypofibrinogenaemia was retarded fibrin formation.
- *Hyperfibrinolysis* can still further reduce the amount of fibrinogen found *in vitro*. Therefore, when severe fibrinolysis is suspected, plasma samples must also be collected in tubes containing fibrinolysis inhibitors.

Interpretation
A low fibrinogen level may be due to:
- Inadequate production due to damaged liver parenchyma.
- Accelerated break-down due to diffuse intravascular coagulation and/or marked increase of fibrinolysis.
- After transfusion, dilution by Maxrodex® or fibrinogen-poor blood (e.g. blood used for preparation of cryoprecipitate).
- Loss by protein-losing enteropathy.
- Hereditary condition or abnormal fibrinogen molecule (fibrinogenopathy).
A high fibrinogen level is found in:
- Diseases showing tissue necrosis and severe inflammatory reactions. A strikingly high fibrinogen content is seen in acute pancreatitis, Hodgkin's disease, secondary amyloidosis, and the active stages of autoimmune diseases.
- Nephrotic syndrome.
- During substitution treatment of haemophilia A with a cryoprecipitate rich in fibrinogen.

2.2.10. THROMBIN TIME

When accompanied by a high sedimentation rate and non-icteric plasma, a spontaneous marked prolongation of the thrombin time is almost pathognomonic for paraproteinaemia.

Principle

Measurement of the rate of fibrin formation in plasma under the influence of limited quantities of thrombin.

Reagents

Thrombin (ROCHE), dissolved in distilled water, 10 N.I.H. U per ml. Quantities for immediate use are held at —20°C in rubber-stoppered glass tubes. Just before use and without allowing it to become too warm, the solution is thawed and part of it diluted 1:1 with distilled water to obtain an additional solution of 5 U per ml.

Technique

The procedure is performed at 37°C. To a tube containing 0.2 ml citrated plasma (pre-heated for 1 minute in a water-bath) add 0.05 ml thrombin solution (not pre-heated) and mix mechanically. The coagulation time is measured with a Kolle hook. In the same way, repeat the determination with the thrombin solution of 5 U per ml.

Normal values

For 10 U per ml: 13 ± 2 seconds.
For 5 U per ml: 24 ± 3 seconds.

Interpretation

Shortening of the thrombin time indicates increased coagulability of fibrinogen or possibly a deficiency of antithrombin III.

Prolongation of the thrombin time occurs in the following forms:

a. Congenital: reduced coagulability of fibrinogen (fibrinogenopathy).

b. Acquired: due to heparin, which means that a heparin contamination must always be kept in mind when taking a blood sample.

c. Due to endogenous circulating anticoagulants:
    - marked elevation of fibrinogen level;
    - marked elevation of gammaglobulin level, either reactive (antithrombin V) or neoplastic (especially in Kahler's disease, in which the paraprotein interferes with the polymerization of the fibrin monomers: antithrombin VI effect);

- degradation products of fibrinogen and fibrin (partially competing with thrombin and partially working, like paraproteins, as
  polymerization inhibitors);
- heparin-like (dialysable?) anticoagulants occurring in Weil's
  disease and in extensive diffuse liver metastases;
- aspecific: in uraemia and hyperbilirubinaemia.

Heparin titration

> To neutralize heparin *in vivo*, only protamine chlo-
> ride should be used.

Principle

The quantity of heparin present in the circulation is estimated on the
basis of the quantity of protamine sulfate necessary to normalize the
thrombin time.

Reagents

a. protamine sulfate or protamine chloride solution (ampoules for
   therapeutic use, usually containing 10 mg per ml).
b. thrombin solution, 10 N.I.H. U per ml distilled water (see page
   189).
c. Michaelis buffer, pH 7.4 (see page 179).

The protamine sulfate solution is diluted with buffer 1:50, 1:100, 1:200,
1:300 and 1:400 (the 1:50 dilution thus contains 0.2 mg protamine
sulfate or protamine chloride per ml).

Technique

The thrombin time is determined after adding 0.05 ml diluted protamine to the 0.2 ml plasma. See further under Determination of the
Thrombin Time (page 189). The procedure should be started with the
1:400 protamine sulfate dilution.

Interpretation

The dilution of protamine sulfate giving a clotting time of just under
30 seconds is used for the calculation of the heparin concentration.
In cases of diffuse intravascular coagulation with circulating degradation products of fibrin or fibrinogen or in cases of hyperbilirubinaemia
and uraemia, etc., in which the thrombin time even without heparin
may be longer than 30 seconds, the neutralization point is reached

Protamine sulfate dilution giving thrombin time < 30 seconds	Amount of protamine chloride required to neutralize heparin (in mg/kg body wt.)
1:400	0.25
1:300	0.33
1:200	0.5
1:100	1
1:50	2

when the protamine sulfate solution gives a distinct and appreciable shortening of the thrombin time and not *per se* a thrombin time just under 30 seconds.

Remarks

The test should of course only be done when a reasonable amount of heparin is present, i.e. when the thrombin time is distinctly longer than 60 seconds.

2.2.11. UREA SOLUBILITY TEST

Solutions and reagents
- 0.05 M $CaCl_2$.
- 5 M urea solution stored in aliquots of 3 ml in the deep-freezer (—20°C).

Technique

To 0.3 ml undiluted citrated plasma, add 0.1 ml 0.05 M $CaCl_2$. After thorough shaking, this mixture must stand for at least 30 minutes at 37°C to give a solid clot. Carefully detach the clot from the wall of the tube and add 3 ml of freshly thawed urea solution. Hold this mixture at room temperature for 24 hours before checking to see whether the clot has dissolved.

Interpretation

If the clot has dissolved, there is a severe deficiency of the so-called fibrin stabilizing factor (factor XIII) (See: Duckert, F., E. Jung, D. H. Shmerling, A hitherto undescribed congenital haemorrhagic diathesis, probably due to fibrin stabilizing factor deficiency. *Thrombos. Diathes. haemorrh.* 5, 179 (1960).)

2.2.12. CLOT RETRACTION

> The clot retraction can be estimated most rapidly from observation of the plasma clot obtained in the determination of the prothrombin time, provided that the determination was made in a platelet-rich plasma.

Principle

In this test the relationship cells: serum: clot provides a basis for the calculation of clot retraction, which is dependent not only on the number and functioning of the thrombocytes but also and equally on the quantity of fibrinogen.

Technique

A conical centrifuge tube (which must be made alkaline again after cleaning with strong acid and rinsed with distilled water or cleaned with steam) containing 5 to 10 ml venous blood is placed in a water-bath at 37°C for 3 hours. The clot is then carefully transferred with a Kolle hook to a second tube, but only after a mark has been made at the serum or blood meniscus. The first tube, which now contains a quantity of erythrocytes pressed out of the clot, is centrifuged for 10 minutes at 1000 *g*. The serum meniscus and the upper level of the erythrocyte sediment are also marked on the tube. The serum is carefully examined and, if necessary, the Ouchterlony test is performed if the sample was collected on fibrinolysis inhibitors (see pages 158 and 228). The erythrocytes are then thoroughly mixed and the clot is brought back into the tube, which is then put back in the water-bath at 37°C. After 24 hours, the entire procedure is repeated. The serum is then held in the refrigerator at 4°C (for screening cryoglobulins).

Calculation

The quantities of serum pressed out of the clot after 3 and 24 hours are determined by simple subtraction of the volumes of the erythrocyte sediment, etc., which are measured as follows. The tube is emptied and rinsed, after which water from a 10 ml pipette is allowed to run into the tube, the amount of water required to reach each mark on the tube being read from the pipette.

The retraction is expressed as a percentage of the serum volume in relation to the total volume calculated with the equation:

$$\text{retraction (\%)} = \frac{\text{serum volume} \times 10{,}000}{\text{total volume} \times (100\text{-haematocrit})}$$

Normal values
After 3 hours   : 78% ± 10%
After 24 hours : 72% ± 13%

Interpretation
Low values are found in severe thrombocytopenia; the correlation between retraction and the platelet count is only moderate, however.

Strongly elevated fibrinogen levels are often accompanied by relatively low values (and *vice versa*).

In paraproteinaemia (Kahler, Waldenström) the retraction can be virtually zero, while the platelet count and bleeding time are normal and there is no distinct haemorrhagic diathesis.

In increased fibrinolysis the clot retraction as such cannot be interpreted. Two examples: a. In liver cirrhosis the retraction often seems normal despite thrombocytopenia, because the fibrinogen content is relatively low and the fibrinolytic activity is relatively high. b. In the defibrination syndrome the clot often seems to be completely dissolved within as little as one hour, but when the blood is poured from the first tube into the second, an already strongly retracted and often miniscule clot is usually found lying on the bottom of the tube.

All the points mentioned under Recalcification Time (page 169) concerning the observations in clot and serum must be taken into consideration.

2.2.13. OUCHTERLONY TECHNIQUE FOR THE QUALITATIVE DE-
TERMINATION OF FIBRINOGEN DEGRADATION PRODUCTS

Materials
- Agar Noble (Difco, Brunschwig Chemie Ltd, Keizersgracht 716, Amsterdam).
- buffered saline, pH 7.4 (to 1 litre physiological saline solution add 10 ml of an aqueous solution of 40.6 g Na_2HPO_4. $2H_2O$ + 6.4 g NaH_2PO_4. $2H_2O$ in 2 litre boiled CO_2- free distilled water).
- sodium azide: 10% solution.
- rabbit antifibrinogen serum.
- aminoblack stain:
      0.5 g   aminoblack
      50   ml distilled water
      40   ml methylalcohol
      10   ml acetic acid (concentrated).
- punch with inner diameter of 3 mm.
- hollow needle with point removed and having the same or a slightly smaller diameter than the punch.
- double-boiler.
- haematocrit tubes (see p 169).

Technique
Make a 1.0% agar solution in buffered saline. The agar dissolves only after being treated for about ½ hour in a double-boiler (provided with a condensation vent). Add 1 ml 10% sodium azide to 100 ml agar. Be sure slides are absolutely level before pipetting 2.5 ml agar onto each slide, and use a pipette with a relatively large opening. Apply agar first along the edges of the slide and wait 5 to 10 minutes for it to gelify at room temperature. Keep any slides not for immediate use at +4°C in a petri dish provided with a piece of moist filter paper. Punch holes in the following pattern:

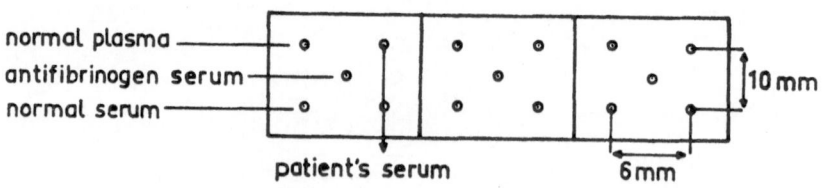

With the hollow needle to which a length of rubber tubing has been attached, the punched-out agar can easily be removed by sucking. Work on a dark background. The holes in the agar are filled exactly to the edge according to the diagram, using non-heparinized haematocrit capillaries. A new capillary should be used for each kind of material and sample. On one slide, three different sera can be tested. When all the holes are filled, keep the slides in a petri dish provided with a moist piece of filter paper for at least 12 hours and preferably for 24 hours at room temperature (absolutely level). Evaluate against dark background and with diffuse light (preferably in a viewing box). If the preparation must be kept, use the following procedure: Rinse out the punch-holes carefully with distilled water and place the prepared slides in a petri dish provided with physiological saline for 24 hours and then washing repeat twice with fresh saline (i.e. for a total of 3 periods of 24 hours). Dry in an incubator at 37°C for 12 to 14 hours, after covering loosely with a flintless filter paper. Stain with aminoblack solution (10-20 min). Rinse with tap water. If the stain has become too dark, bleach with acetic acid.

Interpretation

A positive result means that the serum of the patient contains fibrinogen or fibrin- or fibrinogen degradation products. Remnants of fibrinogen in the serum resemble degradation products and must therefore be removed before the presence of degradation products is judged (see below). It is not possible to distinguish between degradation products of fibrin or fibrinogen with this method.

Elimination of serum fibrinogen

A marked decrease in the coagulability of the blood often results in a residue of clottable fibrinogen in the serum despite the addition of the diluted thromboplastin to the fibrinolysis inhibitors. This occurs particularly in blood from patients treated with heparin or coumarin congeners, or from patients with severe haemophilia or circulating anticoagulants. In cases with a disturbed coagulation mechanism, therefore, the presence of serum fibrinogen should be checked by the addition of 0.1 ml concentrated thrombin solution to 0.1 ml serum. If a clot develops, the serum is defibrinated with 0.4 ml concentrated thrombin solution 60 U/ml to 1 ml serum; because of the dilution with thrombin, however, a weakly positive reaction to degradation products may become negative.

3. ANALYSIS OF TRANSPORTED BLOOD

Under special conditions (contact-free container, rapid transport) and flawless collection of the blood, coagulation determinations can be done reliably in samples shipped to the laboratory.

The proper procedure for collecting blood must be followed rigorously. Therefore, detailed instruction sheets and packaged kits must be available to send to any physician with a patient whose blood requires analysis.

Contents of the kit:
2 disposable plastic syringes (5 ml)
4 disposable needles (19 gauge)
2 ampoules (1 ml) containing sodium citrate (3.2%)
2 polystyrol crystal tubes with cap (empty)
1 polystyrol crystal tube (with cap) containing a pinch of EDTA
1 conical glass tube with rubber stopper
1 request form
1 instruction sheet

An example of an instruction sheet is given on page 197

SHIPMENT OF BLOOD SAMPLES FOR ANALYSIS OF THE
COAGULATION MECHANISM

1. The results of coagulation tests can only be reliable when the
   blood is obtained by flawless venapuncture, is collected in
   plastic test tubes and thoroughly mixed with the citrate
   solution, and does not take more than 6 hours to reach the
   laboratory.
2. First, fill the disposable syringe from the kit with 0.5 ml citrate
   solution (2.3% or 0.1 M; ampoule). Perform the venapuncture with another of the disposable needles. Draw the blood
   up to the 5 ml mark (i.e. 0.5 ml citrate + 4.5 ml blood).
   Leave the needle in place (see under 3). Mix the blood and
   citrate by letting some air into the syringe and tilting the
   syringe back and forth. Transfer the contents of the syringe to
   the plastic tube intended for citrated blood (work cautiously:
   plastic syringes are often difficult to handle). If the first
   attempt is unsuccessful, the spare set can be used.
3. As soon as the citrated blood has been collected, detach the
   syringe from the needle, allow about 5 ml of blood to flow into
   the conical glass tube and then collect 2 ml blood in the tube
   intended for EDTA blood. Withdraw the needle and cover the
   puncture.
4. Fill in the attached form (see p. 202 here).
5. Address shipment clearly.
6. Ship in a way guaranteed to have the sample reach the
   laboratory within 6 hours.

4. ACCURACY OF THE RESULTS

The validity of a given determination is dependent on: 1) variations within the individual, 2) the quality of the venapuncture and the length of time the blood is held, and 3) the experimental error.

Three crucial points must be kept in mind:
- The collection of blood suitable for clotting tests demands great skill and accuracy.
- The accuracy of a determination is to a high degree dependent on the skill and conscientiousness of the technician.
- Every deviational finding should be confirmed by repetition of the test.

The bleeding-time determination is the least accurate (variation coefficient about 25%). The whole-blood clotting time, whether measured by thrombelastography or the recalcification method, also has a large error (variation coefficient about 10%), and therefore each thrombelastogram must be done at least in duplicate and the recalcification time must be determined with two calcium concentrations. The most exact test is the prothrombin time, but even this still shows a variation coefficient of about 5% when applied routinely in daily practice. It is known that short clotting times cannot be measured with a greater accuracy than long clotting times; the experimental error expressed as the coefficient of variation is the same for short and long times determined with the same technique. For statistical calculations, it is therefore preferable to use the logarithms of the clotting time.

When the activities of clotting factors (expressed as % of normal) are calculated from clotting times, the degree of accuracy shown in table 2, expressed as the variation coefficient of the observed activity (a), can be expected.

Table 2. Accuracy of the result of a single determination of clotting factor activities a, expressed as coefficient of variation. (Taken from Van der Meer, J., H. C. Hemker, E. A. Loeliger: Pharmacological aspects of vitamin K_1. *Thrombos. Diathes. haemorrh.* Suppl. 29, 25 (1968)).

Factor II	a	±	15%
Factor VII	a	±	20%
Factor IX	a	±	25%
Factor X	a	±	30%

The accuracy of the result is of course greater the larger the number of measurements on which it is based. This is shown extremely well by the experience acquired in the measurement of the antihaemophilic factors: with the Veltkamp method the experimental error for determinations of the activity of factor VIII or factor IX can be kept down to 6 to 8 per cent (coefficient of variation), an accuracy with which extremely good results are obtained for clinical purposes. It must never be forgotten that in addition to this experimental error there are also variations between individuals (for normal factor VIII activity, for instance, 100 ± 20%) and within each individual. Lastly, the technical quality of blood collection and the length of storage of the sample to be tested influences the accuracy of the final result.

5. FORMS USED IN THE DAILY ROUTINE OF THE LABORATORY

Three forms accompany every sample handled in the laboratory in daily routine:

Request form (figure 1)
Work form (figure 2)
Report form (figure 3)

One copy of the report form is send to the patient's physician, one copy is filed with the request form and the work form. To facilitate retrieval, the patient's name, etc, laboratory data, diagnosis, and advise given are also coded and stored on punched cards.

Haemostasis Laboratory
Request Form
(Please fill in completely)

Requested by: Date:

Patient's name: Department:
Date of birth: File number:
Address   Registration number:
City: Insured with:
Sex:
Family doctor:
Doctor's address:

Clinical data:

Indication for the analysis:
A. Blind biopsy (kidney, liver, etc.)
B. Haemorrhagic diathesis (please specify signs and symptoms)
C. Coagulation investigation as liver-function test.

Blood to be submitted to a complete analysis must be collected by the laboratory technician. In exceptional cases, when the patient cannot come to the hospital, a kit for collecting and shipping samples will be sent on request. Blood of hospitalized patients to be analysed only for fibrinogen content and/or prothrombin time may be collected by the house-staff if the following instructions are carefully followed:
With a plastic disposable syringe containing 0.5 ml sodium citrate 0.1 M (= 3.2%), collect 4.5 ml blood. After drawing some air into syringe, mix well by tilting but do not shake. Send the blood to the laboratory in the syringe (without the needle).

Fig. 1.

Haemostasis Laboratory Work Form		
Name: Sex:		Date:
Street:		Lab. no:
City:		Physician:
Date of birth:		Department:

Diagnosis:

Indication for the analysis:

Determined by:	V.P. Good/Moderate/Poor Time:

Bleeding time:	/ / /	min. sec.

Thrombelastogram: R: K: MA:	Salicylates in urine pos./neg.	Heparin neutralization:
	colour plasma: colour serum:	1:50 1:300 1:100 1:400 1:200

Haematocrit: .... %	Thrombocytes: ...... per mm³ Whole/half chamber counted	ESR

Retraction:
3 hours   24 hours
Volume of cells:
  ''   '' serum:
  ''   '' clot:
 	
       total:
 	
    %
	Recalcification time:
	/
	
	Thromboplastin time
	
	1:1 1:10 1:100
		Thrombin time:
		10U: 5U:

Fibrinolysis time: clotted at:	dissolved at:	duration .... min.

Fibrinogen: 1:10   1:20   1:30   1:40   =   mg%

Fibrinogen degradation products in serum (with inhib. + thr. pl.) pos./neg.

Factors:		Thrombotest dilution curve:		
II	%	Norm. plasma	Patient	plasma
V	%	batch no.:	Thr. test	batch no.:
VII/X	%			
VIII	%	1:2 =	1:2 =	1:2 =
IX	%	1:6 =	1:4 =	1:3 =
X	%	1:10 =	1:6 =	1:4 =
XI	%		1:8 =	1:5 =
XII	%		1:10 =	1:6 =
Normotest	%			
		Inhibitor U.		Factors: %

Sia test: pos./neg.	Urea test pos/neg

Interpretation:

Fig. 2.

Haemostasis Laboratory
Report Form

Name of patient:
Address:
Sex:
Age:

Physician: Date:
Department: Lab. no:

Clinical diagnosis:

Bleeding time (Ivy 1-4 min)   ..
Haematocrit   ..
Thrombocytes (1.5-3.5 × 10⁵/mm³)   ..
Thrombocyte morphology   ..
Retraction (60-95%)   ..
Thrombelastogram r   (15-23 min)   ..
                  k   (7-13 min)   ..
                  ma (41-53 mm)   ..
Recalcification time   ..
Thromboplastin time (Protrombin time) ..
Fibrinolysis (clot lysis time)   ..
Fibrinogen (factor I; 200-400mg%)   ..
Fibrinogen degradation products   ..

Factors:
II   (prothrombin)   ..
II/VII/X   (Thrombotest curve)   ..
II/VII/X   (Normotest)   ..
V   (proaccelerin)   ..
VII   (proconvertin)   ..
VIII   (A.H.F. A)   ..
IX   (A.H.F. B)   ..
X   (Stuart-Prower factor)   ..
XI   (P.T.A. factor)   ..
XII   (Hageman factor)   ..
XIII   (fibrin. stab. factor)   ..
Pathol. circulating anticoag.   ..
Physiol. anticoagulant (A III)   ..

CONCLUSIONS:

Fig. 3.

6. DIAGNOSIS ON THE BASIS OF THE LABORATORY FINDINGS

In combination with all the relevant anamnestic data, the results of laboratory tests can often lead to a (tentative) diagnosis. In the following discussion, the most important laboratory findings in congenital and acquired haemostatic anomalies are listed and discussed point by point in the same sequence, with only brief reference to the pathogenesis.

6.1.   *Hereditary defects of haemostasis*
6.1.1. Haemophilia and haemophilia-like conditions
6.1.2. Thrombocytopenia
6.1.3. Thrombocytopathy

6.2.   *Connatal and congenital defects of haemostasis*
6.2.1. Circulating anticoagulants
6.2.2. Thrombocytopenia, thrombocytopathy

6.3.   *Acquired disorders of haemostasis*
6.3.1. Defective production of factors
6.3.2. Increased consumption of factors
6.3.3. Circulating anticoagulants
6.3.4. Miscellaneous

6.1.   *Hereditary defects of haemostasis*
6.1.1. Haemophilia-like conditions: See table 3 (page 206)
6.1.2. Thrombocytopenia (extremely rare)
a. with eczema and increased chance of infection (Wiskott-Aldrich syndrome, sex-linked)
b. as solitary defect (autosomal)
6.1.3. Thrombocytopathy
a. Glanzmann-Naegeli disease autosomal; homozygotes are affected;
– moderate to severe haemorrhagic diathesis;
– greatly prolonged bleeding time;
– normal thrombocyte morphology, but thrombocytes not aggregated in smear;
– defective clot retraction (two forms: no retraction or retraction distinctly prolonged);
– pathological thrombelastogram (two forms: strongly or moderately reduced *ma*).

b. Soulier-Bernard syndrome: *dystrophie thrombocytaire hémorrhagipare:*
– autosomal;
– greatly prolonged bleeding time;
– moderate thrombocytopenia;
– platelets usually giant forms;
– normal aggregation;
– accelerated disaggregation;
– hyperretractility;
– normal thrombelastogram (or increased *ma*-value).

c. Hardisty-Caen syndrome (deficiency of plasma factor?):
– autosomal;
– haemorrhagic diathesis mild to moderately severe;
– distinctly prolonged bleeding time;
– normal thrombocyte morphology;
– pathological adhesion to collagen;
– normal retraction;
– normal aggregation with ADP.

6.2. Connatal and congenital defects of haemostasis
6.2.1. Circulating anticoagulants
In children of mothers with pathological circulating anticoagulants, the same anomalies are found in the child, since these anticoagulants ($7S_{20}$ gammaglobulins) pass the placenta.

6.2.2. Thrombocytopenia
Disorders of the haemostasis mechanism due to exogenous embryopathy are conceivable. We know persisting thrombocytopenia to occur in combination with other connatal anomalies, possibly with interdependence.

6.3. Acquired disorders of haemostasis
6.3.1. Defective production of clotting factors
a. Liver cirrhosis or chronic hepatitis:
– normal to (slightly) prolonged bleeding time in moderately severe thrombocytopenia (splenogenic);
– often macrocytic red cells in the smear and leucopenia;

Deficiency of	Inheritance	Genetic status	Haemorrhagic diathesis
Fibrinogen (I)	autosomal	homozygote	very mild
Prothrombin (II)	autosomal	homozygote	severe mild
Proaccelerin (V)	autosomal	homozygote	moderate
Proconvertin (VII)	autosomal	homozygote	severe
AHGA (VIII) (Haemophilia A)	sex-linked	hemizygote	severe
		hemizygote	moderate
		hemizygote	mild
		hemizygote	subhaemophilia
	autosomal	heteroz.**	mild
AHGB (IX) (Haemophilia B)	sex-linked	hemizygote	severe
		hemizygote	moderate
		hemizygote	mild
		hemizygote	subhaemophilia
Stuart-Prower factor (X)	autosomal	homozygote	severe
PTA (XI)	autosomal	homozygote	moderate to none
Hageman factor (XII)	autosomal	homozygote	none
FSF (XIII)	autosomal	homozygote	mild to moderate
Bleeding factor * (M. Rita)	autosomal	heteroz.**	mild or severe
Bleeding factor + factor VIII* (M. von Willebrand)	autosomal autosomal	heteroz.** homozygote	mild or severe moderate or severe

*diagnosis must be confirmed by transfusion experiment.

* *trait inherited as a dominant.

Thromboplastin time (human brain)		Clotting time (min)	Bleeding time	Result of specific assay
↗		∽	(↗)	fibrinogen: trace or absent
↗↗	(28/15)	↗	n	1-2 factor II
↗	(19/15)	(↗)	n	5% factor II
↗↗	(95/15)	↗	n	1% factor V
↗↗	(90/15)	n	(↗)	1% factor VII
n		60-150	n	<1% factor VIII
n		25-60	n	1-5%
n		18-25	n	5-25%
n		n	n	25-50%
n		—	n	5-25%
n		45-90	n	<1% factor IX
n		23-45	n	1-5%
n		16-23	n	5-25%
n		n	n	25-50%
↗↗		↗	n	1% factor X
n		↗	n	<1% factor XI
n		30-45	n	<0.1% factor XII
n		↗	n	<0.1% factor XIII clot urea-soluble
n		n	↗ or ↗↗	normal factor VIII activity
n		(↗)	↗ or ↗↗	8-80% factor VIII *
n		(↗)	↗↗↗	1-10% factor VIII *

Legend: n   = normal
(↗) = slightly prolonged
↗   = prolonged
↗↗ = very prolonged

- often elevated ESR, icteric plasma, and positive Sia test;
- normal to distinctly prolonged thrombin time (hypergamma-globulinaemia);
- Thrombotest and Normotest percentages usually not significantly divergent;
- prolonged prothrombin time; Thrombotest time and Normotest time show no reaction to parenterally (i.v. or s.c.) administered vitamin K_1 (except in deficiency such as seen in primary biliary cirrhosis);
- fibrinogen, depending on nature and severity of hepatic inflammation, normal to very distinctly increased in proliferative hepatitis (e.g. early stage of lupoid hepatitis) or with a concomitant disease; distinct decrease occurs only in severe cirrhosis, when the ESR may be elevated due to excessive amounts of gammaglobulin;
- often increased loss of erythrocytes from retracted clot, sometimes with complete clot lysis after 1 to 24 hours, occurring especially after difficult venapunctures or prolonged stasis (tissue activators from capillary bed of lower arm are inadequately neutralized due to deficiency of antiactivators (liver proteins)) or when the blood was collected while or after the patient underwent stress (in reaction to hyperadrenalinaemia there is a discharge of tissue activators that are inadequately counteracted, as in prolonged venous stasis).
b. Acute hepatitis and acute fatty liver occurring in intoxication (P, CCl_4, mushroom toxins, amitriptylin):
- independent of the severity of the disease, normal to moderately prolonged bleeding time and normal to moderately reduced platelet count (splenitis);
- often strikingly low ESR with severely icteric plasma;
- normal to greatly prolonged prothrombin time (no reaction to vitamin K_1);
- usually, moderately prolonged thrombin time (due, among other things, to hyperbilirubinaemia);
- fibrinogen level usually normal (slow turn-over; biological $t\frac{1}{2}$ = 100 hours);
- Thrombotest percentage (especially that determined from dilution curve) higher than Normotest percentage when there is complete failure of liver function (factor VII much lower than factor x due to rapid turn-over (biological $t\frac{1}{2}$ = 3 to 6 hours); Normotest is particularly sensitive for factor VII. Thrombotest-values under 15%

point to severe hepatic-cell necrosis and impending hepatic coma;
- factor v > 30% means a relatively good prognosis and < 10% total liver necrosis (prognosis usually fatal). Factor v activity often exceeds 100% (cholestasis).
c. Vitamin K deficiency:
- bleeding time and platelet count normal unless there is also a deficiency of other vitamins (folic acid and vitamin B_{12});
- icteric plasma in cholestasis; normal colour of plasma in vitamin K deficiency due to prolonged administration of broad-spectrum antibiotics together with intravenous feeding and in coumarin effect; colourless plasma due to iron deficiency in untreated sprue;
- distinctly to greatly prolonged prothrombin time;
- Thrombotest percentages lower than Normotest due to presence of PIVKA (see pages 183, 365);
- Thrombotest dilution curve for determination of PIVKA;
- factor v level normal to elevated (in cases of cholestasis);
- fibrinogen content also normal to increased (in infection or with necrotic tumour).

Remarks
Combined pictures are sometimes seen, i.e. vitamin K deficiency and parenchymal hepatic damage due to prolonged cholestasis (more than 1 to 2 months) and to the primary (xanthomatous) biliary cirrhosis (in which there is severe steatorrhoea, even with incomplete obstruction of the bile ducts).

6.3.2. Increased consumption
a. Diffuse intravascular coagulation:
- Fibrinogen content: reduced (with elevated initial values, the reduction is relative); values < 10 mg% cannot be measured with Clauss's method. When large quantities of fibrinogen or fibrin degradation products are present, this value is even appreciably higher (50 to 100 mg%). In apparently total afibrinogenaemia, a clot (usually small) is often found in what seems to be completely fluid blood when this blood is slowly poured into another tube; when the clot is very small, no thrombelastographic record is obtained. In concomitant hyperfibrinolysis such as is seen in amniotic-fluid embolism, a fibrin residue often cannot be found because the fibrin threads dissolve before they can be observed.

- Prothrombin time is usually only slightly prolonged (decrease in factor v).
- Recalcification time may be shortened in mild forms and always is at the onset of defibrination, due to activity of contact factors and an increase in factor VIII activity. In severe defibrination with severe deficiency of factors v and VIII and in the absence of sufficient fibrinogen, the recalcification time cannot be measured. Special attention must be given to the quality of the small clot formed at measurement of the prothrombin and recalcification times, i.e. does it show spontaneous retraction (platelet function)or does it dissolve (hyperfibrinolysis)?
- Thrombin time is prolonged $1\frac{1}{2}$ to 2 times in chronic and subacute defibrination unless the fibrinogen level (required for the measurement) is very low; individual interpretation is rather difficult, due to the somewhat variable normal value. Thrombin time is greatly prolonged or unmeasurable in acute defibrination. Here again, attention must be paid to possible dissolution of the clot.
- Degradation products of fibrinogen or fibrin are diagnostic criteria for the defibrination syndrome.
- Bleeding time is more prolonged than would be expected from the platelet count, because many of the circulating thrombocytes are 'consumed' ('serum thrombocytes'); thrombocytes are also disabled by circulating fibrin and fibrinogen degradation products;
- Fibrinolysis is increased only in severe cases.
- Colour of the plasma: *pink to burgundy-red* due to free haemoglobin in acute intravascular haemolysis (drowning in fresh water; amniotic-fluid embolism; intoxication with acetic acid *per os* or saponins *per vaginam;* drugs; snake-bite; incompatible ABO blood transfusion); *brown* due to methaemalbumin in recurrent or protracted severe intravascular haemolysis, as seen in paroxysmal nocturnal haemoglobinuria, certain forms of malaria, and thrombotic thrombocytopenic purpura; *icteric to normal* in chronic types of haemolysis.

Pathogenesis of diffuse intravascular coagulation
- Microangiopathy (severe endothelial damage): neoplastic in micrometastases; infectious in meningococcic sepsis or leptospirosis; anoxaemic in blood stasis, e.g. in haemangiomas or in shock (reanimation); immunological in fulminant allergic vasculitis, purpura

fulminans, periarteriitis nodosa, granulomatosis of Wegener (?), and haemolytic uraemic syndrome.
- Increased supply of thromboplastic substances in a normally functioning RES, such as: erythrocyte phospholipid (erythrocytin), which can as mentioned above, give the plasma a reddish brown colour; tissue thromboplastin in lung surgery or cases of cerebral damage due to skull injury; hyperpyrexia (?).
- Reduced clearing of thromboplastic substances from the placenta and amniotic fluid in a blocked RES in pregnancy: foetus mortuus; ablatio placentae; toxicosis of pregnancy; in simultaneous liver pathology such as Sheehan's syndrome (live infant and no placental injury).

Remarks
A strikingly low sedimentation rate is suggestive of the defibrination syndrome. The demonstration of degradation products in the urine is pathognomonic for rejection of a kidney transplant.

b. Deficiency of factor II (described in systemic lupus erythematosus):
Usually accompanied by circulating anticoagulants ('antithromboplastin'). Probably, an immunological complex consisting of prothrombin and an antibody is cleared by the RES, resulting in a loss of factor II.

c. Deficiency of factor x:
A rare complication of amyloidosis, probably dependent on a greatly increased selective consumption of factor x, either in the hepatic cells or elsewhere.

6.3.3. Circulating anticoagulants

a. Paraproteinaemia:
- bleeding time: can be greatly prolonged with normal platelet count (thrombocytes react poorly or not at all with collagen fibres due to coating with paraprotein; or paraprotein 'neutralizes' the bleeding factor);
- clotting time: both the thrombelastographic reaction time and the recalcification time can be slightly prolonged (because paraproteins 'encapsulate' clotting factors and thus cause an apparent clotting-factor deficiency, especially of factor VIII);
- thrombin time: often prolonged, sometimes greatly, especially in Kahler's disease (if polymerization inhibition predominates, there is

hardly any or no repercussion on the prothrombin time or the clotting time);
- clot retraction: often seriously disturbed;
- sedimentation rate: very high;
- Sia test: positive in about one-third of the cases;
- viscosity: plasma and serum give a syrupy impression; after shaking, air-bubbles rise slowly.

Remarks
The acquired syndrome of prolonged bleeding time with low factor VIII activity in paraproteinaemia is mistakenly called acquired Von Willebrand's disease; therapy with fresh plasma or cryoprecipitate has no effect.

b. Auto-immune anticoagulants (anti-tissue-thromboplastin; anti-blood-thromboplastin; anti-factor-VIII; antithrombin):
- Bleeding time: usually normal.
- Prothrombin time: normal to slightly prolonged. The prolongation sometimes becomes distinct when the clotting times are determined with 1:10 and 1:100 dilutions of thromboplastin. The anomaly is caused by anti-tissue-thromboplastin. A selective factor II deficiency may be found at the same time (it is useful to perform a selective factor II determination, because the prothrombin time only becomes distinctly longer at prothrombin levels below 20%).
- Clotting time: normal to extremely prolonged (thrombelastographic reaction time up to 120 min.); with a normal prothrombin time, anti-blood-thromboplastin or anti-phospholipid or an anticoagulant specifically against factor VIII is present. Both anti-phospholipid and anti-factor-VIII influence the result of all determinations of intrinsic clotting factors; but the two types are easily distinguished by determination of the intrinsic factors with concentrated phospholipid solutions: if addition of much phospholipid results in normal activity, an antiphospholipid is present.
- Thrombin time: slightly to greatly prolonged in the presence of circulating antithrombin, e.g. in rheumatoid arthritis.
c. Iso-immune anticoagulants:
- Present in 5 per cent of all haemophilia A cases treated with blood or blood products; exceptional in haemophilia B.

- Severe factor VIII deficiency due to the appearance of a strong anti-factor-VIII after childbirth.

d. Hetero-immune anticoagulants:
- Anti-factor VIII after treatment with animal factor VIII products resulting in a species-specific resistance. The same resistance is seen in patients whose circulation has at one time carried proteins of the same animal species as that from which factor VIII preparations are made (e.g. due to treatment with bovine thrombin foam in dentistry). This resistance may disappear after some years.
- Antithrombin appearing after treatment with animal thrombin preparations.

e. Heparin-like anticoagulants:
- Thrombin time: distinctly prolonged; can for the most part be corrected with protamine chloride. These anticoagulants occur in the terminal stages of extensive liver metastases and are occasionally seen in severe leptospirosis (Weil's disease). Probably also to be included here is the hypocoagulability sometimes seen in the terminal stages of malignant granuloma, in which a pronounced hyperfibrinogenaemia with hepatic steatosis and a moderately prolonged prothrombin time are found.

f. Anticoagulants occurring in vitamin K deficiency (PIVKA), hyperfibrinolysis, and/or the defibrination syndrome, are discussed in detail elsewhere.

6.3.4. Miscellaneous

Uraemia: terminal stages can show not only thrombocytopathy and greatly prolonged bleeding times but also a prolonged clotting time, especially when the fibrinogen content is very high.

Weil's disease:
- strongly icteric plasma;
- prothrombin time normal or prolonged by only a few seconds;
- bleeding time: often greatly prolonged;
- platelet count: normal to moderately reduced;
- clotting time: in severe cases distinctly prolonged (heparin-like anticoagulant);
- thrombin time: distinctly prolonged, partially correctable with protamine chloride;
- fibrinogen degradation products: weakly positive;

– fibrinogen content: usually above 1000 mg%.

Amyloidosis:
– fibrinogen content: often greatly increased;
– prothrombin time: in rare cases greatly prolonged by selective deficiency of factor x;
  Normotest: often higher percentages are found than those obtained with Thrombotest (due to unidentified circulating anticoagulant).

7. RECOMMENDATIONS ON THE BASIS OF LABORATORY FINDINGS

For certain requests for a haemostasis investigation, the report of the results will not be complete without recommendations. The three most frequent reasons for such requests, are:

7.1. Need for biopsy, puncture, or surgery
7.2. Haemorrhagic diathesis
7.3. Thrombophilia.

7.1. *Biopsy, puncture, or surgery*

The primary criterion for the decision of whether or not a biopsy may be performed is the bleeding time according to Ivy. A bleeding time of more than 4 minutes is an absolute contra-indication for a blind biopsy. Further analysis is required only if the bleeding time is normal (inquire about use of anticoagulants and whether there is any possibility of haemophilia).

In *severely disturbed kidney function* a possible clotting disorder may be traceable to an auto-immune anticoagulant. In severe non-specific uraemia, too, clotting disorders may be present, but in such cases the bleeding time is greatly prolonged.

In *liver pathology* (especially in acute forms) the bleeding time may be normal even when there is a distinct clotting disturbance. A clotting-factor level below 30% (Thrombotest curve; Normotest) is an absolute contra-indication for biopsy.

The contra-indications for *sternum puncture* are haemophilia and a severe defibrination syndrome; in doubtful cases, therefore, a fibrinogen determination should be performed. Severe thrombocytopenia is not a contra-indication.

For *bone biopsy*, even more caution must be exercised. A prolonged bleeding time is a relative contra-indication in the evaluation of which the degree of prolongation of the bleeding time plays a role.

For *spleen puncture*, too, thrombocytopenia or thrombocytopathy with prolonged bleeding time form an absolute contra-indication, but this can also be a dangerous operation in the presence of clotting disorders such as a circulating anticoagulant in systemic lupus erythematosus, a defibrination syndrome in leucaemia, or a selective strong depression of the factor v level ($< 20\%$) in myelofibrosis (the factor v deficiency is reflected in a prolongation of the prothrombin time; a prolongation of $1\frac{1}{2}$ times for the prothrombin time determined with human brain thromboplastin means less than 20% factor v).

For *punctures in cavities* (lumbar puncture, pleural and pericardial puncture, ascites puncture, arterial puncture, etc.) performed for diagnostic purposes (thin needle), a haemostasis investigation is less urgent, but a specific anamnesis (haemophilia, anticoagulant treatment) must always be obtained.

For diagnostic punctures and biopsies in the *bronchial tree*, the same remarks hold as for the sternum puncture except that anticoagulant treatment must be considered a contra-indication.

For *operations,* the decision must be made on a differentiated basis, since each operation has its own risk of bleeding. For operations in which the result is dependent on the absence of bleeding (plastic surgery, eye operations, and less urgent vaginal plastic surgery and herniotomy), the operation should be rejected even for limited haemostatic disorders, unless the disorder can be corrected during and after the operation.

The insertion of a Scribner shunt in severe renal insufficiency requires special mention. This operation often involves substantial loss of blood, but is never contra-indicated by a uraemic haemostatic disturbance because in these cases haemodialysis is the therapy of choice.

7.2. *Haemorrhagic diathesis*
7.2.1. *General remarks*
In these cases intramuscular injections, biopsies, excision biopsies, and other surgical procedures are strictly prohibited, both in clotting disorders and thrombocytopenia or thrombocytopathy. A blood loss of 200 ml per hour from a small wound (e.g. tooth extraction) is quite usual in cases of severe haemorrhagic diathesis. This means a transfusion requirement of 12 bottles a day. Mechanical pressure on a bleeding locus (e.g. after sternum puncture or tooth extraction) may give good results. The specific therapy for haemophilia, thrombocytopenia, and vitamin K deficiency is described in detail under other headings (see index).

7.2.2. *Disorders of platelet function*
Congenital thrombocytopathy: The only effective treatment is platelet

transfusion. To prevent iso-immunization, blood transfusions should be limited as much as possible; if unavoidable, use only packed red cells, without buffy coat.

Acquired thrombocytopathy: In medicamentous thrombocytopathy, disturbances due to the drug can remain distinct for several days after the medication has been terminated (for salicylic acid the period (2 to 4 days) is markedly longer than would be expected from its other pharmacotherapeutic effects). These are usually cases of individual oversensitivity of the platelets (inborn error of metabolism?). Therefore, for severe haemorrhage a platelet transfusion is to be considered, since the sensitivity of the donor thrombocytes with respect to the medicament will be different and usually milder. In nephrotoxic (uraemic) thrombocytopathy, the transfusion of compatible platelets also has the effect of staunching bleeding.

7.2.3. Coagulation defects

Congenital coagulation defects: In cases of large blood loss, transfusion is of course indicated, preferably with fresh blood. With normal plasma the deficient clotting factor can be supplemented to a level determined primarily by the biological half-time of the factor in question. Plasma transfusion leads rather rapidly to overloading of the circulation. For vital indications, therefore, a concentrated preparation should be used (cryoprecipitate for substitution of factors I and VIII; PPSB, Prothrombal®, or four-factor concentrate for the substitution of factors II, VII, IX, and X). According to the data in the literature, plasma and if necessary blood transfusion also suffice in cases of deficiency of factors V, XI, and XIII. Cryoprecipitate is also effective in Von Willebrand's disease; like fresh plasma, it stimulates the *de novo* synthesis of factor VIII in the patient, so that in these cases appreciably smaller quantities can be used (about one-third of the quantity required for a patient with haemophilia A). After administration of a loading dose of cryoprecipitate, the treatment can therefore be continued with plasma without danger of overloading the circulation.

Note: For haemophiliacs, a circulating anticoagulant must be excluded before any major operation. During substitution treatment, the blood level attained with the administered clotting factor should be determined twice daily, not only to find out whether the desired level has been reached but also to detect the presence of an anticoagulant as early as possible.

In patients to be treated for the first time with large amounts of blood and/or plasma products, gammaglobulin prophylaxis for serum hepatitis should be considered. The usual dosage is used, the first injection being given intramuscularly during the treatment and the second injection subcutaneously 6 weeks later.

Acquired coagulation defects:

In severe liver parenchymal damage the level of the clotting factors can be held at a safe value by administration of purified prothrombin complex or by the performance of exchange transfusions (if appropriate, with the plasmapheresis technique).

In absolute vitamin K deficiency (obstructive jaundice, sprue, intravenous feeding combined with broad-spectrum antibiotics, gastrocolonic fistula, etc.) the intravenous administration of 1 mg vitamin K_1 is effective for several days. In chronic vitamin K deficiency, 1 mg vitamin K_1 should be given subcutaneously once a week. For relative (coumarin-induced) vitamin K deficiency, the administration of vitamin K_1 offers many difficulties, the object being to avoid activation of the thrombotic process. Carefully considered individual recommendations must be made; vitamin K_1 must not be prescribed for every small haemorrhage. As discussed in detail later (see page 345), the dosage is strongly dependent on the degree of hypocoagulability and on the natural production and resorption of vitamin K. In patients receiving anticoagulant therapy for atherothrombosis, the administration of vitamin K_1 involves appreciably less risk than in patients with a relatively fresh venous thrombotic process. In all cases of bleeding during anticoagulant treatment, the degree of hypocoagulability must be checked; when there is acute danger, however, a sample of citrated blood is taken (0.5 ml 3.2% sodium citrate + 4.5 blood) just before the intravenous injection of 10 mg vitamin K_1, and the determination is made afterwards. In very sick patients or cases with disturbed intestinal function (e.g. intestinal haemorrhage), vitamin K_1 is given intravenously.

Remarks

Intravenous administration of vitamin K_1 must be done very slowly, maximally 1 mg per minute, because over-sensitivity reactions manifested as dyspnoea, cyanosis, and sudden hypotension are sometimes observed.

7.2.4. Combined platelet function and clotting disorders (primary hyperfibrino-(geno)lysis and diffuse intravascular coagulation)

If the condition of the patient demands treatment, heparinization can be applied according to the following scheme:

Loading dose   : 2 mg heparin per kg body wt.
Maintenance dose : 3 mg heparin per kg body wt. daily

Warning

– The administration of heparin directly after an operation is dangerous.
– In ablatio placentae it is not necessary to administer heparin (it is sufficient to compensate for the loss of blood).

After heparinization, heavy loss of fibrinogen should be compensated for with cryoprecipitate (10 donors), and heavy loss of platelets with transfusion of freshly prepared platelets (8 donors).

Exceptional cases

– Post-operatively, hyperfibrino(geno)lysis must sometimes be assumed to have occurred during surgery, e.g. due to shock or transfusion reaction expectable as the result of leucocyte incompatibility in sensitized mothers or in polytransfused patients; the haemostatic plugs dissolve prematurely during the operation, often within 15 to 30 minutes after formation. Severe bleeding, sometimes lasting more than 24 hours, can occur in these cases. Haemostatic investigation usually shows only a somewhat prolonged prothrombin time and a somewhat low fibrinogen level. Blood transfusions should be given in required amounts.
– Amniotic fluid embolism: immediately after collection of blood for haemostatic investigation, 150 mg heparin should be injected through the same needle. In the presence of haemolysis (which can be diagnosed after a 5-minute centrifugation of the citrated blood), 2 g EACA should be administered intravenously. The further dosage of heparin and EACA should be based on the quantity of blood lost and the laboratory data.

N.B. In every delivery room, directions for the procedure to be applied in cases of amniotic fluid embolism should be displayed.

– Metastasized tumours: when there is danger of subcutaneous bleeding, heparin is given as haemostyptic for cosmetic purposes, such as the prevention of disfiguring ecchymoses and haematomas.

7.2.5. *Circulating anticoagulants*

- Paraproteinaemia: In this condition the haemorrhages occur because pathological protein causes thrombocytopathy and coagulopathy in addition to capillary congestion (overfilling of the intravascular space). Rapid improvement of the haemorrhagic diathesis is achieved by reduction of the amount of circulating paraprotein by plasmapheresis; this treatment is highly successful in macroglobulinaemia, in which the 'pool' is relatively small. Ultimately, cytostatics can have the same effect.
- Auto-immune diseases: The anti-lipoprotein anticoagulant seldom causes a severe haemorrhagic diathesis. The level can easily be reduced to acceptable values by plasmapheresis or exchange transfusion. But this is not the case for the much-feared anti-factor-VIII anticoagulant, which gives the same picture as true haemophilia; in these patients exchange transfusion must be followed by administration of a high-potency *(animal)* factor VIII preparation*. Treatment with corticosteroids and/or immuno-suppressives is indicated.
- Iso-immunization (haemophilia A): Use higher doses of cryoprecipitate or administer 10 to 20 times the usual dose of one of the animal preparations.*
- Weil's disease: The anticoagulant disappears upon (peritoneal) dialysis. Bleeding complications arising during dialysis can be restricted by platelet transfusion (indicated only when the bleeding time is extremely prolonged).

7.3. *Thrombophilia*

A predisposition to thrombosis *cannot* be demonstrated with the presently available laboratory methods in the great majority of the cases. However, the anamnesis and laboratory results may contain data that increase the chance that venous thrombosis will occur (risk factors). These are: familial predisposition, varices, thrombosis in the patient's anamnesis, obesity (diabetes), advancing age (> 40 years), immobilization, anaemia, neoplasms, and auto-immune diseases (endothelio-

---

* Can be ordered from Maws, Pharmacy Supplies Ltd., tel. New-Barnet 01-449-5555, Great Britain. After normal working hours, calls will be routed to private numbers.

pathy). Under these conditions, prophylactic anticoagulant therapy should be considered and if possible applied after surgery, in any severe sickness requiring bed rest, and after delivery.

With respect to atherothrombosis, the risk factors must include hypercholesterolaemia, hypertension, diabetes, and smoking.

Local 'thrombophilia' develops with all the artificial prostheses presently in use (Starr-Edwards artificial valve, Scribner shunt, vascular prostheses). In all such cases, long-term prophylactic anticoagulation treatment with coumarin should be given.

Thrombophilic blood dyscrasia can lead to recurrent thromboses, but is rare. Forms known at present are:

a. Thrombocytosis, thrombocythaemia, and possibly elevated platelet adhesivity (cannot yet be definitively determined).
b. Elevated factor VIII level: reactive (especially in anaemia), hyperthyroidism and hyperadrenalinaemia, and shortly after surgery. Apparently, a congenitally high factor VIII activity in the blood also occurs.
c. Deficiency of a physiological anticoagulant, e.g. antithrombin III (including a congenital deficiency of 50 per cent of normal; possibly inherited as a dominant) and fibrinogen (?).
d. Anomaly in the fibrinolytic system; deficiency of activators or increase of anti-activators (reactive?).

> If a thrombophilic blood dyscrasia is suspected (on the basis of unexplained recurrence of thrombosis and/or marked familial predisposition), laboratory investigation should be done.

If a thrombophilic blood dyscrasia is found, anticoagulation therapy should be applied until the treatment for the underlying disease takes effect (e.g. P_{32} in thrombocythaemia). Great caution must be exercised in treating thrombocythaemia with anticoagulants, because there may also be a severe haemorrhagic diathesis based on a platelet function disorder (prolonged bleeding time). In cases of hereditary thrombophilia, anticoagulant theraphy must be applied throughout the patient's life.

DEFIBRINATION SYNDROME

THE ROLE OF FIBRINOGEN AND FIBRIN
DEGRADATION PRODUCTS IN THE BLOOD

H. SCHRIJVER

Plasmatic blood coagulation and hyperfibrino(geno)lysis occur under normal circumstances *in vivo*. Under pathological conditions, however, both intravascular coagulation (called diffuse intravascular coagulation = DIC) and enhanced fibrino(geno)lysis are quite common (26, 31). Under these circumstances thrombi, cleared or formed in the microcirculation, are abolished by the fibrinolytic activity at the site of small vessels *(secondary hyperfibrino(geno)lysis)*. The first products to develop, therefore, result from the degradation of fibrin; but in acute overload of the pulmonary microcirculation, (endothelial?) tissue activator may enter the bloodstream and thus enhance the plasmatic fibrinolytic system, which may break down circulating fibrinogen. *Primary hyperfibrinogenolysis* is rare. It is occasionally observed by the surgeon in case of prostate operations and open heart surgery. Medically, primary hyperfibrinogenolysis is seen especially with cirrhosis of the liver (3). Drugs such as thrombolytic agents, nicotinic acid, and pyrogenics also induce primary fibrinogenolysis.

In secondary as well as primary fibrino(geno)lysis, immunologically indistinguishable fibrin or fibrinogen degradation products (FDP) may be found.

Intravascular coagulation and hyperfibrino(geno)lysis both lead not only to the lowering of the fibrinogen level but also to the consumption of the coagulation factors II, V, and VIII. Thrombocytopenia, however, common in intravascular coagulation, is not seen in primary hyperfibrino(geno)lysis. In practice, since pure primary hyperfibrino(geno)lysis is rare, the demonstration of FDP in the blood usually means the presence of intravascular coagulation. FDP counteract the adhesion aggregation and viscous metamorphosis of the thrombocytes (1, 5, 16, 18, 19); in other words, there is an inadequate capillary haemostasis. Consumption coagulopathy, especially a shortage of platelets, factor V,

224

and factor VIII, enhances the severity of the haemorrhagic diathesis. Moreover, FDP inhibit thrombin (8, 21, 29, 30) and the polymerization of the fibrin monomers (13).

FDP are sometimes demonstrable in the urine (12) and this also holds for transsudates and exudates (2). Clearance most probably occurs in the reticuloendothelial system, with different speeds for breakdown products having different molecular sizes. For instance, the clearance rate of FDP having high molecular weight was assessed at a t$\frac{1}{2}$ of about 80 hours, and of those with a low molecular weight at a t$\frac{1}{2}$ of about 20 hours (11) in a woman in childbed (the normal half-life of fibrinogen is about 100 hours (10)).

DIC is a syndrome associated with many diseases (9, 17, 23, 32) and generally develops when clot-promoting (thromboplastic) substances enter the circulation, or when there is stasis of blood or, thirdly, in patients suffering from (micro-)angiopathy. Examples of clot-promoting substances entering the circulation are especially frequent in obstetrics (27), including amniotic fluid embolism, solutio placentae, intra-uterine foetal death, toxicosis, and moles. Shock and giant cell haemangioma (28) are examples of DIC due to bloodstasis. Formation of microthrombi primarily due to angiopathy is seen in fulminant gram-negative infections (7), virus infections (24), purpura fulminans (15), the haemolytic-uraemic syndrome (33), sunstroke (25), metastatic malignant carcinoma (6), melano-sarcoma (22), myeloid leucaemia (4), etc.

Only in case of amniotic fluid embolism can immediate heparin treatment possibly save a life (page 240; (14)). In cases of chronic DIC anti-coagulants are given in order to prevent excessive bleeding. Heparin is preferable to coumarin preparations, because heparin inhibits thrombin formation more completely. Intensive coumarin treatment may also give good results, however. During treatment with heparin, the FDP disappear. Initially, the heparin is given intravenously; later, subcutaneous injections can also be used.

Epsilon-amino-caproic acid has a favourable effect only on primary hyperfibrinogenolysis; in the presence of DIC it is contra-indicated except in acute cases when it is combined with heparin (page 240). Corticosteroids block the reticulo-endothelial system and hence hinder clearance of FDP; therefore, in cases with severe haemorrhagic manifestations corticosteroids are not recommendable.

226   H. SCHRIJVER

SUMMARY

Degradation products of fibrinogen and fibrin found in the blood of
patients suffering from diffuse intravascular clotting are mainly the result of secondary hyperfibrinolysis. Primary hyperfibrinogenolysis is
seen only rarely. Pathogenesis, laboratory findings, and treatment are
briefly discussed.

REFERENCES

1. Barnhart, M. I., D. C. Cress, R. L. Henry, J. M. Riddle, Influence of fibrinogen split
   products on platelets. *Thrombos. Diathes. haemorrh.* 17, 78 (1967).
2. Benz, J. J., Clotting factors and fibrinogen split products in the extravascular space.
   Thrombos. Diathes. haemorrh. 19, 226 (1968).
3. Brodsky, I., L. H. Dennis, Evaluation of fibrinolysis in hepatic cirrhosis; relation of
   serial thrombin time and euglobulin lysis time. *Amer. J. clin. Path.* 45, 61 (1966).
4. Cooperberg, A., Acute promyelocytic leukemia. *Canad. med. Ass. J.* 97, 57 (1967).
5. Cronberg, S., Effect of fibrinolysis on adhesion and aggregation of human platelets.
   Thrombos. Diathes. haemorrh. 19, 474 (1968).
6. Dam, J. van, A. Hensen, E. A. Loeliger, C. H. W. Leeksma, Defibrinatie-syndroom behandeld met heparine. *Ned. T. Geneesk.* 109, 894 (1965).
7. Dennis, L. H., R. J. Cohen, S. H. Schachner, M. E. Conrad, Consumptive coagulopathy
   in fulminant meningococcemia. *J. Amer. med. Ass.* 205, 183 (1968).
8. Gormsen, J., B. Laursen, Fibrinogen break-down products and clotting parameters.
   Thrombos. Diathes. haemorrh. 17, 467 (1967).
9. Hardaway, R. M., Syndromes of disseminated intravascular coagulation. Charles C.
   Thomas, Springfield, Illinois (1966).
10. Hart, H. Ch., De biologische halveringstijd van 131 J-fibrinogeen. Thesis, Utrecht (1966).
11. Hemker, H. C., N. Fekkes, A. Hensen, H. Schrijver, E. A. Loeliger, *Quantitation of cir-
    culating fibrinogen breakdown products in intravascular clotting*. Diffuse Intravascular Clotting,
    F. K. Schattauer-Verlag, Stuttgart 226 (1966).
12. Herschlein, H. J., D. F. Steichele, Immunochemischer Nachweis von Fibrinogenderi-
    vaten im Urin bei Verbrauchskoagulopathien. *Thrombos. Diathes. haemorrh.* 19, 248 (1968).
13. Hirsch, J., A. P. Fletcher, S. Sherry, Effect of fibrin and fibrinogen proteolysis products
    on clot physical properties. *Amer. J. Physiol.* 209, 415 (1965).
14. Hoedt, H. Th. E., Een geval van vruchtwaterembolie, behandeld met ε-amino-capron-
    zuur. *Ned. T. v. Verlosk. en Gyn.* 62, 331 (1962).
15. Hollingsworth, J. H., D. N. Mohler, Microangiopathic hemolytic anemia caused by
    purpura fulminans. *Ann. Int. Med.* 68, 1310 (1968).
16. Jerushalmy, Z., M. B. Zucker, Some effects of fibrinogen degradation products (FDP)
    on blood platelets. *Thrombos. Diathes. haemorrh.* 15, 413 (1966).
17. Jordan, F. L. J., Diffuse intravasale stolling. *Ned. T. Geneesk.* 112, 2010 (1968).
18. Kopeć, M., A. Budzynski, J. Stachurska, Z. Wegrzynowicz, E. Kowalski, Studies on the
    mechanism of interference by fibrinogen degradation products (FDP) with the platelet
    function role of fibrinogen in the platelet atmosphere. *Thrombos. Diathes. haemorrh.* 15,
    476 (1966).
19. Larrieu, M. J., S. Inceman, V. Marder, Action des produits de dégradation du fibrino-
    gène sur les fonctions plaquettaires. *Nouv. Rev. franç. Hémat.* 7, 691 (1967).

20. Lasch, H. G., D. L. Heene, *Diagnosis of intravascular coagulation and fibrinolysis. Platelets: Their role in hemostasis and thrombosis.* F. K. Schattauer-Verlag, Stuttgart 351 (1967).
21. Lipinski, B., Z. Wegrzynowicz, A. Z. Budzynski, M. Kopeć, Z. S. Latallo, E. Kowalski, Soluble unclottable complexes formed in the presence of fibrinogen degradation products (FDP) during the fibrinogen-fibrin conversion and their potential significance in pathology. *Thrombos. Diathes. haemorrh.* 17, 65 (1967).
22. Loeliger, E. A., Fibrinogenmangel mit hämorrhagischer Diathese bei einem metastasierenden Melanom. *Schweiz. med. Wschr.* 87, 1588 (1957).
23. McKay, D. G., *Disseminated intravascular coagulation.* Hoeber Medical Division, Harper & Row, New York, (1965).
24. McKay, D. G., W. Margaretten, Disseminated intravascular coagulation in virus diseases. *Arch. Intern. Med.* 120, 129 (1967).
25. Meikle, A. W., J. R. Graybill, Fibrinolysis and hemorrhage in a fatal case of heat stroke. *New Engl. J. Med.* 276, 911 (1967).
26. Merkskey, C., A. J. Johnson, G. J. Kleiner, H. Wohl, The defibrination syndrome: clinical features and laboratory diagnosis. *Brit. J. Haemat.* 13, 528 (1967).
27. Neef, J. C., G. J. H. den Ottolander, *Coagulation disorders in obstetrics.* Proc. Dijkzigt Conf. Excerpta med., Amsterdam (1966).
28. Propp, R. P., W. B. Scharfman, Hemangioma-thrombocytopenia syndrome associated with microangiopathic hemolytic anemia. *Blood,* 28, 623 (1966).
29. Steichele, D. F., Defekte Thrombusstruktur und Hemmung der Thrombusbildung bei Defibrinierungsblutungen infolge ungerinnbarer Fibrinogenderivate. *Thrombos. Diathes. haemorrh.* 17, 543 (1967).
30. Triantaphyllopoulos, D. C., C. R. Muirhead, Formation of anticoagulants by digesting fibrin with thrombin. *Thrombos. Diathes. haemorrh.* 19, 397 (1968).
31. Verstraete, M., J. Vermylen, A. Lust, Diagnosis and treatment of disseminated intravascular coagulation. *Folia med. neerl.* 10, 164 (1967).
32. Vreeken, J., Pathologische intravasale bloedstolling. *Ned. T. Geneesk.* 109, 897 (1965).
33. Wehinger, H., H. U. Zollinger, W. Schenck, W. Künzer, Hämolytisch-urämisches Syndrom (Gasser). *Klin. Wschr.* 46, 874 (1968).

QUANTIFICATION OF SPLIT PRODUCTS

N. FEKKES

A. MANCINI TECHNIQUE (8); A SINGLE RADIAL AGAR DIFFUSION TECHNIQUE

Material
Agar Noble (Difco; see page 194)
Phosphate buffer

(pH 7.4) –	NaCl	8 g
	KCl	0.2 g
	$Na_2HPO_4.2H_2O$	1.15 g
	KH_2PO_4	0.2 g
	Distilled water	to 1000 ml.

Petri dishes (plastic), (8.5 cm in diameter (URBANTI, RHENOVA, Nieuwe 's-Gravelandseweg 72, Bussum, The Netherlands).
Microlitre syringe, 10 ml (Hamilton & Co., Whittier, Calif., U.S.A.).
Punch and needle without point (see page 193).

Procedure
Dissolve 0.8 g% agar in phosphate buffer (see above). Pipette 12 ml hot agar solution into glass centrifuge tubes, cork, and place in water bath at 56°C. When the agar solution has cooled to this temperature, add 0.1 ml anti-fibrinogen serum, mix well, and pour the contents of the tube into an absolutely level petri dish. Cover, and allow the agar to gelify. Punch holes in the agar according to the mould (page 229) and remove the punched-out agar as described in the Ouchterlony technique (page 195).

With the microlitre syringe, bring 10 μl of the material to be tested into each of the punch-holes in the agar (to obtain sharp, easily read rings, the material should be diluted to concentrations between 3 and 30 mg%. Cover the agar with liquid paraffin to prevent it from drying out, and place it absolutely level in an incubator for 48 to 72 hours. Under diffuse light, photograph the precipitation rings by placing the petri dish directly on photosensitive paper.

For measurement of the diameter of the rings, the best results are obtained with use of a stage grid.

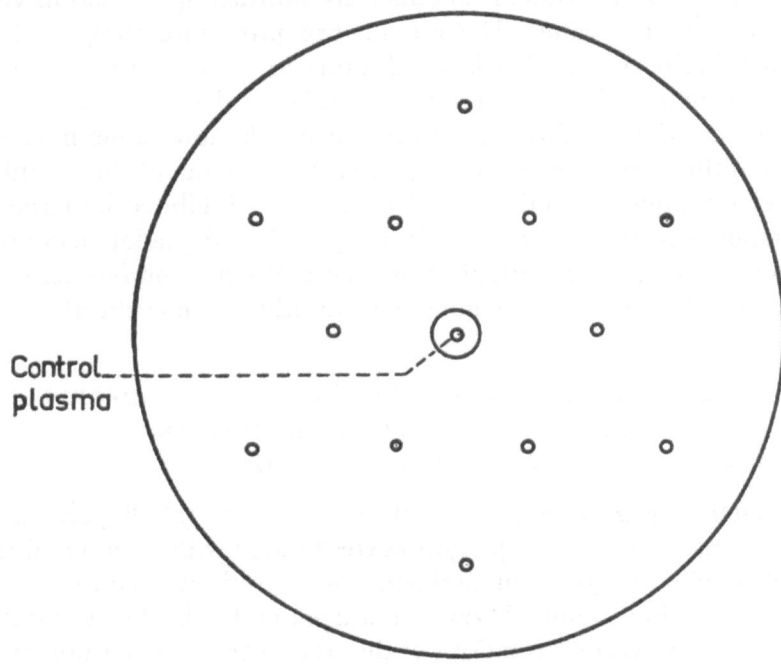

Control plasma

Interpretation

The antigen placed in the punch-holes diffuses into the surrounding agar, leading to a circular concentration gradient. At a given distance from the punch-holes, there will be an antigen concentration with a relationship to the constant antibody concentration in the agar such that precipitation occurs. The surface of the precipitation ring is directly proportional to the concentration of the applied antigen. The values can be read from a standard curve based on a dilution series of normal pooled plasma with a known fibrinogen content, the results being interpreted as corresponding to a given quantity of fibrinogen. This does not mean that the amount of degradation products may be directly equated with these values, since the size of the precipitation area is not solely dependent on the concentration of the material applied. At equal concentrations, the degradation products with smaller molecules will give a larger precipitation area than fibrinogen.

This technique can be used to determine not only the concentration of immunologically reacting degradation products in serum but also the fibrinogen concentration in plasma. In the presence of breakdown products, the latter value is obtained by subtracting the serum value from the plasma value. The gravimetric procedure (weight of the washed fibrin clot) or biochemical procedure (measurement of the nitrogen content of the washed clot) should give identical results.

The Clauss method (page 186) results in false low values in case of severe diffuse intravascular coagulation, because the fibrinogen-fibrin conversion under the influence of thrombin is inhibited by large degradation products of fibrin and fibrinogen; these degradation products seem to compete with normal fibrinogen molecules and interfere with the polymerization of fibrin monomers (antithrombin VI effect).

B. MERSKEY TECHNIQUE (7); A TANNED RED-CELL HAEMAGGLUTINATION INHIBITION IMMUNOASSAY (TRCHII) *

This method was originally described by Boyden (2). Boyden makes use of a suspension of sheep erythrocytes treated with tannin and then labelled with the relevant antigen. The sensitized erythrocytes are added only after pre-incubation on antigen and a fixed concentration of antibody to various dilutions of the test serum, to determine up to which dilution agglutination occurs. This titration method is very sensitive. The smallest measurable quantity lies between 4 and 8 micrograms/ml. For Merskey's modification of this technique, human group O erythrocytes are used. The sensitivity of the modified technique is 5 to 10 times greater than that of the Boyden method. The (as in the original TRCHII) human group O erythrocytes are tanned but not formalinized, and the procedure is performed on a blood-grouping plate. If held at +4°C, the sensitized cells can be stored for three to four weeks. The frozen cells are good for at least four months. The test can be completed within an hour, even starting with frozen cells. The smallest measurable quantity of fibrinogen or fibrin/fibrinogen degradation products is 0.2 to 0.5 micrograms/ml.

* Details of the technique have been taken from the original paper (preprint) through the courtesy of the author. Publication in the *Proc. Soc. exp. Biol.* (1969).

Materials
1. Human group O cells, preferably from blood collected in ACD solution (20 ml/3 ml). Blood collected in sodium citrate or EDTA is also suitable. The cells can be stored for several days at 4°C in ACD solution before sensitization.
2. Buffers:
    a. Phosphate-saline buffer, pH 6.4-1 volume 0.15M phosphate buffer + 1 volume normal saline.
    b. Phosphate-citrate buffer, pH 6.4-1 volume 0.15M phosphate buffer + 1 volume 0.1M sodium citrate.
3. ACD solution formula A.
4. Glycerol-citrate-glycerol USP, 5% trisodium citrate.
5. Antiserum to human fibrinogen, diluted in phosphate-citrate buffer
6. Human or bovine serum albumin.
7. Standard normal plasma-pooled normal citrated plasma containing 50 units of Trasylol*/ml, stored in aliquots at —20°C.
8. Blood grouping plate. Transparent (perspex) plates with rounded wells measuring 1.6 mm in diameter and 1.6 mm deep, were used in these studies.

Methods
a. Sensitization of cells
1. Wash cells 3 times in 20 times the volume of phosphate-saline buffer.
2. Mix equal volumes of 2% cell suspension in phosphate-saline buffer and 1:20,000 dilution of freshly prepared tannic acid in the same buffer.
3. Incubate for one hour at room temperature, stirring with a magnetic stirrer.
4. Wash cells 3 times in 20 times the volume of phosphate-citrate buffer.
5. Mix equal volumes of 4% cell suspension in phosphate-citrate buffer and 1:250 dilution of normal citrated plasma in the same buffer.
6. Incubate 1 hour at 37°C, mixing occasionally.
7. Wash cells 3 times in 20 times the volume of phosphate-citrate buffer.

* Preparation A 128 (proteinase inactivator), Farbenfabriken, Bayer, A. G., Leverkusen, Germany.

8. Before use, suspend cells at 4% concentration in phosphate-citrate buffer.

9. To prepare cells for storage at 4°C, suspend them at 4% concentration in phosphate-citrate buffer containing 0.05% human serum albumin and 0.1% sodium azide. Before use, wash once and resuspend cells in phosphate-citrate buffer.

10. To prepare cells for storage at —20°C, centrifuge 2.0 ml of a 6.5% suspension of cells in phosphate-citrate buffer and discard supernatant. At 37°C, add glycerol citrate 40% (4 volumes glycerol, 6 volumes citrate) drop by drop to the red cells (a total of 0.5 ml for each ml of original suspension), shaking after each drop is added. The cells are stored at —20°C. Remove the glycerol at 37°C after storage by adding warm glycerol citrate (30%, 20% 10%, 5%, and 2%) at 5-minute intervals in amounts equal to the total volume at that time. Centrifuge the mixture, discard the supernatant, and resuspend the cells at 4% concentration in phosphate-citrate buffer.

11. Control cells sensitized in the same way with thrombin-treated normal serum (instead of plasma) are also prepared. These should show no agglutination with the antiserum.

b. Test method

1. Determine concentration of antiserum to be used. Prepare doubling dilutions of antiserum (0.1 ml volume) on the blood-grouping plate; add 1 drop (0.025 ml) of cells. The antiserum concentration used in the test should be 2 to 3 doubling dilutions less than that causing good agglutination in 15 minutes, i.e., if a 20,000 dilution causes good agglutination, use 1:5000 in the test.

2. Prepare dilutions of standard normal plasma in phosphate-citrate buffer directly in the blood-grouping plate; doubling dilutions (0.1 ml volumes) are prepared using an automatic pipette. The dilution range should be 1:200 to at least 1:50,000.

3. Prepare similar dilutions of the test sample. The starting dilution will depend on the antigen concentration anticipated.

4. Add 1 volume of antiserum to each well; e.g. antiserum diluted 1:6000 is used.

5. Allow antibody-antigen mixture to stand 30 minutes at 4°C. Add one drop (0.025 ml) sensitized cells to each well, mix by gently rotating the blood-grouping plate, and leave at room temperature.

6. After 30 minutes, read the results. The inhibition produced by dilution of the unknown sample is compared directly with the standard curve, giving the result immediately. The antigen-antibody reaction is relatively stable after a 30-minute pre-incubation, though less time may be required. Results can be read within 15 to 30 minutes after the cells are added. If the standard curve and the unknown sample were set up at the same time, results are directly comparable 5 or 10 minutes after addition of the red cells. Changes are negligible after 30 minutes. The standard normal plasma in a 1:6400 or higher dilution usually inhibits agglutination. If this plasma contains 320 mg% fibrinogen, each dilution would represent:

$$320 \times \frac{1,000}{100} \times \frac{1}{6400} / \mu g/ml = 0.5 \ \mu g/ml$$

A similar degree of inhibition by a 1:50 dilution of an unknown sample would indicate that it contains 25 $\mu g/ml$ of fibrinogen or split products.

REFERENCES

1. Bang, N. U., Normal and abnormal fibrin polymerisation. *Thrombos. Diathes. haemorrh.* (Stuttg.) Suppl. 13, 131 (1963).
2. Boyden, S. V., The adsorption of proteins on erythrocytes treated with tannic acid and subsequent hemagglutination by antiprotein sera. *J. exp. Med.* 93, 107 (1951).
3. Clauss, A., Gerinnungsphysiologische Schnellmethode zur Bestimmung des Fibrinogens. *Acta haemat.* 17, 237 (1957).
4. Fahey, J. L., E. M. McKelvey, Quantitative Determination of Serum Immunoglobulins in Antibody-Agar plates. *J. Immunol.* 94, 84 (1965).
5. Ferreira, H. C., L. G. Murat, An immunological method for demonstrating fibrin degradation products in serum and its use in the diagnosis of fibrinolytic states. *British J. Haemat.* 9, 299 (1963).
6. Hemker, H. C., N. Fekkes, A. Hensen, E. A. Loeliger, Quantitation of circulating fibrinogen breakdown products in intravascular clotting. Diffuse intravascular clotting and peptides active in clotting and vascular function. Trans. St. Moritz Conf. (1965), *Thrombos. Diathes. haemorrh.* Suppl. 20 (1966).
7. Merskey, C., P. Lalezari, A. J. Johnson, A rapid, simple, sensitive method for measuring fibrinolytic split products in human serum. *Proc. Soc. exp. Biol.* 131, 871 (1969).
8. Mancini, S., J. P. Vaerman, A. C. Carbonara, J. F. Heremans, A single radial diffusion method for the immunological quantitation of proteins. *Protides of the Biological Fluids* Proc. 11th Colloquium Bruges (1963).
9. Ouchterlony, Ö., Antigen- Antibody Reactions in Gel. *Acta path. microbiol. Scand.* 26, 507 (1949).
10. Rümke, Ph., Personal communications.
11. Seligmann, M., V. Marder, Application des techniques immunochimiques a l'étude du fibrinogène et de ses produits de dégradation par la plasmine. *Nouv. Rev. franç. Hémat.* 5, 345 (1965).

TREATMENT OF HAEMORRHAGIC DIATHESIS

GENERAL CONSIDERATIONS CONCERNING
TREATMENT OF HAEMORRGHAIC DIATHESIS

E. A. LOELIGER

The four major defects in the haemostatic mechanism may be arranged according to the magnitude of the problem in daily practice as follows:

- vitamin K deficiency
- defective platelet function
- hereditary coagulation disorder
- diffuse intravascular clotting

Vitamin K deficiency is mostly iatrogenic, i.e. induced by coumarin congeners. In The Netherlands '*Randstad*' (the urban coastal complex stretching from Amsterdam to Rotterdam) the frequency of patients treated in order to prevent atherothrombotic recurrences amounts to about 0.5 per cent of the population. The prevalence in the elderly male population approximates 5 per cent, and the total number of patients receiving long-term anticoagulant treatment approaches 30,000. In case of effective treatment (thrombotest values 5% to 13%) the incidence of haemorrhagic complications is 1 in 10 to 15 treatment years. Hence, in the '*Randstad*' population 2,000 to 3,000 iatrogenic bleeding complications are to be expected a year. The total number of coumarin-induced haemorrhages, however, is substantially larger, because of the many patients receiving short-term treatment or pure prophylaxis. Fortunately, bleeding complications are generally not serious and, if necessary, can be easily controlled by the potent antidote of coumarin congeners, *vitamin K_1*. Bleeding is, however, only one, and probably a minor, indication of the use of vitamin K_1. Except for cases of manifest bleeding, vitamin K_1 is used much more often prophylactically, when the coagulation check reveals dangerously low hypocoagulability. An adequate individual dosage of vitamin K_1 is difficult, to determine, but can be arrived at more easily since Van der Meer clarified some important points regarding the pharmacological aspects

of vitamin K_1 in man (3). Relevant findings are presented in Chapter
IV, page 345.

The second important achievement in the field of treatment of
haemorrhagic diathesis during the last ten years is *platelet transfusion*.
Although certainly less important for general practice, it is applied in
many hospitals almost daily. Bosch has developed the technique of
transfusion in our department (1), and Eernisse has introduced the
method in the routine practice of the Leiden Blood Bank.

On the basis of Van Rood's work on histocompatibility (7), Eernisse has worked out a procedure to be followed in case of isoimmunization against platelets. Relevant information is to be found in a short
survey given on page 242.

The third and most important contribution to progress in the field of
therapeutics is the introduction of easily available coagulation factor
concentrates for *replacement therapy in haemophilia*. Because of the less
well known clinical picture and the importance of this type of treatment, and also with respect to all other coagulation factor deficiencies,
some general remarks will provide a preface to the contributions
specific to haemophilia A (page 261) and haemophilia B (page 251).

Haemophilia is the well-known sex-linked hereditary coagulation
defect. The defect on the x-chromosome results in a defective synthesis
of factor VIII or factor IX. Factor VIII deficiency is called haemophilia A
or classical haemophilia, and the deficiency of factor IX haemophilia B
or Christmas disease.

The number of haemophiliacs is still slowly increasing, because of
better life expectancy provided by improved forms of treatment. Frequency is roughly one patient in 5,000 to 10,000 persons. About four-
fifths of the patients lack factor VIII and only about one-fifth factor IX. A
double defect is extremely rare. There are, however, different types of
severity in both groups. More than half of the haemophiliacs belong to
the mild type, in which the activity of factor VIII or factor IX lies between 5 and 25 per cent of normal. These patients display, under the
conditions of normal daily stress, only minor or no signs of haemorrhagic diathesis, while in case of major trauma or surgery they often
show potentially fatal bleeding complications, similar to those known
for haemophiliacs suffering from the severe or moderate type (< 1 per
cent and 1 to 5 per cent factor activity, respectively).

In view of the incidence of haemophilia, all of us, sooner or later
will be confronted with the need for transfusion therapy in emergency

cases. The aim then will be to substitute for the lacking factor in blood, i.e. to attain and maintain a level of antihaemophilic factors sufficient for normal haemostasis and wound healing. This means a level of more than 25 per cent, and preferably 40 to 80 per cent during the first days after severe trauma. For the achievement of this goal, large amounts of coagulation factors are needed, since the disappearance rate of the transfused factor is rather high.

The two factors behave very similarly in this respect, so that the amount to be transfused in haemophilia VIII does not differ substantially from that in haemophilia B when similar levels are aimed at. The amount of coagulation factors to be transfused, expressed in terms of freshly drawn normal plasma, is 1 to 4 litres per day.

After the initial loading dose, the daily amount of coagulation factors needed to maintain a given level can be calculated, when the dose is to be given in a constant drip infusion, with the following formula:

$$H = 17 \times P \text{ (plasma volume in litres)} \times L \text{ (desired increase of level)}.$$

Table 1. Dosage scheme for adult with haemophilia A

	ml net plasma	
	haemophilia A	haemophilia B
loading dose	1500	2000
daily dose (constant drip-infusion)		
1st – 4th day	2500	1700
5th – 10th day	1400	1275
11th– 14 th day	1000	850
total dose	23,900	20,000

From table 1 it is seen that a higher dosage is proposed for haemophilia A than for haemophilia B. This difference is based on the clinical experience that safe haemostasis in haemophilia A may possibly require higher coagulation factor levels. The reason for this may be that in haemophilia A only a single coagulation factor is transfused, whereas in haemophilia B not only factor IX but the whole complex, which includes factors II, VII, and X, is transfused; and the increase of activity of factor X (often up to 2-3 times normal) may contribute substantially to the total haemostatic activity of blood. Another reason why haemophilia A generally needs more intensive substitution may be the presence of an inactive factor VIII molecule (defective production) present in the circulation of almost all haemophilia A patients that (competitively) inhibits thrombin formation; such a defective molecule is only rarely found in haemophilia B (6).

With regard to factor VIII concentrates, the practical problem has been solved since cryoprecipitate fraction from freshly prepared citrated human plasma proved to be satisfactory in almost all respects (4). No circulatory overload need be feared, even when the level of factor VIII in patients must be maintained at between 50 and 100 per cent of normal for as long as 10 days. Nor will there be a fibrinogen overload, which may limit the use of the formerly applied fraction I according to Cohn, or of fraction I-O according to Blombäck (5). The preparation of cryoprecipitate is so easy that it can be executed by all hospitals and centres with blood-processing facilities. In The Netherlands, besides the Central Laboratory of the Red Cross Blood Transfusion Service at least ten other centres are producing many thousands of cryoprecipitates annually.

For factor IX concentrates, the problem of substitution has also been solved. Since 1962 it has been possible to prepare factor IX concentrates that are highly suitable for clinical use (2). We think that the procedure recently developed by Bruning will make production possible at many centres involved in blood processing.

The preparation for surgical treatment in the haemophiliac, especially of type A, includes a thorough search for a circulating anticoagulant. Only a high potency factor VIII concentrate can break through the barrier of these anticoagulants. Such preparations containing factor VIII concentrated 500 to 1000 times in protein basis will soon be available.

As the last and fourth acquisition, *heparin treatment in diffuse intravascular clotting* should be mentioned, although the indications are relatively rare (see pages 220, 224) and have scarcely any bearing on general practice. In our hospital we do not encounter this problem more than once a month. The goal of heparin administration is the arrestation of increased intravascular consumption of platelets and clotting factors in order to restore normality. An increase of the haemorrhagic diathesis present in patients with diffuse intravascular clotting must be avoided. Clinical experience has shown that this goal can be achieved under the condition of painstaking coagulation control, preferably by means of thrombelastography, until the normal haemostatic homeostasis has been attained. The following scheme may be useful in practice:

Loading dose (intravenous; 5 min)	2 mg (=200 I.U.) per kg body weight
Maintenance dose (constant intravenous drip-infusion)	3 mg (= 300 I.U.) per kg body weight per day
Optimal prolongation of coagulation time	$1\frac{1}{2} — 2\frac{1}{2}$ times the normal value

In case of overt haemorrhagic complications with severe blood loss, heparin has to be infused at a much higher rate than in cases without blood loss; the most striking example of this is amniotic fluid embolism, where the blood loss can easily amount to 1 to 2 litres per hour and the heparin dosage required may reach values of 40 mg per hour (12 mg/kg per day). Moreover, heparin treatment, after a safe therapeutic haemo-static level has been achieved, should preferably be combined with cryoprecipitate infusion (a single dose prepared from 10 donors) and platelet transfusion (a single dose prepared from 8 donors).

As the final remark in this introduction to the presentation of more detailed information, it must be stressed that none of the so-called hae-mostyptic drugs, which are often so fervently propagated by the pro-ducers, has ever proven to be of any real help, either prophylactically or in case of emergency, with the exception of *antifibrinolytics*. Indications for these drugs, however, are rare: major operations in patients dis-playing leucocyte isoimmunization or chronic hepatitis and/or liver cirrhosis are the only indications we consider of importance, because the intrinsic fibrinolytic activity may dangerously increase after an antigen-antibody reaction and in case of insufficient clearing of fibri-nolysis activators (relased from tissues) by the liver. The benefit ob-tained by administration of antifibrinolytic drugs in prostatectomy, though statistically proven is only of minor practical importance and may be accompanied by an increase of thrombo-embolic complica-tions. And as antidote to thrombolytic agents they are not yet required and will probably not often be needed in the near future.

REFERENCES

1. Bosch, L. J., W. R. Faber, J. J. van Rood, M. Vervloet, Thrombocyten overlevingsduur en thrombocyten transfusies. *Ned. T. v. Geneesk.* 107, 2010 (1963).
2. Loeliger, E. A., A. Hensen, M. J. Mattern, J. J. Veltkamp, P. F. Bruning, H. C. Hemker, Treatment of haemophilia B with purified factor IX (PPSB). *Folia Med. Neerl.* 10, 112 (1967).
3. Meer, J. van der, H. C. Hemker, E. A. Loeliger, Pharmacological aspects of vitamin K_1. A clinical and experimental study in man. *Thrombos. Diathes. haemorrh.* Suppl. 29 (1968).
4. Meijer, K., J. G. Eernisse, J. J. Veltkamp, H. C. Hemker, E. A. Loeliger, Treatment of haemophilia A with purified factor VIII obtained from human plasma by cryoprecipitation. *Folia Med. Neerl.* 10, 49 (1967).
5. Meijer, K., *Substitutie van factor VIII bij haemophilie A. Een vergelijkende studie van fractie 1-0 en cryoprecipitaat.* Thesis, Leiden (1968).
6. Roberts, H. R., J. E. Grizzle, W. D. McLester, G. D. Penick, Genetic variants of hemophilia B: Detection by means of a specific PTC inhibitor. *J. Clin. Invest.* 47, 360 (1968).
7. Rood, J. J. van, J. G. Eernisse, The detection of transplantation antigens in leucocytes. *Seminars in Haematology*, 5, nr. 2 (1968).

PLATELET TRANSFUSION IN PATIENTS WITH PLATELET ISO-ANTIBODIES

J. G. EERNISSE

Platelet transfusion has become a routine therapy for thrombocyto-penic patients in many hospitals. In every blood bank or hospital where a sufficient number of donors can be bled, platelet concentrates can be prepared easily and the otherwise unaffected units of blood can be transfused to other patients.

The method of preparation of a platelet concentrate from fresh ACD blood taken either in bottles or in plastic bags involves two centrifu-gations (figure 1).

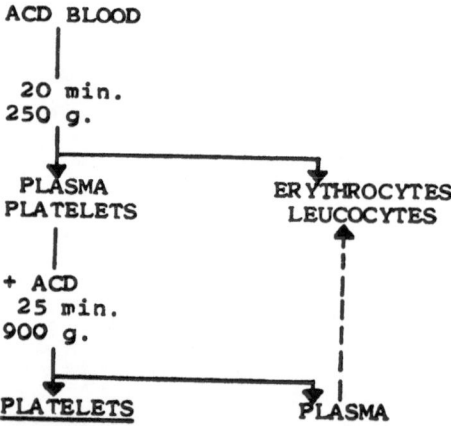

Fig. 1. The procedure for the preparation of a platelet concentrate.

Although the method works quite satisfactorily when bottles are used, there is of course the risk of contaminating their contents at the moment when needles have to be introduced in order to suck off the plasma or to return it to the red cells. Moreover, plastic bags allow a higher speed of centrifugation, which, especially in the second step, will speed up the process.

About one-fifth of the amount of ACD normally used in a bottle of blood must be added to the platelet-rich plasma in order to prevent irreversible clumping of the platelets after centrifugation (4).

The rationale for a platelet transfusion is summed up in table 1.

Table 1. Disease states in which a platelet transfusion may be helpful, and the various factors influencing the result of such a transfusion.

	Platelet transfusion
Rationale:	prophylaxis and/or treatment of bleeding tendency caused by aplastic thrombocytopenia hereditary thrombocytopathy
Determinants:	dosage blood volume spleen size iso-immunization

A few comments are necessary. Only thrombocytopenia resulting from a failure of production caused by toxins, chemotherapy, or otherwise can be remedied by platelet transfusion. Rapid breakdown of the patient's platelets, as in Werlhof's disease, will also affect the transfused platelets, and no increase in platelet numbers lasting for more than a few hours can be expected.

In thrombopathia such as the disease of Glanzmann-Naegeli, the haemorrhagic diathesis can be overcome by the transfusion of normal donor platelets, in contrast to the far more frequent cases of thrombopathia caused by paraproteinaemia. In the latter, the function of the transfused platelets will likewise be impaired by the paraproteins. Only after reduction of the amount of paraproteins by plasmapheresis or cytostatic therapy can a platelet transfusion – if still necessary at that moment – be helpful.

As is shown in table 1, the effect of a platelet transfusion depends upon a number of factors:
Dosage and blood volume taken together amount to the following: The yield of donor platelets is about 60 per cent, i.e. 75×10^9 platelets from 500 ml of blood. In a recipient with a blood volume of 5 litres, this should give a rise of the platelet count amounting to 15,000 per μl. However, recovery in the recipient is normally only about 50 per cent, resulting in a rise of only 7,500 platelets per μl (3).

The processing of 8 bottles of fresh ACD blood, which is our standard procedure for an adult patient, should be followed by a rise of the platelet count of 60,000 to 80,000 per μl. For children, smaller amounts can be given. Because of the rather short life-time of the platelets (8-10 days, Aas and Gardner), the effect of the transfusion will have disappeared after 4 to 5 days and the transfusion may then have to be repeated. Transfusion of far greater amounts of platelets will hardly be of benefit for longer than 4 to 5 days and is therefore useless.

The size of the spleen plays an important role in the recovery of transfused platelets in the circulation of the recipient. The normal recovery of about 50 per cent can be attributed entirely to the presence of a spleen of normal size. After splenectomy, recovery will be 100 per cent (3). On the other hand, in recipients with an enlarged spleen recovery will be less than 50 per cent and will be roughly proportional to the extent of enlargement of the organ. This pool of sequestered platelets, however, is constantly exchanged with the platelets in the circulation (2). The low platelet count found in most patients with an enlarged spleen has to be attributed to this same phenomenon of sequestration of an abnormally large proportion of their platelets in the spleen.

Iso-immunization poses a special problem. In most cases in which a long-term treatment with platelet concentrates is given, the patients develop iso-antibodies towards platelets, resulting in a rapid breakdown of the transfused platelets. These antibodies are probably elicited by the leucocytes present in the concentrates, and act specifically with antigens present on both leucocytes and platelets (5). Detection of these

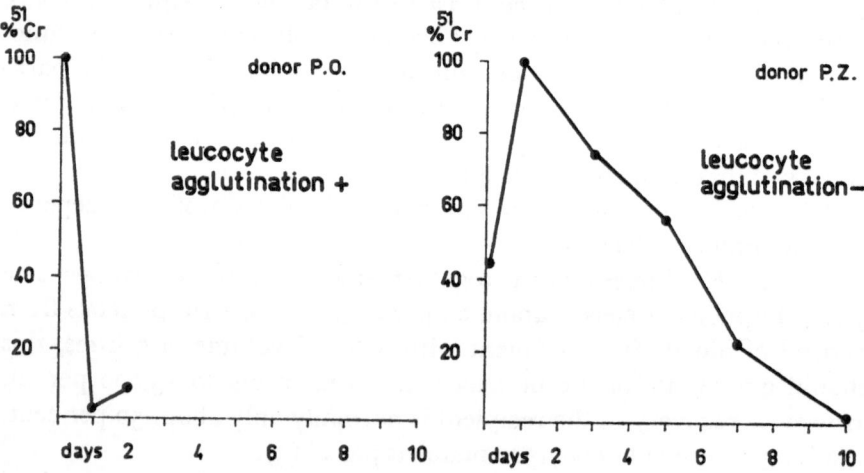

Fig. 2. Survival of ⁵¹Cr labelled platelets in a recipient with leucocyte antibodies. Positive agglutination test with leucocytes from donor P.O. and shortened survival of his platelets, negative test with donor P.Z. and normal platelet survival (Bosch).

antibodies is much easier in serologic tests with leucocytes than with platelets, and they are therefore referred to as leucocyte antibodies. Leucocyte (c.q.platelet) iso-antibodies can also be formed after blood transfusions, as well as during pregnancies in more or less the same manner as erythocyte iso-antibodies causing the haemolytic disease of the newborn.

Transfusion of platelets in which the specific antigen is lacking will just be as effective as the transfusions given before the iso-antibodies had developed. Their survival is normal, as shown in figure 2.

Compatible platelets can be found in various ways: by determining the total antigenic pattern of the leucocytes of the patient and of the possible donors (preferably brothers and sisters of the patient) and selecting those with the same pattern, or by doing cross-match tests between serum of the patient and leucocytes of the possible donors and using the platelets of those who show a negative reaction. Usually, one has to perform plasmapheresis (or rather thrombopheresis) on these donors to obtain sufficient numbers of platelets.

The possibilities and difficulties mentioned here were all encountered during the treatment of two patients.

Case I.

A 34 year old woman had been treated with chloramphenicol for chronic bronchitis, and had received 30 grams of the drug in about 4 months. After this treatment her bone-marrow became aplastic and the platelet count dropped to 5,000 – 15,000 per μl. The resulting haemorrhagic diathesis necessitated blood transfusion, and the patient was admitted to the Leiden University Hospital for further treatment with platelet transfusions. As is shown in figure 3a, the platelet count could be kept at a reasonable level by the administration of a platelet concentrate every 3 or 4 days. During this time the patient did not show any signs of the bleeding tendency. After 4 weeks the therapy was discontinued for a longer period in order to evaluate the patient's own production of platelets, which did not show any improvement: the platelet count fell to 2,000 per μl, purpura and bleeding from the mucous membranes of the nose and the gums reappeared, and transfusion of platelet concentrates had to be resumed.

After the first transfusion a reasonable rise of the platelet count was observed, but later transfusions were followed by a poor result. Very large concentrates prepared from 48 and 24 units of blood resulted in a

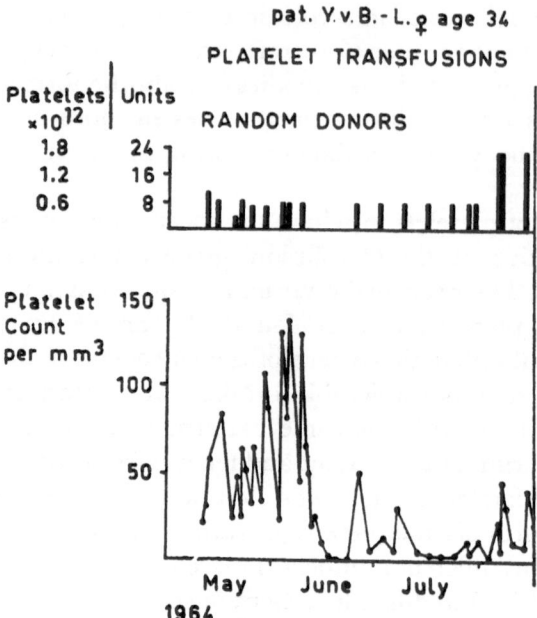

Fig. 3a. Results of repeated transfusions of platelets from unrelated donors in a patient with thrombocytopenia caused by chloramphenicol (Case 1).

rise of the platelet count comparable to that seen after a transfusion of only 5 or 6 units. It was clear that the patient had become immunized, and leucocyte antibodies with anti-8a specificity were indeed found in her serum. The test was negative with the leucocytes of her nearest relatives: father, mother, 2 brothers, and 4 sisters. The treatment with platelet concentrates was continued with these 8 relatives as donors. By plasmapheresis, two of them were bled four times in each session at weekly intervals. Results with these compatible platelets were good for another 5 weeks. Then the platelet count rose to a level to be expected after a transfusion of only 4 units. At that time, another leucocyte antibody (anti-4a) could be detected in the patient's serum. Three of the donors were 4a-negative, and with their help the treatment could be continued. In view of the possibility that in the end the patient might become immunized by and against their incompatible antigens as well, splenectomy was considered as a last resort: after splenectomy the patient's own production of platelets would be fully available to the circulation and it was hoped that the level reached would be such as to prevent bleeding. After an extra loading dose of platelets, splenectomy was performed without any complications. As can be seen from figure 3b, the platelet level reached after transfusion of the same number of platelets was significantly higher than before splenectomy. Although the platelet count dropped to between 10,000 and 20,000 per μl, the patient did not show signs of a haemorrhagic diathesis. About a year after onset, spontaneous recovery set in and the patient has since been well (figure 3c).

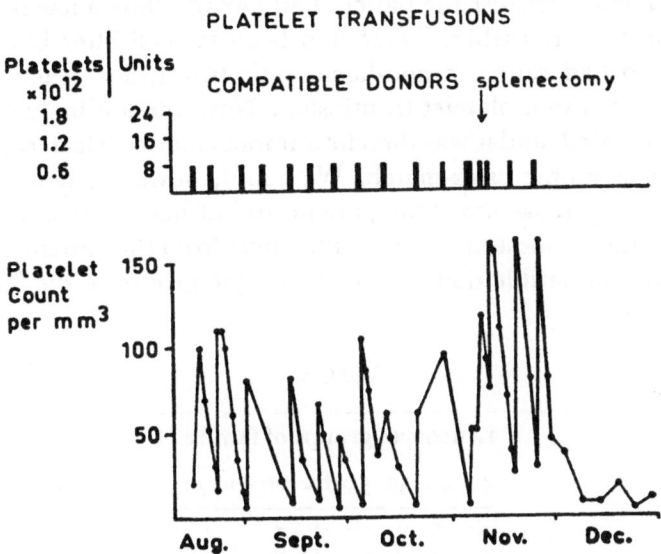

Fig. 3b. As fig. 3a, but now after transfusions of compatible platelets obtained by plasmapheresis. Donors were nearest relatives of the patient.

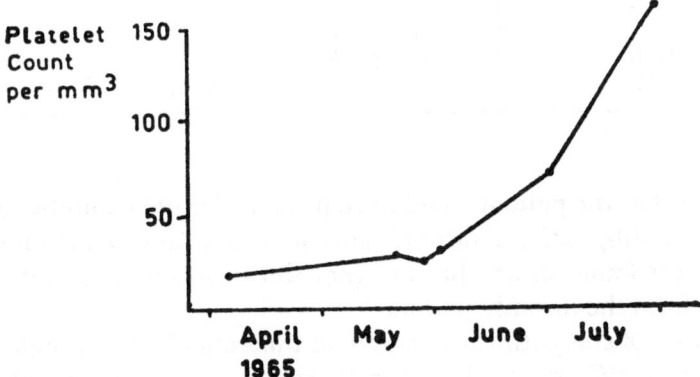

Fig. 3c. Further course in the same patient.

Case II.

A 20 year old girl with a known diagnosis of hereditary thrombocyto-
pathia (Morbus Glanzmann-Naegeli) was admitted to the Department
of Gynaecology of the Leiden University Hospital because of a rapidly
growing tumour in the lower abdominal region. An operation was clearly
indicated, but was impossible in view of the prolonged bleeding time.
This could not be reverted to normal with platelet transfusions from
random donors, because the patient had already shown leucocyte antibodies three years earlier. These had been formed after blood transfusions, and had caused a non-haemolytic transfusion reaction and a
febrile reaction to a platelet transfusion. Now the antibody could not
be demonstrated, and it was therefore impossible to select compatible
donors by a simple cross-match. We could, however, determine the
leucocyte antigen pattern of the patient and of her relatives and select
those with the smallest number of differences from the patient's pattern,
as possibly compatible donors. The leucocyte groups of the family are
shown in table 2.

Table 2.

	4a	4b	5a	5b	6a	6b	7a	7a'	7b	7c	7d	8a	9a	
	Leucocyte groups of family H.													
father	+	+	+	+	+	+	−	−	+	+	−	+	+	
mother	+	+	+	+	+	+	+	+	+	−	−	+	−	
pat. C.H.	+	+	+	+	+	−	−	−	+	+	−	+	−	
sister V.-H.	+	+	+	+	+	+	+	−	+	−	−	+	+	
sister P.-H.	+	+	−	+	+	+	+	−	+	+	−	+	+	
sister H.H.	+	+	+	+	+	−	−	−	+	−	−	+	−	
brother J.J.H.	+	+	−	+	+	−	+	+	+	−	−	+	−	cr.m.
brother J.H.	+	+	−	+	+	−	+	+	+	+	−	+	−	(+)

It is clear that the patient could have produced quite a number of antibodies: anti-6b, anti-7a, anti-7a', anti-7d and or anti-9a. An identical
pattern was found in one brother (not shown in table 3), but he also
suffered from the thrombopathia.

Selection of compatible donors could theoretically be brought about
by successive ^{51}Cr survival studies. There were, however, a number of
disadvantages to this procedure:

1. The time involved. A normal survival curve would have to be followed to the point of complete disappearance of platelet activity. Superposition of a curve of rapidly decreasing activity upon a normal one would make interpretation of the results rather difficult.

2. Immunization might be caused by the platelet survival study itself.

The other approach would have been to do a plasmapheresis on as many of the relatives in as short a period of time as possible and do the operation as soon as a good haemostasis was obtained. The latter scheme was adopted, and as the first pair the two sisters (P.-H. and V.-H.) with the greatest discrepancy in the leucocyte antigen pattern were chosen for plasmapheresis. In case of a good effect on haemostasis, differentiation between these two would be made possible by a ^{51}Cr survival study of the platelets of one of them. The result was negative: the bleeding time was unaffected and the ^{51}Cr survival time was less than 24 hours. The next day, plasmapheresis was performed with sister H.H. and brother J.H. as donors. A ^{51}Cr survival study was impossible for technical reasons. Bleeding time was clearly influenced by the platelet transfusions, and this effect was still present the next morning. It was decided to repeat the plasmapheresis with these two donors and perform the operation immediately after the transfusion.

At operation, the tumour could be removed without difficulties. Bleeding was negligible except in an area of about 3×4 cm where the tumour had adhered to the broad ligament. This area was ligated and the abdomen was closed. During the evening it became clear that the patient was still bleeding intra-abdominally, and blood transfusions had to be administered. Plasmapheresis was again performed with the brother as platelet donor. After the transfusion, bleeding time was still greatly prolonged.

Obviously, the wrong donor had been chosen and the normalization of the bleeding time had been due to the transfusion of platelets from the sister H.H. only. This sister was then used again as platelet donor for two days following the operation, and the bleeding time, although still prolonged, could be kept within reasonable limits. Addition of platelets from the mother did not contribute to this result, as shown by their very short ^{51}Cr survival time. Before the transfusion on the third post-operative day, the bleeding time was much prolonged and was hardly influenced by the platelet transfusion. The ^{51}Cr survival study did not give a clear-cut answer to the question of whether or not the sister's platelets survived normally. Since the condition of the patient was excellent, no further platelet transfusions were administered (table 3).

Table 3. Schematic representation of platelet transfusions and the resulting bleeding times in Case II.

'Plasma'-pheresis donor			Bl. time (min.)	'Plasma'-pheresis donor			Bl. time (min.)
Mon.	P.-H.	3×		Wed.	J.H.	4×	> 25
	V.-H.	3×					
		Cr⁵¹O		Thurs.	H.H.	4×	14
Tues.	H.H.	4×			mother	4×	11
	J.H.	4×	9/20	Fri.			10/12.5
Wed.			12/18		H.H.	3×	
	H.H.	2.5×			mother	3×	9/13
	J.H.	4×	8/10			Cr⁵¹O	
	Operation			Sat.			32
					H.H.	3×	19/31
Wed./Thurs. shock, 3 blood transf.						Cr⁵¹ normal?	

The history of the first patient shows that platelet transfusions from random donors can be given successfully in non-immunized patients. However, one has to expect iso-immunization, and from then on transfusion of compatible platelets is necessary. Even then, as shown by both patients, immunization may occur. If surgical treatment is indicated, this should not be postponed any longer than is strictly necessary.

REFERENCES

1. Aas, K. A., F. H. Gardner, Survival of blood platelets labelled with chromium. *J. clin. Invest.* 37, 1257 (1958).
2. Aster, R. H., J. H. Jandl, Platelet sequestration in man. *J. clin. Invest.* 43, 843 (1964).
3. Bosch, L. J., *Studies on platelet transfusion in man.* Thesis, Leiden (1965).
4. Bosch, L. J., W. R. Faber, J. J.. van Rood, M. Vervloet, Thrombocytenoverlevingsduur en thrombocytentransfusies. *Ned. T. v. Geneesk.* 107, 2010 (1963).
5. Rood, J. J. van, A. van Leeuwen, J. G. Eernisse, E. Frederiks, L. J. Bosch, Relationship of leukocyte groups to tissue transplantation compatibility. *Ann. N. Y. Acad. Sci.* 120, 285 (1964).

PURIFICATION AND CLINICAL APPLICATION OF THE FOUR FACTORS OF THE PROTHROMBIN COMPLEX

P. F. BRUNING

Purified factor IX preparations such as the French PPSB (abbreviation of *P*rothrombin, *P*roconvertine, *S*tuart factor, and anti-haemophilia *B* factor) which has been clinically applied since 1960, make it possible to perform major operations on haemophilia B patients. The table on page 253 shows the plasma concentrations of factor IX required for the prevention or treatment of severe haemorrhages in haemophilia B patients, as well as the quantities of whole plasma to be administered daily in a given case.

The scarcity of these concentrates limits their use. Because national needs were far from met by the production in France (7), England (1) and the U.S. (3, 5, 6, 8), the preparation of factor IX concentration was started in The Netherlands. In Nijmegen, the French method is being applied on a small scale (2). The Central Laboratory of the Red Cross at Amsterdam has introduced a product called the four clotting factor concentrate (9), which is prepared according to a method developed there and somewhat resembles the American method. In Leiden over the past two years we have developed a method to produce a factor IX concentrate, called Prothrombal, in the simplest possible way by a technique that can be performed by any blood-bank staff. The Amsterdam and the Leiden methods are both based on the citrated plasma remaining after cryoprecipitation, so that packed red cells, platelet suspension, albumin, and gammaglobulin are also available for clinical application without the use of special procedures.

The French method, which like the two just-mentioned procedures uses an adsorption technique, requires EDTA blood as starting material, which means that the erythrocytes and platelets cannot be administered to the patient without restriction, because of the undesirable characteristics of EDTA. Furthermore, the French method, like the Oxford me-

thod, is technically too complicated for small-scale production. Figure
I shows the simple procedure for the preparation of the Leiden factor
IX concentrate (Prothrombal) schematically. After cryoprecipitate has
been obtained from the standard donor blood, i.e. citrated blood, the

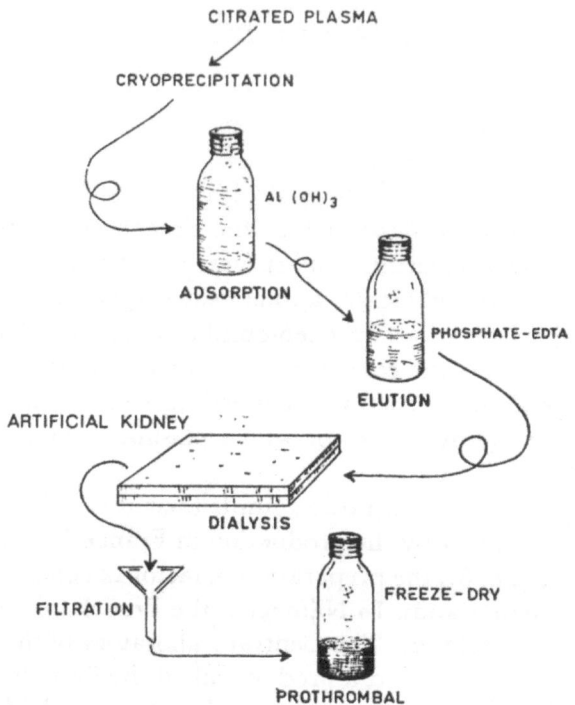

Fig. 1. Scheme of preparation of Prothrombal.

so-called prothrombin complex is removed from the plasma by adsorption to aluminum hydroxide. The aluminum hydroxide remains in
suspension for only a few minutes before it is spun off, after which the
coagulation factors are eluted with a phosphate solution to which a
small amount of EDTA is added. This EDTA serves to prevent possible
thrombin formation in the preparations by calcium ions. The phosphate
concentration is reduced to a clinically acceptable value by dialysis
with a simplified artificial kidney according to Kiil for 5 hours. After
sterilizing filtration, the preparation is freeze-dried; it is then highly
soluble. Short-lasting adsorption is essential for a good factor IX yield,
since aluminum hydroxide, in addition to adsorption promotes denaturation of coagulation factors. Strict conditions must be maintained

for the procedure to be certain of a sterile product that will be well tolerated by patients. Every batch is tested in animals as to pyrogenic, toxic, or cardiovascular effects.

Table 1

Prothrombal				
	Factor	II	VII/X	IX
in vitro yield	%	50	106	72
in vivo yield	%			approx. 20

Table 1 shows the yield obtained *in vitro* and *in vivo* (factor IX) with our method. For factor IX, there appears to be an appreciable difference between the yield obtained *in vitro* and *in vivo*, the latter having been calculated from the findings in three patients with severe haemophilia B (factor IX <1% of normal). From the preliminary experience in six patients, which demonstrated excellent tolerance and a satisfactory yield, we felt justified in asking an orthopaedic surgeon (B. van Linge, Annakliniek, Leiden) to perform a major arthrodesis operation on one of our severe haemophilia B patients (GBM 1565/86) under protection of Prothrombal for the definitive correction of a *pes equinus* which this young man had developed as the result of a haemorrhage in the *musculus gastrocnemius*. For the dosage of the preparation, which was administered as a continuous drip infusion, we based ourselves on the extensive experience accumulated between 1960 and 1968 in Leiden with the administration of the French PPSB, as shown in table 2 (4).

Table 2

Loading dose $\qquad$ $H = P \times L \times 10$
Daily required substitution dose $\qquad$ $H = 17 \times P \times L$
$\quad$ in which H = net plasma equivalent in ml
$\qquad\quad$ P = plasma volume in litres
$\qquad\quad$ L = desired rise of the blood level in per cent

the constant 17 $\quad$ is derived from $\quad \dfrac{0.693 \times 24 \times 2 \times 1000}{20 \times 100}$

in which $\;$ 0.693 = ln 2
$\qquad\quad$ 24 = duration of the infusion in hours
$\qquad\quad\;\,$ 2 = multiplication factor for calculation of the virtual distribution space of factor IX
$\qquad\;\;$ 20 = biological half-life of factor IX in hours

The results are shown in figure 2. The haemostatic effect was excellent.

Figure 2 also shows the levels of factors II, VII, and X in the patient's plasma. It must be kept in mind here that the factor IX concentrate contains not only factor IX but also the other factors of the so-called

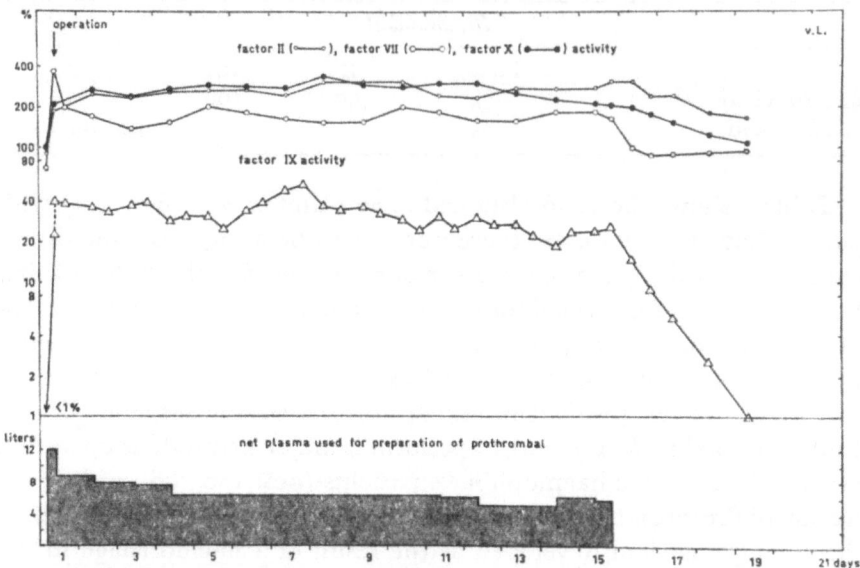

Fig. 2. Results of infusion of Prothrombal. Patient GBM 1565/68, 21 year old male, factor IX < 1 per cent of normal, plasma volume 2,9 liters; *arthrodesis* for *talipes equinus*.

prothrombin complex. The indication range for the application of this concentrate is therefore as wide as shown in table 3.

Tabel 3. *Indications for factor* II-VII-IX-X-*concentrate*

I	congenital deficiencies
II	vitamin K deficiency
	.relative (coumarin-induced)
	.real
III	liver insufficiency
	.hepatitis
	.postnatal
	.intoxication

In practice, the most important application of Prothrombal concerns the substitution treatment for severe haemorrhages in haemophilia B or vitamin K deficiency, especially that induced by coumarin derivatives. Figure 3 illustrates the latter indication. The prothrombin time determined in a 25 year old man (GBOE 1175/68) with chronic pancreatitis was about 174 seconds (normal: 14 seconds) at admission. From

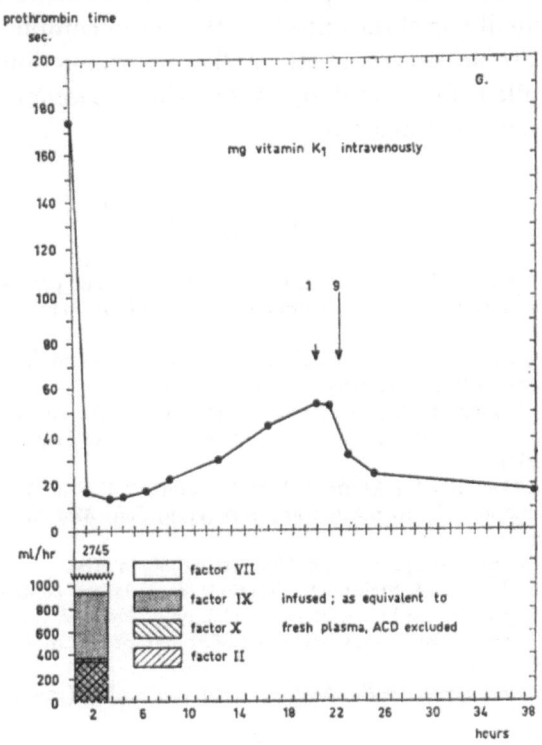

Fig. 3. Results of infusion of Prothrombal. Patient GBOE 1175/68, 25 year old male, plasma volume 2.5 liters; severe vitamin K deficiency.

figure 3 it can be seen that with a quantity of Prothrombal prepared from 3.15 net plasma, the prothrombin time can be returned to normal within minutes. Due to the rapid biological disappearance of factor VII, the effect is short-lasting. The intravenous administration of 10 mg vitamin K_1 then results again in anal – beit much slower – normalization of the prothrombin time. It is clear that in emergency cases, such as intracranial bleeding following administration of coumarin, simultaneous administration of concentrated prothrombin complex and vitamin K_1 given intravenously can provide safe haemostasis rapidly and lastingly.

Conclusions

When purified prothrombin-complex preparations are available, the prognosis *quoad vitam et sanationem* of haemophilia B patients is appreciably improved. These preparations also offer far better prospects when severe haemorrhages threaten patients with deficiencies of factors II, VII, or X individually or of the entire prothrombin complex.

A rapid and simple procedure for small-scale production of a purified preparation, called Prothrombal, is described. Dosage scheme and clinical experience are presented.

REFERENCES

1. Bidwell, E., J. M. Booth, G. W. R. Dike, K. W. E. Denson, The preparation for therapeutic use of a concentrate of factor IX, containing also factors II, VII and X. *Brit. J. Haemat.* 13, 568 (1967).
2. Haanen, C. A. M., R. L. McShine, A. Kunst, Preparation and clinical use of factor IX concentrate PPSB(according to Soulier). *Vox Sanguinis* (in press).
3. Hoag, M. S., F. F. Johnson, A. J. Robinson, P. M. Aggeler, In vivo observations with concentrates containing clotting factors II, VII, IX and X. *Proc.* XII *Congress Int. Soc. of Haemat. New York* (1968).
4. Loeliger, E. A., A. Hensen, M. J. Mattern, J. J. Veltkamp, P. F. Brunning, H. C. Hemker Treatment of haemophilia B with purified Factor IX (PPSB). *Folia Med. Neerl.* 10, 112 (1967),
5. Pert, J. H., *ibidem.*
6. Shanbrom, E., *The hemophilias*; Int. Symp. New York 1968, in press.
7. Soulier, J. P., Ch. Blatrix, M. Steinbuch, Fractions 'coagulantes' contenant les facteurs de coagulation adsorbables par le phosphate tricalcique. *Presse Méd.* 72, 1223 (1964).
8. Tullis, J. L., M. Melin, P. Juriçian, Clinical use of human prothrombin complexes; *New Engl. J. Med.* 273, 667 (1965).
9. Vreeken, J. J., *Jubileum Symposium Bloedtransfusiedienst*, Amsterdam (1968).

FOUR-CLOTTING-FACTOR CONCENTRATE

J. VREEKEN

Since the end of 1967, the clotting factors of the prothrombin complex (factor VII, Christmas factor, prothrombin, and factor X) have been prepared in the Central Laboratory of the Netherlands Red Cross Blood Transfusion Service according to a method described by Deggeller (1). The preparation can be made from ordinary ACD-plasma, from which other plasma derivates can also be produced; for the production of the concentrate, the plasma of 16 donors (8 litres plasma) is pooled.

From this pool, 7 ampoules of the concentrate are made. The product is sterilized by passing it through a bacteria filter. The clotting factors are adsorbed onto DEAE-cellulose, eluted, and then freeze-dried. After drying, the product is suitable for transport throughout the country. Before use, the dried product must be dissolved in 10 ml water. The substance dissolves quickly, giving a clear solution with a light-blue colour due to the presence of caeruloplasmin in the product. So far, we have processed 850 litres of plasma in this way. The preparation can be used for patients with congenital deficiencies of the clotting factors II, VII, IX, and X.

In some patients with a severe parenchymatous liver disease and a decreased value of these clotting factors, a temporary correction can be useful in connection with a surgical procedure or to stop bleeding, especially when this occurs in the digestive tract and gives rise to hepatic coma. Lastly, for overdosed coumarin-treated patients the concentrate – when given in an appropriate dose – can induce an immediate correction of the defect.

This is especially useful for patients in whom correction by vitamin K would take too much time (e.g. cerebral haemorrhages). The expected concentration of the factors, after the preparation has been dissolved, is 5000% (the concentration of normal plasma being 100%); the values obtained (means of 30 determinations) were for prothrombin, 2600% (yield 52%; standard deviation 550%); for factor VII, 1900% (yield

38%; standard deviation 500%); for factor IX, 3300% (yield 66%; standard deviation 560%); and for factor x, 2400% (yield 48%; standard deviation 580%).

The clot-promoting activity of 1 ampoule of the 4-clotting-factor concentrate is equivalent to 350 ml fresh plasma in haemophilia B (Christmas disease) and to 220 ml fresh plasma in factor VII deficiency. We have never seen conversion of prothrombin to thrombin in the concentrate. A small amount of factor xa, however, may occasionally be found in the product. Concerning factors ixa and viia, we have insuffi-

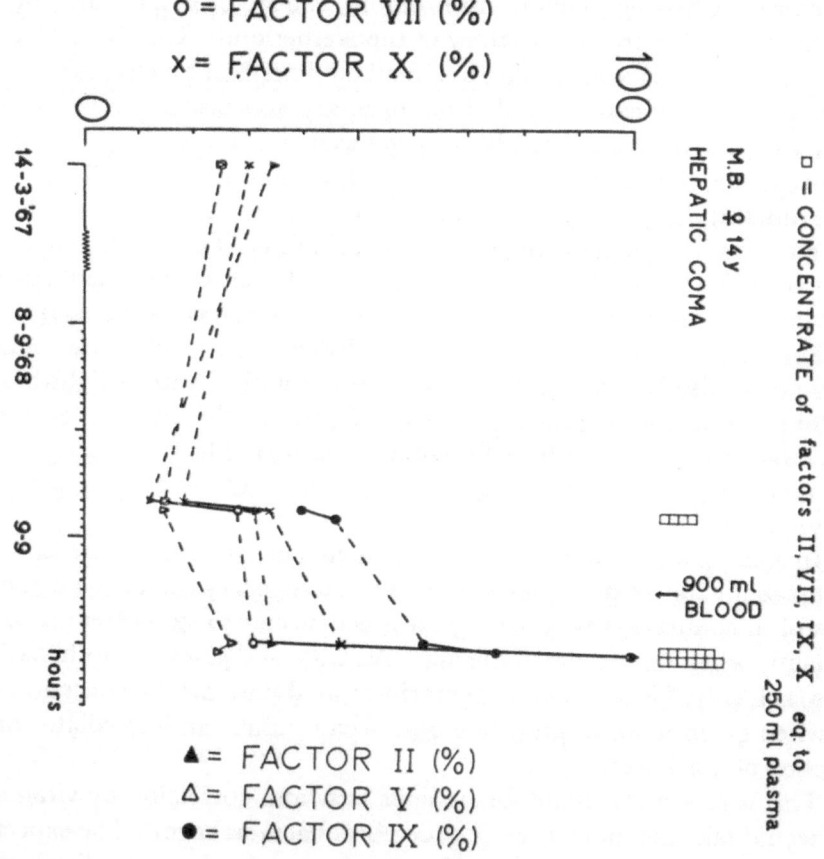

Fig. 1. Increase in the clotting factors of the prothrombin complex in a patient with hepatic cirrhosis after administration of 3 ampoules followed by 11 ampoules of the 4-clotting-factor concentrate. Note that the correction of factors VII, x, and II is complete, whereas the correction for factor IX is almost complete.

cient information. The concentrate was tolerated well; however, an occasional febrile reaction was observed.

Using our product, Cohen (2) found biological half-life times of 56 hours for factor II and 52 hours for factor X in two non-bleeding patients with congenital deficiencies of these factors. This is about the same as the times mentioned in the literature for comparable preparations.

An example of the application of the concentrate in a patient with hepatic coma at the final stage of juvenile hepatic cirrhosis is shown in figure 1. After administration of 11 ampoules of the concentrate factor VII, the prothrombin and factor X levels returned to normal and factor IX rose to 72%.

REFERENCES

1. Deggeller, K., Panel discussion on 'Optimal use of human blood' held May 31, 1968 on the occasion of the 25th anniversary of the Netherlands Red Cross Blood Transfusion Service. *Vox Sang.* (in press) 1969.
2. Cohen, O., Panel discussion on 'Optimal use of human blood' held May 31, 1968 on the occasion of the 25th anniversary of the Netherlands Red Cross Blood Transfusion Service. *Vox Sang.* (in press) 1969.

PREPARATION AND CLINICAL APPLICATION
OF CRYOPRECIPITATE

KLAZINA MEIJER AND J. J. VELTKAMP

Cryoprecipitate represents an important acquisition for the treatment of haemophilia A patients, not only because it makes it possible to bring the factor VIII level to any desired value without danger of overloading of the circulation but also because it can be prepared so easily. Blood is collected in a plastic double-bag system by means of a vacuum pump. After centrifugation in a cooled centrifuge, the plasma extractor is used to transfer the plasma to the supplementary bag, which is then submerged in a mixture of dry ice and alcohol (-50° to -60°C) for about 15 minutes before being placed in the refrigerator (4°C) until the next day (original method according to Pool (4) or thawed in a waterbath at about 6°C in a period of about 90 minutes (modification of Brown and Hardisty (1)). The cryoprecipitate is found in the thawed plasma as a clumpy sediment. After centrifugation, the plasma is allowed to flow back to the erythrocyte concentrate and the bags are separated. When required for use, the contents of the appropriate number of bags are dissolved in a citrate-saline solution and pooled.

We have prepared cryoprecipitate routinely since 1965. Originally, the product was mainly used for the evaluation of the preparation itself. We found a yield *in vitro* amounting to 46 per cent factor VIII, a fibrinogen to factor VIII ratio of 0.8, and a purification on protein basis of 14 times. One cryoprecipitate derived from the donation of one blood donor corresponds to about 90 ml fresh net plasma.

The results of transfusion experiments were used to calculate the disappearance rate of factor VIII. The curve shows a distinctly biphasic course. The $t\frac{1}{2}$ of the first phase, i.e. the equilibration between intra- and extra-vascular spaces, amounted to 4 hours; the $t\frac{1}{2}$ of the second phase, i.e. the biological degradation of factor VIII, amounted to 14 hours.

It was also demonstrated that in patients with a limited factor VIII production, i.e. the types indicated as 'moderate and mild', there is no depression of production during and after transfusion of the cryoprecipitate. The curves for patients of the 'severe' and the 'moderate-mild' types show virtually the same course when the calculations are based on the same average plasma volume. The blood level desirable for haemostasis is therefore the sum of the amount circulating in the patient

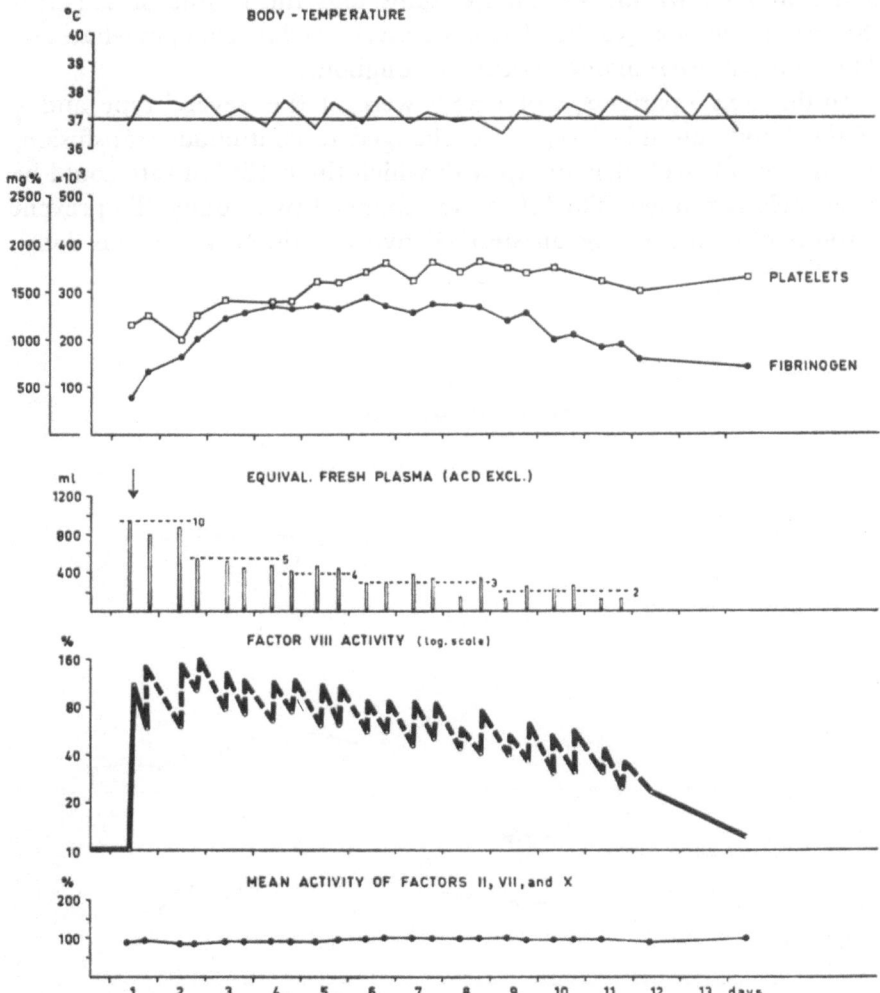

Fig. 1. Data concerning treatment and clinical course of a patient suffering from haemophilia A operated upon for an inguinal hernia. Arrow indicates operation.

as the result of his own production and of the increase achieved by transfusion (2, 3).

Our first total substitution with cryoprecipitate (in a 6 year old boy requiring a herniotomy) was performed with intermittent administration, with which an average factor VIII content of 50 to 60 per cent was reached. In a period of 11 days, substitution was performed with a total of 92 cryoprecipitates. As can be seen from figure 1, the fibrinogen content remained within acceptable limits and the factors of the prothrombin complex and the platelet count showed no changes whatever. The temperature remained normal throughout.

In the next 6 patients, 2 of whom were of the 'severe' type and 4 of the 'moderate-mild' type, we changed to continuous transfusion, making use of an electric pump with which the perfusion rate could be accurately regulated. The infuse was changed twice daily. To prevent thrombophlebits, 20 mg unesterified hydrocortisone was given daily,

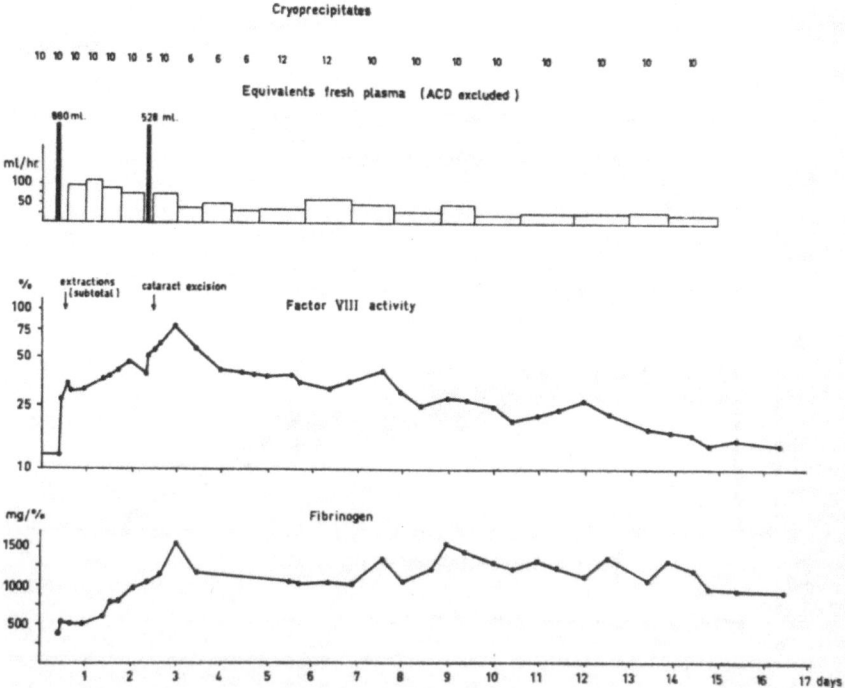

Fig. 2. Clinical and laboratory data obtained during substitution therapy of patient A.J.L.: dental extraction and cataract operation.

and to prevent clotting in the infusion needle, 10 mg heparin was added to the cryoprecipitate solution daily.

The dosage of cryoprecipitate was calculated with an appropriate equation and, when necessary, adjusted on the basis of the daily check.

Patient 1 (figure 2) was a 57 year old man belonging to the mild type and having a factor VIII production of 10 per cent. He was admitted for extraction of several teeth and a cataract operation. After a loading dose of 10 cryoprecipitates, the factor VIII level rose to 26 per cent, after which 9 teeth were extracted. The factor VIII level was then maintained at about 40 per cent. Two days after the extractions, an intracapsular

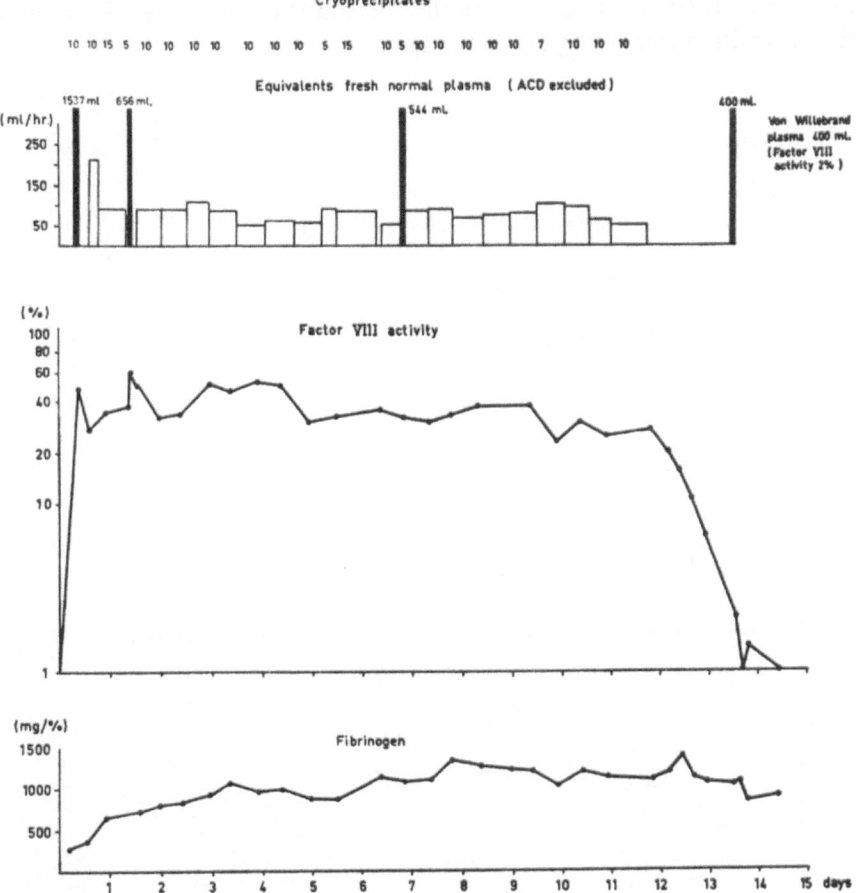

Fig. 3. Clinical and laboratory data of patient H.P.R.: dental extraction.

cataract extraction was performed on the left eye after administration
of an extra dose of 5 cryoprecipitates. Recovery was entirely uneventful. This patient received a total of 175 cryoprecipitates over a period
of 13 days.

Patient 2 (figure 3) was a 37 year old man suffering from the severe
form of haemophilia A who required extraction of all his teeth. After
the administration of 10 cryoprecipitates, 18 teeth were extracted, the
alveolar cavities being filled with Spongostan and then sutured. Two
days later, the remaining 13 teeth were extracted. Three days later, a
painful haematoma developed at the site of an alveolar fracture. During
the bleeding, the factor VIII level proved to be 30 per cent. The further
course was uneventful. Over a 12 day period the patient received substitution with a total of 235 cryoprecipitates.

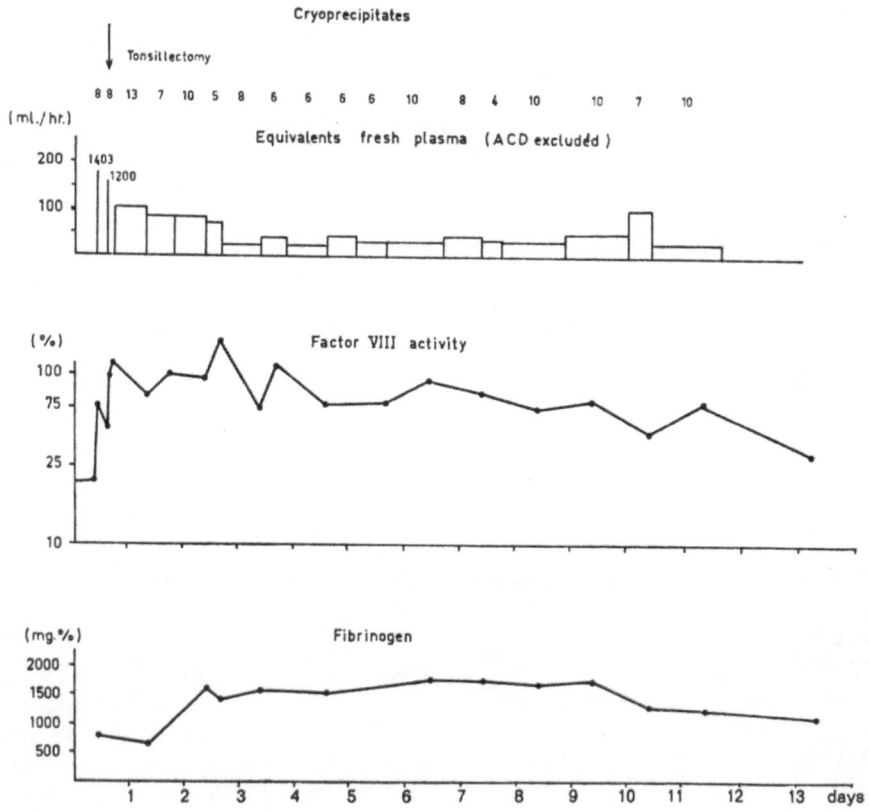

Fig. 4. Clinical and laboratory data of patient J.G.L.O.: tonsillectomy.

Patient 3 (figure 4) was a 47 year old man belonging to the mild type with a factor VIII production of about 20 per cent, admitted for a tonsillectomy. Pre-operatively, he received 10 cryoprecipitates, the factor VIII level rising to 70 per cent. During the further period of substitution the factor VIII level averaged 50 per cent. Over a period of 11 days the pa-

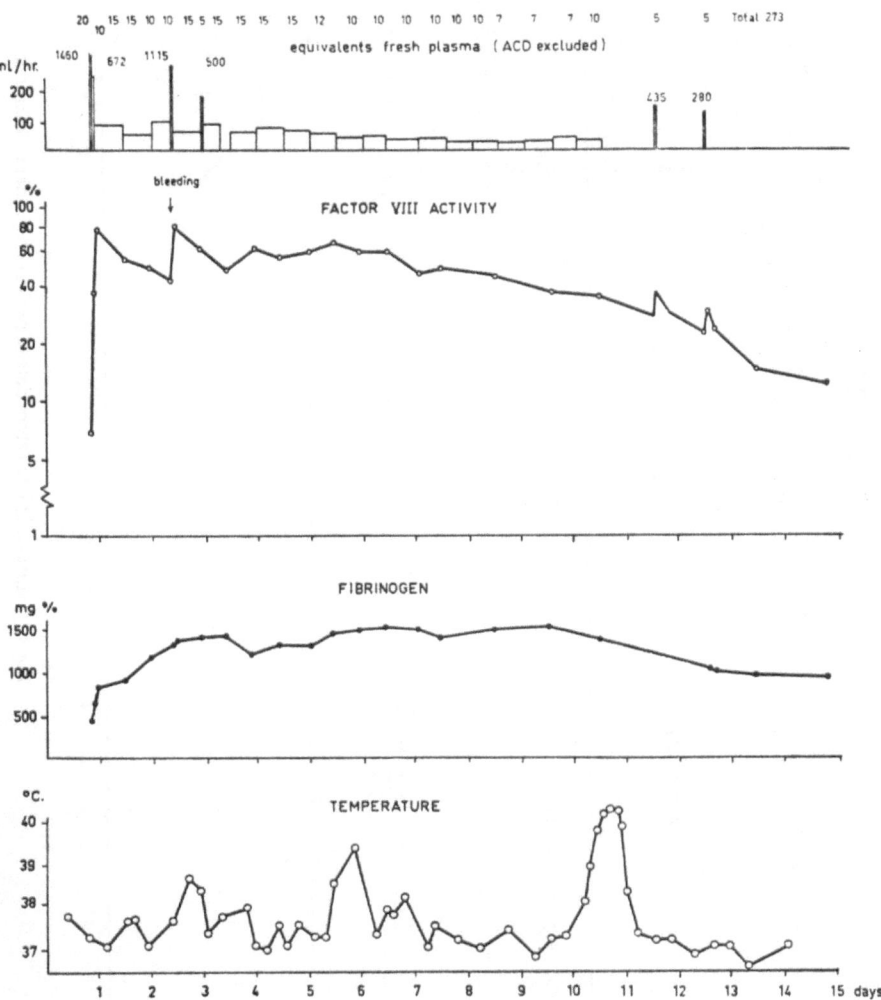

Fig. 5. Clinical and laboratory data of patient J.M.: appendectomy.

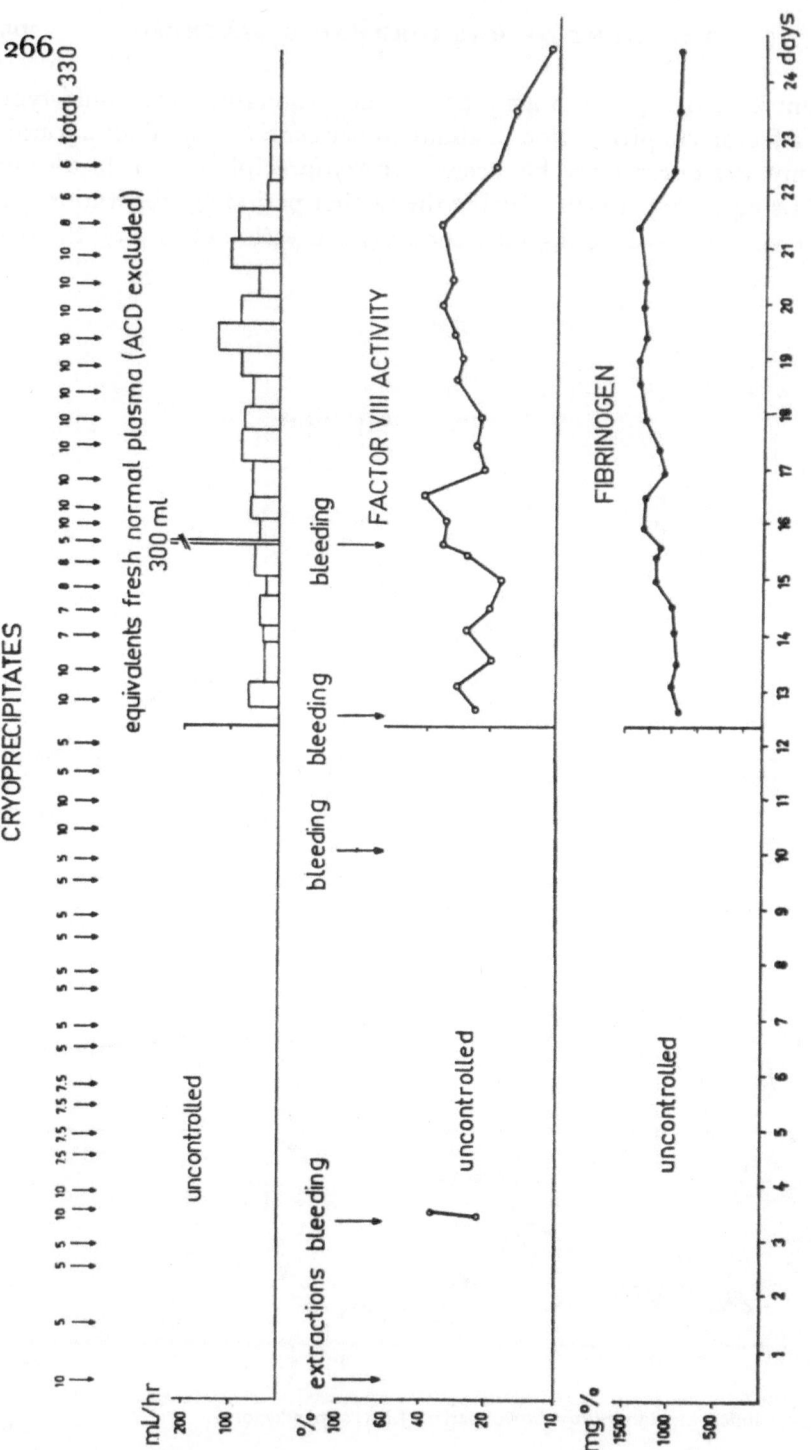

Fig. 6. Clinical and laboratory data of patient H.V.: dental extraction.

tient received a total of 142 cryoprecipitates. No complications occurred.

Patient 4 (figure 5), a man of 45 years, had a factor VIII production of about 7 per cent. He was operated upon for an acute appendicitis. On the third post-operative day the wound bled slightly and a small haematoma formed. At this time, the factor VIII level was 40 per cent. The substitution dosage was temporarily increased, after which the bleeding stopped. The substitution was continued over a period of 12 days, with a total of 273 cryoprecipitates.

Patient 5 (figure 6) was a young man of 19 years belonging to the mild type, with a factor VIII level of 6 per cent, who was admitted for the extraction of 4 carious teeth. He was initially given intermittent substitution with 2 daily doses of 5 cryoprecipitates, with which factor VIII levels between 20 and 30 per cent were reached. Three of the wounds healed rapidly, but on the 11th day at the site of the fourth extraction a haematoma developed which extended submucously into the maxillary sinus. An alveolar fracture could not be demonstrated. Continuous substitution was then applied with 20 cryoprecipitates per day, during which the factor VIII level remained around 30 per cent, or somewhat lower than was to be expected. In agreement with this relatively low level, there was incidental slight bleeding. The dosage of cryoprecipitate could not be increased due to an inadequate supply. A circulating anticoagulant (which would have been highly improbably in a patient producing factor VIII) was not demonstrated. It seems possible that during the development and resorption of the haematoma there was an increased consumption of factor VIII. Further healing of the wound was uneventful. Over a period of 24 days the patient received a total of 330 cryoprecipitates.

Patient 6 (figure 7) was a 15 year old boy suffering from severe haemophilia A who had been operated upon elsewhere for appendicitis. He had received inadequate substitution post-operatively, resulting in a severe haemorrhage in the area of the wound a week after the operation. After admission to our department, substitution with cryoprecipitate resulted in a factor VIII level of about 40 per cent. On the fifth day after admission, the incompletely healed wound became infected and the patient's temperature rose to 39°C; treatment with antibiotics was successful. The administration of cryoprecipitate was stopped on the

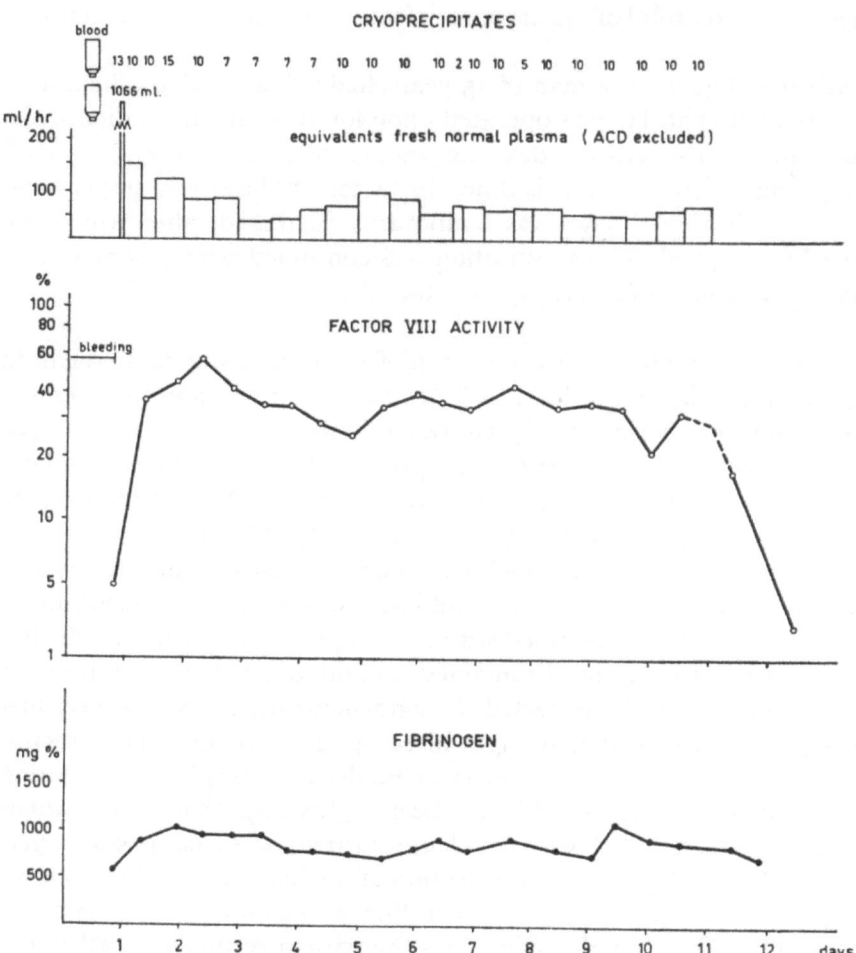

Fig. 7. Clinical and laboratory data of patient E.O.: appendectomy.

13th day after admission (21st post-operative day). A few days later, after the patient had vomitted, a haematoma developed in the area of the wound. Substitution was resumed for 6 days. The haematoma emptied spontaneously, and further healing was uneventful. A total of 308 cryoprecipitates were used.

Conclusions

To investigate the applicability of the equation (2) used in the calculations, for each period of substitution the average of the observed values for the plasma of the individual patients was determined and compared with the expected increase (calculated with the equation) above the patient's own level. The equation proved to be generally applicable, but the individual discrepancy between the two values was rather large in some cases. This means that during substitution *the factor* VIII *activity in the patient's plasma must be determined at least twice a day to be certain that the substitution is adequate.* This practice also gives the assurance of prompt detection of any resistance caused by the appearance of a circulating anticoagulant.

The course after hospitalization of these patients shows, once again, that the haemostatically safe level must amount to at least 40 per cent, certainly during the first few post-operative days.

The continuous administration of cryoprecipitate is preferable to intermittent substitution. With the former, in the first place, a new infusion does not have to be introduced twice daily. Secondly, it can be calculated that the required amount of cryoprecipitate for continuous administration amounts to about 80 per cent of the amount required for intermittent perfusion. This difference arises from the fact that with twice-daily administration the loss of factor VIII *in vivo* due to the biological degradation is appreciably greater than the loss associated with continuous perfusion, for which the loss *in vitro* over a 12 hour period of perfusion was found to be about 20 per cent.

In summarization of the foregoing it may be said that cryoprecipitate represents an easily prepared factor VIII concentrate with a good haemostatic effect and virtually no side-effects. Continuous administration deserves preference on economic as well as technical grounds. A few cases of serum hepatitis were observed.

REFERENCES

1. Brown, D. L., R. M. Hardisty, M. H. Kosoy, C. Bracken, Antihaemophilic globulin: Preparation by an improved cryoprecipitation method and clinical use. *Brit. med. J.* 2, 79 (1967).
2. Meijer, K., J. G. Eernisse, J. J. Veltkamp, H. C. Hemker, E. A. Loeliger, Treatment of haemophilia A with purified factor VIII obtained from human plasma by cryoprecipitation. *Folia med. neerl.* 10, 49 (1967).
3. Meijer, K., *Substitutie van factor* VIII *bij haemophilie* A. Thesis, Leiden 1968.
4. Pool, J. G., A. E. Shannon, Production of high-potency concentrates of anti-hemophilic globulin in a closed-bag system. *New Engl. J. Med.* 273, 1443 (1965).

SOME REMARKS CONCERNING THE PRODUCTION
AND ADMINISTRATION OF CRYOPRECIPITATES

J. VREEKEN

In the Central Laboratory of the Netherlands Red Cross Blood Transfusion Service, cryoprecipitates are not prepared from freshly with-
drawn blood but from plasma obtained by so-called 'plasma campaigns'.
The evening before production of the precipitate, the blood is collected
somewhere in the country. It is stored overnight at 4°C and the next
morning cryoprecipitates are produced in the usual way. Each batch
derives from 1 litre of plasma (4 donors). After freeze-drying of the
product it can be kept at 4°C, and is suitable for distribution throughout the country.

Cryoprecipitates for the treatment of haemophilia A and Von Willebrand's disease have been produced by the Central Laboratory since
1966. In 1967, about 2,700 4-donor-cryoprecipitates were produced,
and in 1968 the number increased to about 6,000. This increase may
be expected to continue in the coming years.

Before use, the preparation must be dissolved in 50 ml water. Since
the yield of factor VIII is about 45%, the clot-promoting activity of our
cryoprecipitates in haemophilia A is equivalent to 450 ml fresh plasma.
However, the yield of the product is rather variable. The standard
deviation is 150 ml fresh plasma. One must realize, however, that the
measurement of factor VIII activity in concentrates is not very reliable,
at least in our hands. The preparations usually dissolve rather quickly
after addition of the water, but sometimes small particles of undissolved
material remain. Therefore, we always administer the preparation
through the filter system of a transfusion apparatus. The activity of the
preparation is always good when a sufficient amount is given and provided that there is no anticoagulant against factor VIII in the patient's
blood. When the AHG level is kept over 30% (as measured with our
methods), one can expect an uneventful post-operative course in patients with haemophilia A. Therefore, the treatment of the patients de-

pends upon a sufficient supply of the material and on the possibility of measuring blood levels of factor VIII.

The following adverse reactions have been observed: in some cases a spasm of the blood vessel used for transfusion is seen, and after prolonged transfusion of the precipitate the risk of thrombophlebitis is higher than with more indifferent solutions. Sometimes febrile reactions are observed; these are mostly of short duration and do not necessarily recur after renewed infusion of the precipitate.

Taking the usual frequency of serum hepatitis into account, we could have expected at least 100 cases of this complication after administration of cryoprecipitates derived from 26,800 donors. So far, only one case of serum hepatitis has been reported, but no systematic follow-up for hepatitis was made. Nevertheless, it seems probable that the frequency of hepatitis after donation of this product is lower than would have been expected. It seems possible that polytransfused patients, for whom this therapy is mainly used, are rather immune with respect to this complication.

In recent years there has been a shift in the rapidity with which substitution therapy is given to haemophiliacs. Because of the ease of treatment, patients are coming in earlier with minor bleedings, and as a result the idea of prophylactic treatment of all haemophiliacs arises. However, it must be realized that in The Netherlands there are about 1000 haemophiliacs who would then need annually 365,000 4-donor-cryoprecipitates (each patient receiving 1 cryoprecipitate per day) deriving from 1,460,000 donations a year, whereas at present we only obtain about 380,000 bottles of blood per year. It seems clear that we do not have sufficient blood for the systematic prophylactic treatment of haemophiliacs.

In the U.S., preparations with a very high concentration of factor VIII have been produced (1). But more important than the concentration of factor VIII in a preparation is the yield of the production. A high percentage of factor VIII in a preparation with a low yield can benefit only a few patients. Viewed on a large scale, the increase of the yield is more important than the concentration.

When there is a shortage of human material, the use of animal antihaemophilic globulin for selected patients over a short period of a few days is still to be considered. This saves human material, and makes it possible to obtain very high levels of factor VIII for a certain time. Of course, the possibility of hypersensitivity reactions and thrombocytopenia must be kept in mind, as well as the fact that after some time resistance to this preparation always develops. It is, however, possible to give factor VIII of the same animal more than once in a lifetime, provided there is a rather long interval between treatments.

An example of the possibilities of treatment with material containing factor VIII is provided by the history of a 25-year-old patient with a pseudotumour of the right ileum (figures 1 and 2). This tumour had destroyed a large area of bone and given rise to a fracture; the operation was performed by Prof. W. van Enst (2) under protection of animal factor VIII and non-freeze-dried cryoprecipitate. The post-operative course was uneventful except for a small bleeding during the change from porcine to human material. Two years later, another pseudotumour had developed on the left femur, again causing destruction of the bone (figures 3 and 4). At the second operation porcine AHG was given, and although urticaria developed, a sufficiently high level of factor VIII could again be maintained for a few days. After this substitution therapy had been followed by freeze-dried human cryoprecipitate, the level of factor VIII during the period in which freeze-dried precipitate was administered was about the same as that during treatment with the cryoprecipitate that had not been freeze-dried, as can be seen from figure 5.

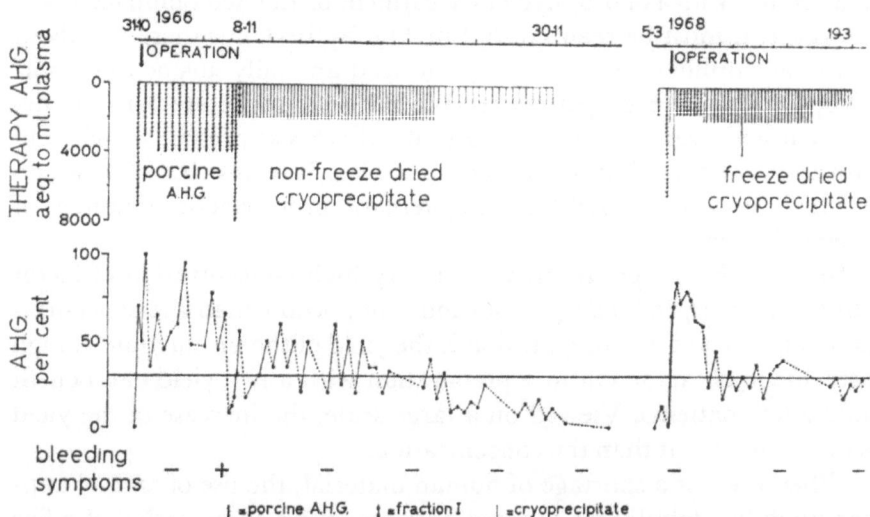

Fig. 5. Substitution therapies applied in a patient with haemophilia A, who was operated upon twice, for two different pseudo-tumours. Note the AHG-levels with freeze-dried and non-freeze-dried cryoprecipitate and the levels obtained with porcine AHG given on two different occasions.

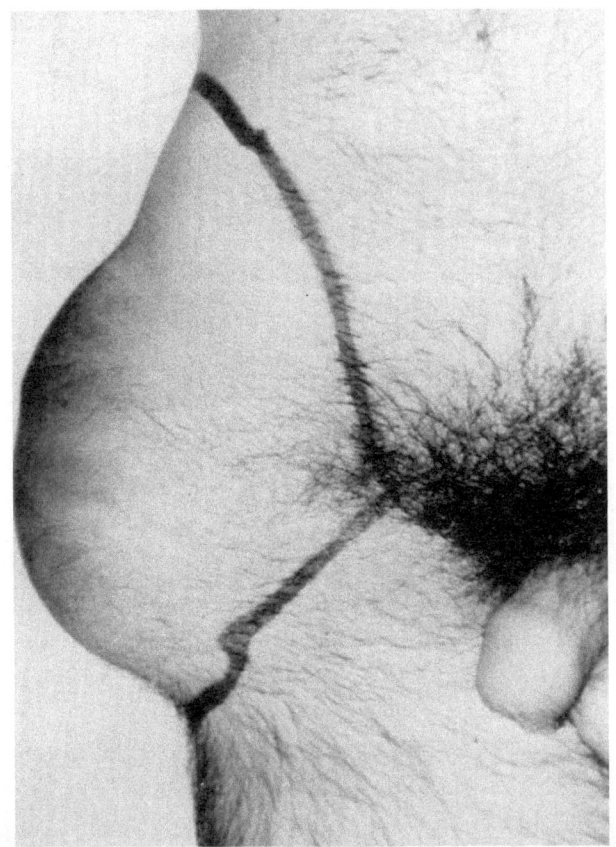

Fig. 1. External aspect of a large pseudo-tumour in a patient with haemophilia A.

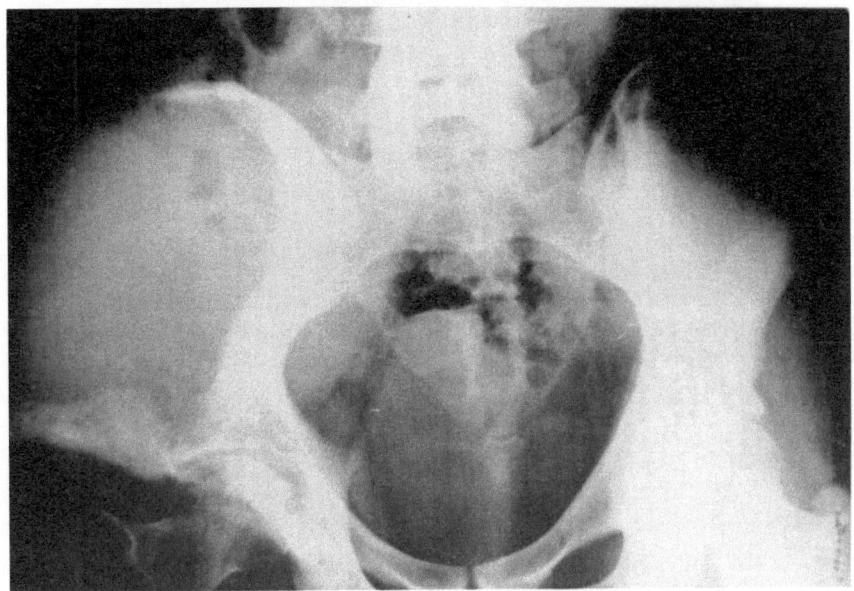

Fig. 2. Roentgenologic aspect of the tumour in Fig. 1. Note that the major part of the right os ileum has disappeared. There is a fracture of the bone.

Vreeken, Some remarks

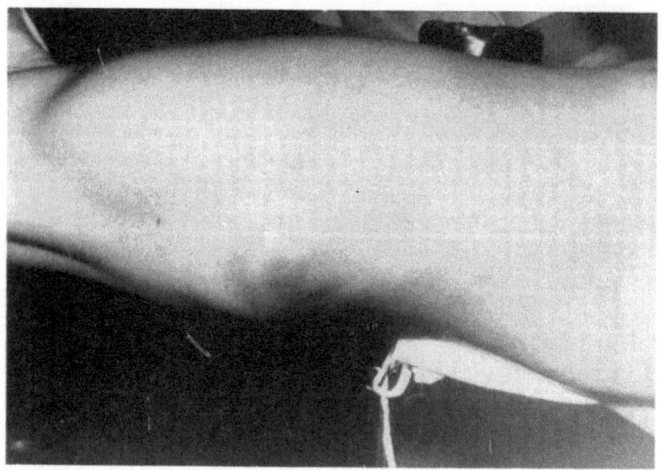

Fig. 3. External aspect of another pseudo-tumour of the left femur in the same patient.

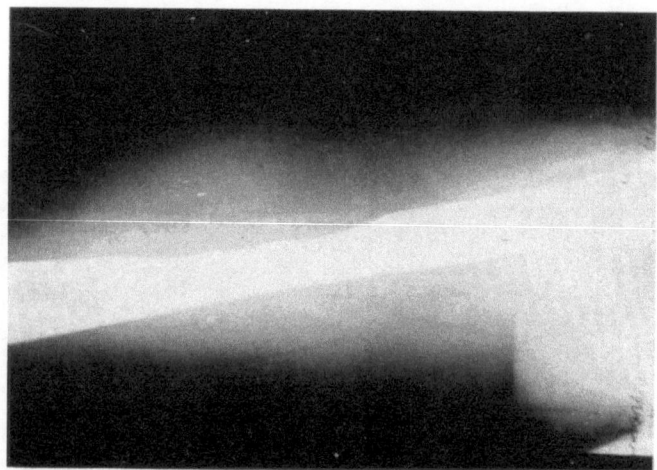

Fig. 4. Roentgenologic aspect of the tumour in Fig. 3. Note that the cortex of the os femur has disappeared over a considerable distance.

REFERENCES

1. Shanbrom, E., Panel discussion on 'Optimal use of human blood' held May 31, 1968 on the occasion of the 25th anniversary of the Netherlands Red Cross Blood Transfusion Service. *Vox Sang.* (in press) 1969.
2. Heijdenrijk, P. A., J. Vreeken, De behandeling van een grote pseudotumor in het os ileum bij een patient met ernstige haemophilie A. *Ned. T. Geneesk.* 112, 90 (1968).

GENETIC COUNSELLING IN HAEMOSTATIC DISORDERS

J. J. VELTKAMP

Genetic counselling in hereditary bleeding disorders mainly concerns haemophilia, since the other disorders i.e. thrombocytopathy of Glanzmann-Naegeli and the inherited coagulation-factor deficiencies of factors II, V, VII, X, and XI are rare and show autosomal inheritance. Only homozygotes for these pathologic genes have a tendency to bleed, and genetic advice would be relevant only with respect to an intrafamilial marriage.

Genetic counselling for the haemophilias is not only more necessary but is also much more complicated than for the other bleeding disorders. Firstly, the haemophilic patient and his relatives must be informed about the mode of inheritance of haemophilia. Many haemophiliacs refrain from procreation because they do not want to transmit the haemophilia gene through their daughters. Others express confidence in the future progress of treatment. A decision of this kind should in any case be made in full awareness of the hereditary mechanism involved. The biggest problem we encounter in this respect is presented by the female relatives of the haemophilic patient, perhaps his sisters or a girl cousin, who from childhood have witnessed the suffering of the bleeder and do not want to have haemophilic children themselves. Most of them want to know whether or not they are carriers, so they can take contraceptional measures if necessary.

We started an investigation into proven carriers five years ago, because at that time no unequivocal data permitting reliable genetic counselling were available. The only information we had was that as a group, carriers of haemophilia show a subnormal activity of factor VIII or IX. The pitfall in these investigations proved to be the large experimental error and the considerable biologic variation shown by the clotting factor within the individual. It thus became evident that the requirements for genetic counselling in potential carriers are: 1. a reliable factor VIII and IX assay with a small experimental error (5 to 10%), and 2. knowledge of the biologic variation within the individual.

As can be seen from table 1, repeated investigation reduces the influence of the biologic variation within the individual; a threefold investigation, performed on three independent occasions, narrows the limits of the outcome reasonably well.

Table 1. 95% confidence intervals of activity of factors VIII and IX (in per cent of normal) expected on the basis of repeated investigations in a haemophilia carrier displaying 50 per cent and a normal individual displaying 100 per cent activity of that clotting factor.

Number of	factor VIII		factor IX	
investigations	Carrier	Normal	Carrier	Normal
1	34–74	75–134	37–68	76–131
3	40–63	84–118	42–60	86–117
10	44–56	91–110	45–55	92–109
∞	50	100	50	100

The levels of factors VIII and IX in the normal population and in a population of definite carriers were determined (figures 1 and 2). A considerable overlap in activities, given here as log activity, was found in the normals and the carriers. The carriers of haemophilia show a wider population variation than the normals.

A mechanism to explain this wide variation was put forward by Lyon. Lyonization also provides an explanation for dosage compensation, i.e. why males with one x-chromosome have the same bloodlevel of enzymes produced on the x-chromosome as females with two x-chromosomes (double dosed). According to the Lyon hypothesis, one x-chromosome in each female cell is inactive, and can be seen as a Barr body. This inactivation takes place early in embryonic life, and the daughter cells show the same inactivation pattern. So if all abnormal x-chromosomes in a carrier were to be inactivated by chance, we would find a normal factor VIII or IX level. If all the normal x-chromosomes are inactivated, the individual will have haemophilia herself. Indeed, many carriers display signs and symptoms of true haemophilia, even of the severe type; others have completely normal coagulation-factor levels. In G-6-PD deficiency, which is also a sex linked trait, carriers can be detected by the demonstration of two populations of red cells, one fully normal and one fully enzyme-deficient, which respectively represent the cells with inactivation of the defect x-chromosome and the cells with inactivation of the normal x-chromosome. Unfortunately, this approach cannot be applied to the cells producing factors VIII and IX, and we must therefore make the discrimination between normals and carriers on basis of the level of factor VIII or factor IX.

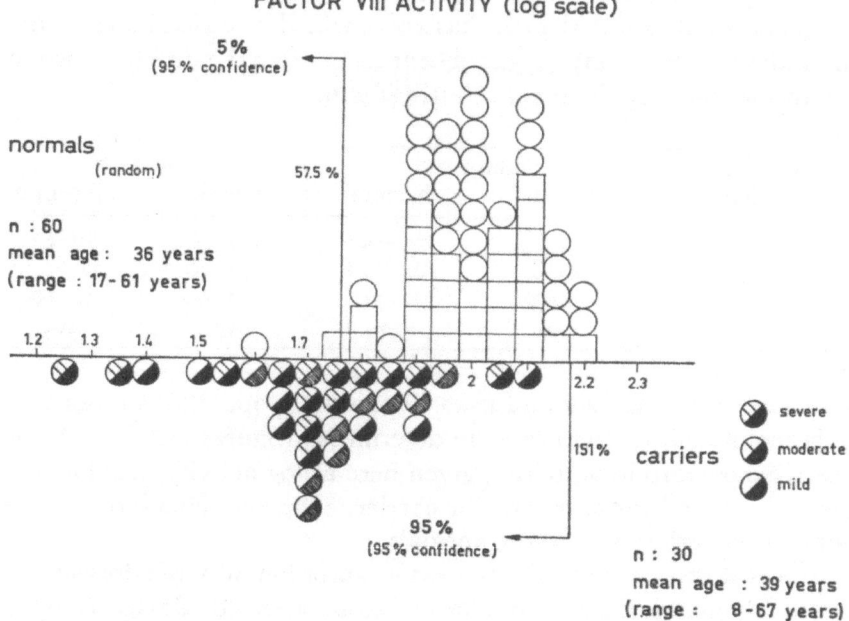

Fig. 1. Grouped frequency histogram of factor VIII activity as assessed in haemophilia A carriers and normals, plotted on logarithmic scale, class intervals being 0.05 and class boundaries .025 and .075, respectively. The upper part shows values obtained in normals on one occasion, squares indicating men and circles women; in the lower part, each circle represents the average value obtained in a carrier tested on different occasions. Half-shaded circles refer to daughters of haemophiliacs.

In figures 1 and 2, tolerance limits have been drawn to mark the 5 per cent lowest normal values and the 5 per cent highest carrier values. Below this limit we will find the carriers that can be detected with a mean confidence of 95 per cent. For the potential carriers of haemophilia A, for instance sisters of haemophiliacs who thus have a 50 per cent genetic chance of carriership, the proportion that can be detected is 17/30 (17 below the limit of the total of 30), or 32 per cent. This means

64 per cent of the true carriers in this group. The exclusion of carriership is only possible in 2.5 per cent of the potential carrier population. For carriers of haemophilia B the percentage of detectable carriers in the group with 50 per cent genetic chance is 39 per cent, whereas 21 per cent will prove to be normal. We suspect that these figures for haemophilia B are a little too optimistic, however, because the basic

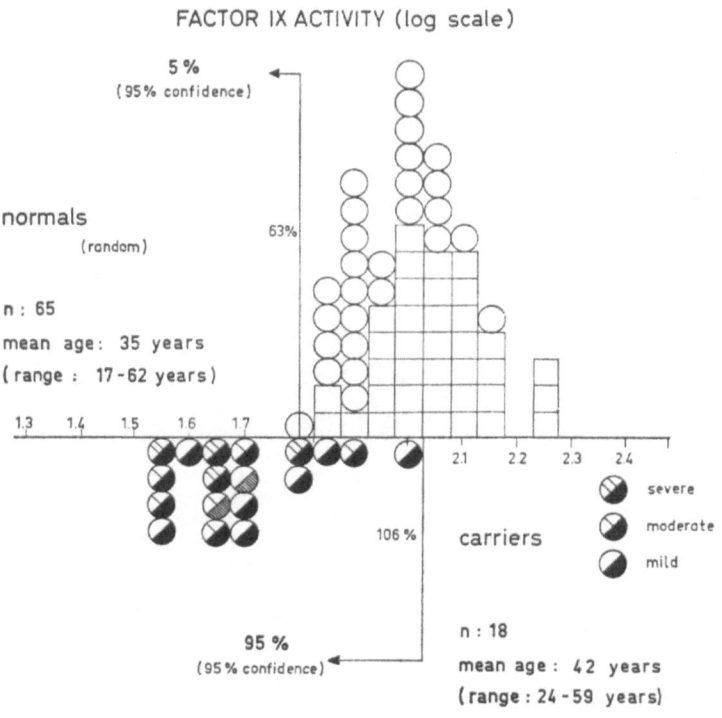

Fig. 2. Results obtained in haemophilia B carriers and normals, grouped as in figure 1. The values for both carriers and normals represent the result of only one test.

material of definite carriers in this study was relatively small and 8 of them belonged to the same family. Nevertheless, it remains possible that at the moment that Lyon's postulated inactivation of female x-chromosomes occurs, more mother cells of the factor-IX-producing cells are present than mother cells of factor-VIII-producing cells. The effect of the *random* inactivation would then be less marked and the carriers values will be grouped more closely around their average value.

The estimation of the individual chance of carriership is based in the first place on the genetic chance of carriership and in the second place on the outcome of the factor VIII or IX assay. The theorem of Bayes can be used to calculate the chance that a given individual belongs to the normal or to the carrier population, when mean values and variances of those populations are known. Curves, based on this formula, for direct reading of the chances of carriership are given in figures 3 and 4.

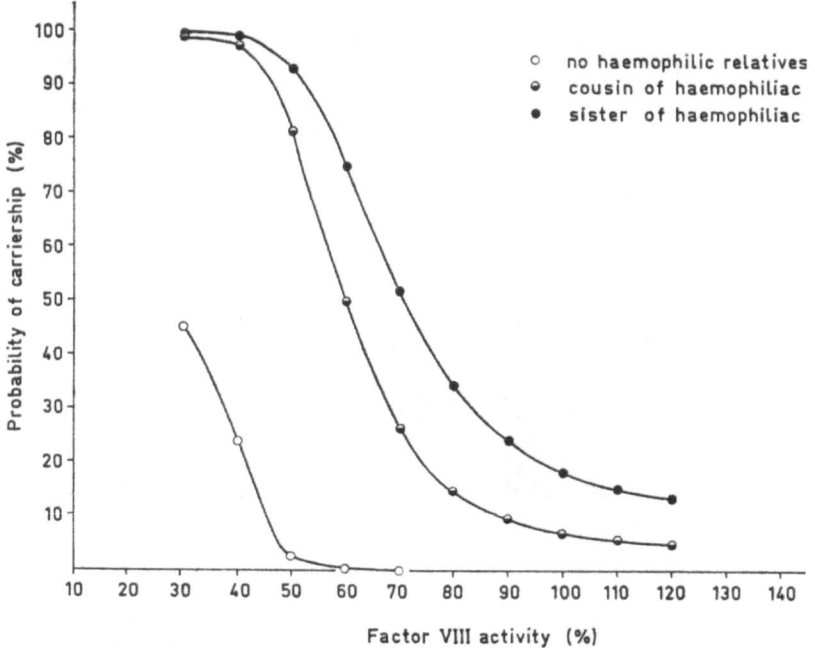

Fig. 3. Curves for reading probability of carriership of haemophilia A for individuals with a known factor VIII activity, at three different levels of genetic chance.

The essentials for genetic counselling in haemophilia are:

1. Thorough explanation of the mode of inheritance and complicating mechanism.
2. Reliable assay procedures for assessment of the clotting factors VIII and IX.
3. Knowledge of the variation in the levels of factors VIII and IX in the normal and definite-carrier population.

4. Repeated investigations (three at the least) to minimize the effect of the biologic variation within the individual.
5. Thorough explanation of the meaning of probabilities in general as well as in relation to the result obtained.
6. Absolute freedom of decision with respect to procreation for the individual who asks advice.

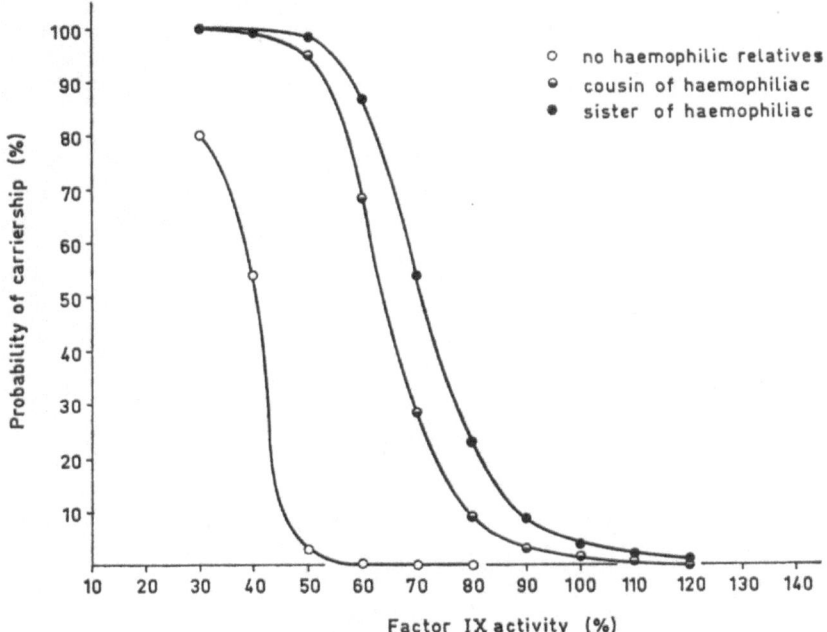

Fig. 4. Curves for reading probability of carriership of haemophilia B for individuals with a known factor IX activity, at three different levels of genetic chance.

REFERENCES

1. Veltkamp, J. J., E. F. Drion, E. A. Loeliger, Detection of the carrier state in hereditary coagulation disorders. *Thrombos. Diathes. haemorrh. I,* 19, 279 (1968), *Thrombos. Diathes. haemorrh. II,* 19, 403 (1968).

CHAPTER III

BLOOD COAGULATION CONTROL IN ORAL
ANTICOAGULANT TREATMENT

GENERAL CONSIDERATIONS ON A
COUMARIN-INDUCED HYPOCOAGULABILITY
AND ITS CONTROL

E. A. LOELIGER

Vitamin K antagonists comprising 4-hydroxy-coumarin and indandion derivatives induce a reduction in the rate of synthesis of the four coagulation factors II, VII, IX, and X, as can be judged from a decrease in the respective activities in the blood. Coagulation factor synthesis is thought to be blocked at the site of action of vitamin K_1 as the result of an interchange of physiological vitamin K with the coumarin congener molecule.

All coumarin congeners induce the same response of the four coagulation factors to an *initial loading dose* (2). If a high initial loading dose is given, synthesis is completely blocked and the rate of decrease of each of the four factors depends wholly on its biological half-life. Factor VII disappears the most rapidly (biological $t\frac{1}{2}$ = 6 hours), prothrombin (factor II) the slowest (biological $t\frac{1}{2}$ = 60 hours). The rate of decay, however, does not solely depend on the nature of the coagulation factor; it is also considerably influenced by the metabolic condition of the patient. In hypothyroidism, catabolism is decreased and there is a consequent decrease in the disappearance rate, whereas in hyperthyroidism and febrile states there is a considerable increase in the rate of disappearance (9, 12).

In daily practice, maximum disappearance rates are induced only when short-acting coumarin congeners are given in doses many times larger than the maintenance dose. Long-acting preparations seldom lead to a maximum response, because their initial loading dose is relatively small and an excessively high dose would induce undesired overshooting.

Under the influence of a *constant maintenance dose,* a stable depression of the production rate is achieved and the four factors show a constant and mutually similar degree of lowered activity, under optimum conditions down to an average value between 15 per cent to 20 per cent of normal (10, 11). The relatively high factor IX level found in elderly people is a phenomenon of age; a relatively low factor X activity, as measured by conventional methods, is due to the entrance of an anti-coagulant into the circulation upon administration of vitamin K anta-gonists. The high concentration of factor II reported by investigators who use a thrombin generation test for the assessment of prothrombin could be due to the fact that this anticoagulant (a protein analogous to prothrombin) may slowly acquire thrombin-like properties (1, 7); it is known that the level of the staphylocoagulase-reacting factor – which is biochemically indistinguishable from prothrombin – is increased after the intake of coumarin congeners (16). Since the finding of this circulating anticoagulant, which was provisionally called preprothrombin (4, 5) and is now more generally termed PIVKA (protein induced by vitamin K absence or antagonists) (6), we know that the result of a *coagulation check* in cases of coumarin-induced hypocoagulability depends on the sensitivity of the test system not only for quantitative variations of fac-tors II, VII, and X, but also for the presence of this circulating anticoa-gulant. Thrombotest, which is now widely used, is particularly sensi-tive to both the depression of coagulation factors and the presence of the anticoagulant, whereas the prothrombin time assay procedures, especi-ally when performed with commercially available rabbit-brain throm-boplastin preparations, lack this sensitivity. As a result of the action of the inhibitor, the thrombotest activity in patients on long-term (stable) anticoagulant treatment is reduced to half the value expected from the level of the coagulation factors present in their plasma (see pages 322, 365).

Some general remarks concerning the intensity of hypocoagulability to be aimed at during anticoagulant treatment, the so-called *thera-peutic range*, may serve to conclude this introduction. Hypocoagulability, as defined by this range, on the one hand powerfully counteracts the progression of thrombosis and on the other does not produce a danger-ous haemorrhagic diathesis. By trial and error, this therapeutic range has now been defined rather clearly (8, 13, 14, 15). The establishment of such a therapeutic range, however, depends on very close supervision of the patient, such as is realized by the program of the Netherlands Thrombosis Services. Under optimal conditions, short-acting coumarin congeners also appear to be useful in long-term anticoagulant treat-ment, although hypocoagulability is more constant when a long-acting preparation is used. (3). It must be realized, however, that the safety of the treatment is equally dependent on a delicately graduated dosage of the anticoagulant and, when necessary, of its antidotum *vitaminK*$_1$.

REFERENCES

1. Biggs, R., A. S. Douglas, The thromboplastin generation test. *J. Clin. Path.* 6, 23 (1953).
2. Esch, B. van der, E. A. Loeliger, De werking van coumarine-preparaten op de bloedstolling bij hoge initiële dosering. *Verslag 3e Conf. Thrombosediensten Ned. Roode Kruis*, Zeist, p. 26 (1960).
3. Fekkes, N., J. J. Veltkamp, E. A. Loeliger, *Acenocoumarin and phenprocoumon in long-term anticoagulant treatment. A controlled trial.* To be published.
4. Hemker, H. C., J. J. Veltkamp, A. Hensen, E. A. Loeliger, On the nature of prothrombin biosynthesis. *Nature*, 200, 589 (1963).
5. Hemker, H. C., J. J. Veltkamp, A. Hensen, E. A. Loeliger, Preprothrombin, a circulating anticoagulant in coumarin treated and vitamin K-deficient patients. Proc. Gleneagles Conf. of the Int. Comm. for the Nomenclature of blood clotting factors, 1963. *Thrombos. Diathes. haemorrh.* Suppl. 13 (1964).
6. Hemker, H. C., E. A. Loeliger, Kinetic aspects of the interaction of blood-clotting enzymes. III. Demonstration of the existance of an inhibitor of prothrombin conversion in vitamin K-deficiency. *Thrombos. Diathes. haemorrh.* 19, 346 (1968).
7. Josso, F., *Personal communication.*
8. Loeliger, E. A., A. Hensen, F. Kroes, L. M. van Dijk, N. Fekkes, H. de Jonge, H. C. Hemker, A double-blind trial of long-term anticoagulant treatment after myocardial infarction. *Acta Med. Scand.* 182, 549 (1967).
9. Loeliger, E. A., B. van der Esch, H. C. Hemker, M. J. Mattern, The biological disappearance rate of prothrombin, factors VII, IX, and X from plasma in hypothyroidism, hyperthyroidism, and during fever. *Thrombos. Diathes. haemorrh.* 10, 267 (1964).
10. Loeliger, E. A., B. van der Esch, M. J. Mattern, A. S. A. den Brabander, Behaviour of factors II, VII, IX, and X during long-term treatment with coumarin. *Thrombos. Diathes. haemorrh.* 9, 74 (1963).
11. Loeliger, E. A., A. Hensen, M. J. Mattern, H. C. Hemker, Behaviour of Factors II, VII, IX, and X in bleeding complications during long-term treatment with coumarin. *Thrombos. Diathes. haemorrh.* 10, 278 (1964).
12. Meer, J. van der, H. C. Hemker, E. A. Loeliger, Pharmacological aspects of vitamin K$_1$. *Thrombos. Diathes. haemorrh.* Suppl. 29 (1968).
13. Poller, L., Methods for the laboratory control of short-term anticoagulant therapy. *Acta haemat.* 28, 168 (1962).
14. Rozenberg, M. C., H. Kronenberg, B. G. Firkin, 'Thrombotest' and prothrombin time: A controlled clinical trial. *Aust. Ann. Med.* 14, 3 (1965).
15. Sevitt, S., D. Innes, Prothrombin-time and thrombotest in injured patients on prophylactic anticoagulant therapy. *Lancet*, I, 124 (1964).
16. Soulier, J. P., O. Prou-Wartelle, Etude comparative des taux de cofacteur de la staphylocoagulase (C.R.F.) et des taux de facteur II dans diverses conditions. *Nouv. Rev. Franç. Hémat.* 6, 623 (1966).

THE NETHERLANDS THROMBOSIS SERVICE

F. L. J. JORDAN

In 1949, a seminar was held at the Department of Medicine of the Utrecht University Hospital, on the problems with which the physician is faced in connection with new trends in medicine. Oral anticoagulant therapy was one of the topics discussed, at a time when this type of therapy had only recently been developed in the U. S. A.. Even then, the problem with which we are still dealing today, namely the reliable laboratory evaluation of blood, was mentioned. Few facilities were available at that time, only the bigger hospital having a coagulation laboratory. As a consequence, many patients who needed anticoagulants could not be given this form of treatment.

To fill this gap a 'Thrombosis Service' was founded by the University Hospital of Utrecht in July 1949. At the request of the general practioner, an experienced nurse visited the patient in his home to withdraw blood for laboratory tests. Ambulant patients were asked to come to the hospital during office hours. This made it possible to treat many unhospitalized patients properly. I will not enter here into such technical details as the organization of the service, the convenience offered to the patients and their physicians, and the additional advantage of fewer demands for admittance, thus diminishing the shortage of hospital beds. These problems are fully covered by earlier publications (1, 2).

In view of the needs on a nation-wide scale, negotiations were opened with the Netherlands Red Cross Organization, which agreed to participate in the creation of many 'Thrombosis Services' throughout The Netherlands.

Initially, the scientific board of the Red Cross Thrombosis Services advised the use of a modification of Quick's method. Later, the Thrombotest of Owren came under discussion, on which Dr. de Vries reports (page 314).

The Netherlands Thrombosis Service lends itself pre-eminently to controlled studies in large numbers of patients; for instance, the search for optimal anticoagulation, i.e. for effective hypocoagulability with an acceptable rate of bleeding complications; and the problem of how long the treatment should be continued. Continuation over too long a period of time exposes the patients to risks, but the same holds true for too short a period. In this respect myocardial infarction in particular has given rise to a serious controversy. Two Thrombosis Services in The Netherlands have carried out investigations on this point, which has made it possible to arrive at an answer to this question (pages 336 and 339).

Intercurrent diseases and the drugs used to combat them seem to be of growing importance in the elucidation of complications arising during anticoagulant therapy. As a consequence, every bleeding must be seen as an indication for a thorough investigation of the organ system concerned. Such investigation can lead to the detection of many abnormalities in an early stage, thus greatly benefitting the patient. A separate seminar would be required to discuss the whole field of diseases and drugs influencing the dose of anticoagulants. The unique part played by the liver in blood coagulation will be discussed later (page 361).

Even if, as we hope and expect, the future brings a form of treatment of thromboembolic processes not dependent on laboratory tests, which will make thrombosis services superfluous, for the present we must continue to the problem of coagulation tests, for patients suffering from haemorrhagic diathesis, liver disease, and many other pathological conditions.

REFERENCES

1. Jordan, F. L. J., The 'Thrombosis Service' at Utrecht. *Proc. 1st Int. Congr. Thromb. Embol.* Karger, Basel (1954).
2. Jordan, F. L. J., Organization of the 'Thrombosis Service' in the Netherlands. *Thrombos. Diathes. haemorrh.* 2, 527 (1958).

LABORATORY TESTS

Prothrombin time

THE MANCHESTER COMPARATIVE REAGENT

A NATIONAL REFERENCE STANDARD FOR ANTIGOAGULANT THERAPY

L. POLLER AND JEAN THOMSON

The scheme for providing uniform anticoagulant treatment with the Manchester Comparative Reagent (MCR) has been in operation for six years. It provides a service incorporating the majority of hospital centres in England, and a proportion in Scotland and Wales. It aims to give a standard for commercial and home-made tissue extract thromboplastin (4). The scheme has recently been endorsed by the British Committee for Standardisation in Haematology, and all hospitals have been encouraged to use it.

Table 1. Average results obtained with different thromboplastins from a group of patients, individual plasma specimens showing more marked variation (table 2) (3).

Reagents	mean prothrombin activity%	mean prothrombin ratio
Standard (Manchester Comparative Reagent)	32	1.9
Simplastin	63	1.2
Geigy	49	1.4
Ortho	49	1.3
Diagen (dried)	58	1.5
Difco	37	1.3
Dade	29	1.4
Thrombotest	23	1.7

Before our scheme was introduced, individual hospital pathologists had no yardstick to standardise successive batches of their own home-made reagents or favourite commercial extract. Not only is there still considerable difference between the different commercial extracts, but considerable inter-batch variation. Human brain extracts are widely used in Britain and are the most popular. There are good grounds for the belief that human brain is the most satisfactory reagent for measuring

Table 2. Activity (in %) obtained in four patients.

Reagents	Patient No.			
	1	2	3	4
Manchester Comparative Reagent	34	16	32	32
Thrombotest	22	9	24	16
II, VII, X	32	10	29	21
Simplastin	70	60	100	78
Acuplastin	100	32	50	42
Geigy	65	45	50	55
Stayne	30	19	28	30
Diagen (dried)	56	24	35	46
Difco	45	19	30	30
Dade	30	15	26	28

human extrinsic system blood clotting factors because of its species specificity.

The prothrombin time ratio is a measure of the sensitivity of a reagent to the coagulation defect produced by oral anticoagulants. No commercial Quick test thromboplastin gives as good prothrombin ratios as our human brain standard, and in our recent survey nearly all human brain preparations made at the individual hospitals were far superior to the commercial extracts (see table 3). Many commercial

Table 3. The results of a recent national survey in which a variety of thromboplastins were used (5). The term prothrombin ratio has been used, and we calculated the figures corresponding to 1.7 and 3.0 found with the Manchester reagent at the 72 hospitals participating in the study.

Type of tissue extract	No. of Hospitals	Prothrombin ratio = 1.7 (33% prothrombin activity) with Manchester Comparative Reagent	Prothrombin ratio = 3.0 (15% prothrombin activity) with Manchester Comparative Reagent
Human brain thromboplastin	38	1.7	2.9
Simplastin	10	1.3	1.9
Geigy	6	1.6	2.6
Difco	4	1.4	2.1
Diagen	6	1.4	2.6
Stayne	6	1.4	2.1
Ortho	2	1.2	1.6

extracts are particularly insensitive to factor VII depression. Human brain also has advantages as a standard, because of the large bulk of material that can be manufactured at one time, particularly with our methods of production (see page 294). This allows us to obtain enormous quantities of reagent in a single batch. It may be possible, however, to manufacture animal tissue extracts of adequate sensitivity, but this has not yet been done commercially. One group of hospitals that participates in our standard scheme does in fact produce an admirable home-made rabbit brain preparation, superior to any commercial extract. There is no reason, therefore, why our standard scheme based on human brain could not be applied abroad where human brain reagents are not available, provided that the standard is shown to be of adequate sensitivity. A lyophilised preparation of our material could be used as a standard for this also. The existence of a functioning national scheme may thus pave the way for an international standard to provide uniform anticoagulant treatment.

The service is a two-tier one, as illustrated by figure 1.

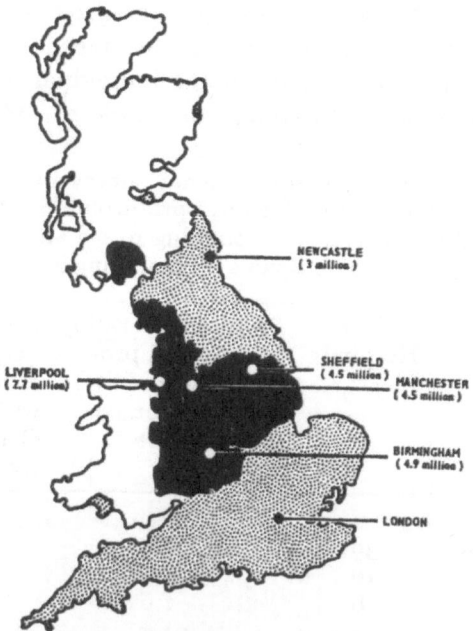

Fig. 1. Service areas for the MCR thromboplastin.
a. A routine supply scheme covering area in black, with a population of 15 millions.
b. The standard scheme in clotted areas covers the rest of the country with relatively few hospitals receiving routine supplies.

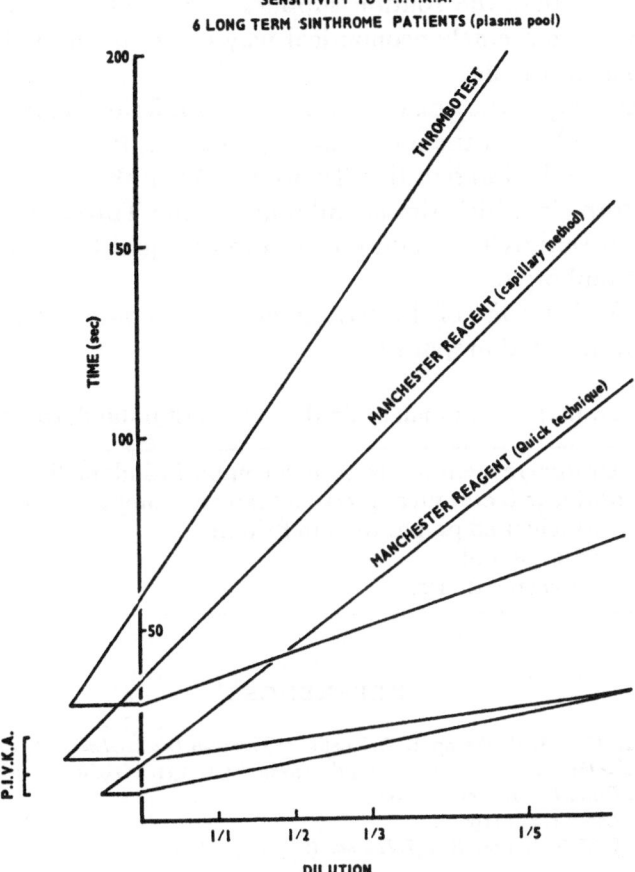

SENSITIVITY TO P.I.V.K.A.
6 LONG TERM SINTHROME PATIENTS (plasma pool)

Fig. 2. Sensitivity to PIVKA demonstrated by the use of an animal brain thromboplastin (Thrombotest) and a human brain thromboplastin (the Manchester Reagent) in plasma from 6 patients on long-term Sinthrome anticoagulant therapy.

The Manchester standard reference scheme does not change the existing system of testing and reporting at the individual hospitals. It does provide a check on the variations of successive batches of homemade or commercial preparations as well as a constant check on deterioration, which happens sooner or later with all types of thromboplastin. In this way we have linked up with a number of well-established local schemes. The standard scheme also allows the use of the same therapeutic range as that employed in a number of current therapeutic trials. The national standard scheme uses an extremely small quantity of reagent, less than the routine supplies of a single large hospital. It is therefore an extremely economical way of producing uniformity of control on a large scale.

The sensitivity of the MCR to PIVKA (1) is not inferior to that of Thrombotest, although with the unmodified Quick test, the Manchester reagent appears to be less sensitive (figure 2). When the MCR is used in its capillary form, in which similar dilutions to the Thrombotest method are used, its sensitivity to PIVKA is seen to be equal to or greater than that of Thrombotest.

Finally, I give a list of the advantages of a human brain thromboplastin as a standard preparation:

Table 4. Advantages of human brain thromboplastin standard (MCR)

---

1. A most sensitive reagent to the human coumarin-indanedione effect.
2. More sensitive to factor VII depression than any commercial product.
3. The most widely used preparation in Britain.
4. Available in large bulk.
5. Constant between batches.

REFERENCES

1. Hemker, H. C., J. J. Veltkamp, E. A. Loeliger, *Thrombos. Diathes. haemorrh.* 19, 346 (1968).
2. Poller L. *The theory and practice of anticoagulant treatment*, p. 131. Wright - Bristol (1962).
3. Poller, L., *Brit. Med. J.* 2, 565 (1964).
4. Poller, L., *Lancet* 1, 491 (1967).
5. Poller, L., J. M. Thomson, *Brit. J. Haemat.* (in press) (1968).

PREPARATION OF A SALINE EXTRACT OF HUMAN BRAIN THROMBOPLASTIN (Poller 1962; 2)

A brain should be obtained at autopsy within 24 hours of death.

The superficial vessels and meninges are completely removed and the cerebellum is discarded. The brain is thoroughly rinsed in distilled water to remove all traces of blood and then cut into thin slices.

The brain is macerated for 2 minutes in 1500 ml normal saline preheated to 45°C, using a mixer or alternatively a blender.

The resulting emulsion is then incubated at 37°C (water-bath) for 30 minutes, stirring occasionally. It is then placed at 4°C in the refrigerator and left overnight for maximum extraction.

The emulsion is then centrifuged in 500 ml blood bottles at 2,000 r.p.m. for 15 minutes in a refrigerated centrifuge at a temperature of 4°C.

The supernatant is then collected and it should appear slightly turbid. Each brain yields approximately 800-1000 ml of saline extract. A satisfactory extract should give a pro-thrombin time of 10-12 seconds with normal pooled plasma.

The extract can be stored either:

In a deep-freezer at -20°C where it will remain stable and keep its activity for several months. Repeated thawing and freezing is detrimental. A reserve stock is kept deepfrozen. (In the absence of a homogenizer of the type mentioned, perfectly satisfactory prepara-tions can be made with a slightly more laborious technique. The brain is cut into small slices and placed in a large mortar; it is then pounded with a pestle, warm saline being added in increasing amounts up to 1500 ml of normal saline, and after adequate pounding the thick emulsion is decanted and centrifuged as in the above method).

Or at 4°C after adding 0.5 per cent phenol to the extract. In this way it will remain stable for several weeks, but it must not be frozen.

After storing for two weeks, at -20°C, during which maximum activation occurs, the saline extract is ready for assay, after phenol has been added.

At least six human brains are used in each pool.

DISCUSSION

Stormorken: I should like to ask Miss Thomson about the batch-to-batch control of thromboplastin preparations. We refer to a pool of plasma from 30 normal donors. The preparation of a stable standard plasma reflecting normality is difficult and time consuming, and we have not yet succeeded in producing it on a large scale. On the other hand, we have prepared a Primary Standard for both the Normotest and the Thrombotest that can be stored for years. So we use a double check, one to the Primary Standard and the other to the Normal Plasma. Dr. Tryding, in Sweden, found an average value of 98 per cent Normotest in a large normal material.

Thomson: Each batch of thromboplastin is monitored by comparing it to the preceding batch. We use a saline dilution curve and a pool of at least six normal plasmas with which we check the therapeutic points. The thromboplastin is also monitored against coumarin plasmas from patients within the therapeutic range. If there is a difference between batches of plus or minus one second, it is adjusted accordingly. We do not find great inter-batch variation. We do not use our standard dried plasma for testing batches of reagent; it is used as a check on technique at the different hospitals.

Stormorken: A pool of six normal plasmas is not necessarily adequate, because it may display any value between 80 and 120 per cent. If there is activation in only one of the six samples, the entire pool will be activated.

Thomson: Activation does not matter a great deal with our reagent because, unlike Thrombotest, it is not very contact sensitive.

Loeliger: Our normal pooled plasma standard is prepared from 30 persons with a mean age of 30 years and equal numbers of males and females. We have checked ten Thrombotest batches with this plasma pool and have obtained results identical to those indicated by the Oslo group.

Owren: Dr. Thomson's statement that human brain preparations are just as sensitive to inhibitors as Thrombotest is not consistent with our findings. We have found higher values with the Manchester Comparative Reagent than with Thrombotest when testing coumarin plasma, also with techniques securing equal dilutions of the test plasma in the final reaction mixtures. This confirms our statement that thromboplastin prepared from human brain is less sensitive to the PIVKA inhibitor than thromboplastin prepared from ox brain.

Thomson: We have shown previously that the lower percentage results with Thrombotest are not due to greater sensitivity to coumarin-affected clotting factors but to excess adsorbed plasma in the Thrombotest technique. If the Quick test results are read from an adsorbed plasma curve instead of a saline curve, the percentages are similar. As far as PIVKA is concerned our reagent appears just as sensitive when used with a Thrombotest-like technique.

LABORATORY TESTS

Thrombotest

THE HISTORY OF THROMBOTEST

P. A. OWREN

We have in recent years witnessed a revolution in laboratory investigations, characterized by an ever-increasing number of tests and computerized automated systems for greater speed, productivity, and economy. An essential aspect of this steadily growing outflow of test results is that the data presented are meaningful and can be used by the clinician to improve diagnosis and therapy. This fortunately holds for most tests, but laboratory data for the purpose of guiding anticoagulant therapy have for years been neither meaningful nor comprehensive or reliable.

In order to be meaningful, these methods should measure those essential changes that are relevant to the guiding of anticoagulant therapy, in such a way that treatment would be both safe and efficient. This means that the method applied should reflect exactly those properties that govern the haemostatic function on the one hand and the antithrombotic affect on the other hand. Only when such methods are available is it possible to define the optimal therapeutic level of hypocoagulability that will assure safe navigation between Scylla and Charybdis, giving maximal therapeutic effect with minimal risk.

When anticoagulant therapy with dicumarol was introduced into clinical medicine more than 20 years ago, Quick's prothrombin time test was generally adopted for its control. In retrospect, it is interesting to notice that specific determination of prothrombin by the two-stage method was found to be misleading by resulting in a high incidence of bleeding complications. Quick's test obviously reflected other factors besides prothrombin, which were unknown at that time. This test is still in widespread use, but has been modified by substituting different commercial and laboratory prepared tissue extracts for the original rabbit brain thromboplastin of Quick. It has been recognized for many years now that different thromboplastins give highly different results, and the need for standardization of thromboplastins and methods has been stressed repeatedly. We are still far from a general and successful solution of this problem. The subject has been under study for several years by the working party on the standardization of the one-stage prothrombin time, which was appointed by the International Committee on Haemostasis and Thrombosis. Annual progress reports by Biggs and Denson (1, 2, 3), based on continuing international cooperative study, illuminates the chaotic situation which has been created by the use of different and poorly standardized thromboplastins giving different results from one laboratory to another and from one batch of the reagent to another. Thrombotest and its British twin the 'two-seven-ten reagent' were the only exceptions giving reproducible results. With other thromboplastins, differences of up to 3 to 4 times the lowest recorded activity were found by testing of the same plasma in different laboratories. Taken into consideration that criteria for the therapeutic level has also varied from one place to another, it is not surprising that bleeding complications have varied from an incidence of more than 100 to below 1 per 100 treatment years, and the therapeutic effect from zero to impressively good results.

The story of the Thrombotest method goes back to my studies on factor v deficiency in 1943-45. I then devised a modification of Quick's prothrombin time test, which was later termed the P & P (prothrombin-proconvertin) method (8, 9, 10). Rabbits were not available in our country at that time, and I therefore substituted human brain for rabbit brain as a source of thromboplastin. Secondly, I introduced adsorbed ox plasma as an additional reagent for securing an optimal concentration of factor v and fibrinogen in the reaction mixture under all conditions. This modifications has several advantages. I shall only mention that diluted test plasma could be used, whereby the all-over sensitivity was increased as illustrated by the steeper correlation curve (figure 1).

When I introduced dicumarol therapy in Norway in 1948, I first did a study comparing Quick's prothrombin time test and the P & P method. After controlling some hundred patients over some months I discarded Quick's method for several reasons. Most important was the finding that different batches of acetone-treated rabbit brain tended to give different results at testing of the same plasma, the same finding as reported by Biggs and Denson in more elaborate studies. Other drawbacks were the lower sensitivity, the specified calcium concentration for recalcification became inoptimal at abnormal hematocrit values and reproducibility required performance of the test within one-half hour after drawing the specimen, a requirement which is often difficult to satisfy in the average laboratory. The correlation curve for transforming prothrombin times in seconds into percentage activity had to

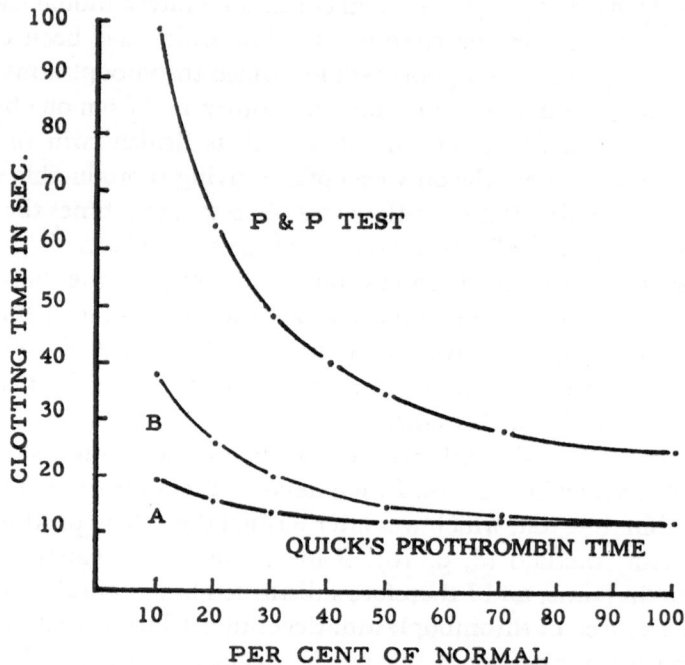

Fig. 1. Correlation curves for converting clotting time in seconds into per cent of normal. The curves are prepared by testing serial dilutions of a normal standard plasma. For the prothrombin time test, adsorbed normal plasma should be used as a diluent. (Curve A). The use of saline for dilution (Curve B) leads to false prolongation of the prothrombin time for higher dilutions, because of inoptimal concentrations of factor v and fibrinogen. For the P & P method (and Thrombotest) saline can be used, because factor v and fibrinogen are provided for by adsorbed ox plasma.

be prepared with adsorbed plasma as diluent and not with saline, because serial dilutions with saline gave a false prolongation of the prothrombin time in higher dilutions due to deficient concentrations of factor v and fibrinogen.

We used the P & P method for about 10 years in thousands of patients, but I was not completely satisfied with the results. We observed slight differences between results based on different batches, but more

Table 1. Patients who experienced bleeding complications and had a prolongation of the bleeding time as a sign of overdosage, but who nevertheless showed therapeutic levels with the P & P method and different prothrombin time methods.

Patient No.	Type of bleeding	Bleeding time in min.	P & P %	Prothrombin times in sec.			
				Human brain	Rabbit brain	Geigy	Simplastin
1	Haematuria	18	12	34	25	27	25
2	—"—	25	13	37	24	30	28
3	Ecchymosis	20	14	36	28	34	26
4	Bruises	13	15	35	25	33	27
5	Haematuria	30	10	36	30	35	30
Normal plasma				15	12	16	14
Therapeutic range				30–37	24–30	32–40	28–35

important was the observation that bleeding complications occasionally occured at P & P levels in the therapeutic range of 10-25 per cent which we used at that time. Some of these patients had a prolongation of the Borchgrevink bleeding time as a definite sign of overdosage. We also checked these same patients with Quick's prothrombin time test, using different thromboplastins, and all these tests gave values that are generally assumed to be quite safe (table 1). Consequently, anticoagulant therapy seemed to produce changes in haemostasis that were not picked up by any of these methods. These disturbing observations led to renewed investigations on thromboplastins and methodology, and resulted in the Thrombotest method.

At that time, we believed, like others, that many bleedings were caused by a deficiency of factor IX (antihaemophilia B factor) in addition to the depression of the extrinsic clotting system. We actually also found excessively low values of factor IX in some patients with bleeding complications. I therefore tried to develop a method which would be sensitive to the depression of factor IX under these circumstances. The P & P method was modified by introducing a thromboplastin preparation with low activity, in order to slow down the extrinsic clotting system, and a cephalin preparation with high activity, in order to increase the rate of the intrinsic system. It was actually found that this system had a certain sensitivity to the severe depression of factor IX in patients subjected to acute overdosage.

The second modification, which has since been found to be more important, concerned the technique of preparation of the thromboplastin.

Table 2. Incidence of haemorrhagic complications in different studies, using different methods for control. The average maintenance dosage used in the study of Borchgrevink (P & P method) and in the study at the Institute for Thrombosis Research (Thrombotest) were 110 mg and 109 mg, respectively. The incidence of bleeding complications, however, were 7 and 0.7, respectively.

Authors		Method	Bleedings per 100 patient treatment years	
Pastor, Resnick & Rodman	(1961)	Simplastin	140	Total
Wright & Tullock	(1954)	Link-Shapiro	39	,,
Bjerkelund	(1957)	P-P, 20%	7.5	,,
Borchgrevink	(1960)	P-P, 19%	7.0	,,
Institute for Thrombosis Research	(1963)	T-T, 15%	0.7	,,
Roos & Joost	(1965)	T-T, 11%	6.0	,,
Loeliger	(1965)	T-T, 8%	10	,,

We were aiming at preparing a completely uniform thromboplastin both physicochemically and also with respect to the biological activity. The latter object was reached by purification and complete removal of residual traces of serum clotting factors and clotting intermediates from the crude extract. Clinical studies to compare the new method, called the Thrombotest method, and the P & P method revealed that Thrombotest was superior to the P & P method in heralding bleeding complications. In groups of patients treated to the same level of intensity, as evaluated from an identical average maintenance dosage, the incidence of bleeding complications was reduced from about 7 to below 1 bleeding episode per 100 treatment years (table 2). By testing patients at low levels we found correlation between the Borchgrevink bleeding time and the Thrombotest value (figure 2). In large clinical series, the incidence of bleeding episodes has been found to be well correlated with the mean Thrombotest value (figure 3). Empirically, it may be concluded, therefore, that the Thrombotest method is sensitive to those specific changes that determine bleeding tendency. What, then is responsible for these changes?

It certainly is not factor IX as was generally assumed before factor X was discovered. When methods became available for measuring factor X, we found that this factor was disproportionately reduced in patients stabilized on anticoagulant therapy. The Thrombotest results closely followed the recorded factor X activity, which again correlated with bleeding time and clinical bleedings. We therefore concluded that low factor X activity is the most frequent cause of bleeding complications

in stabilized patients. Loeliger (6) objected to this conclusion because he found all factors depressed in parallel during anticoagulant
therapy. These controversial results seem to be explained by the
very important discovery of Hemker, Veltkamp, Hensen and Loeliger

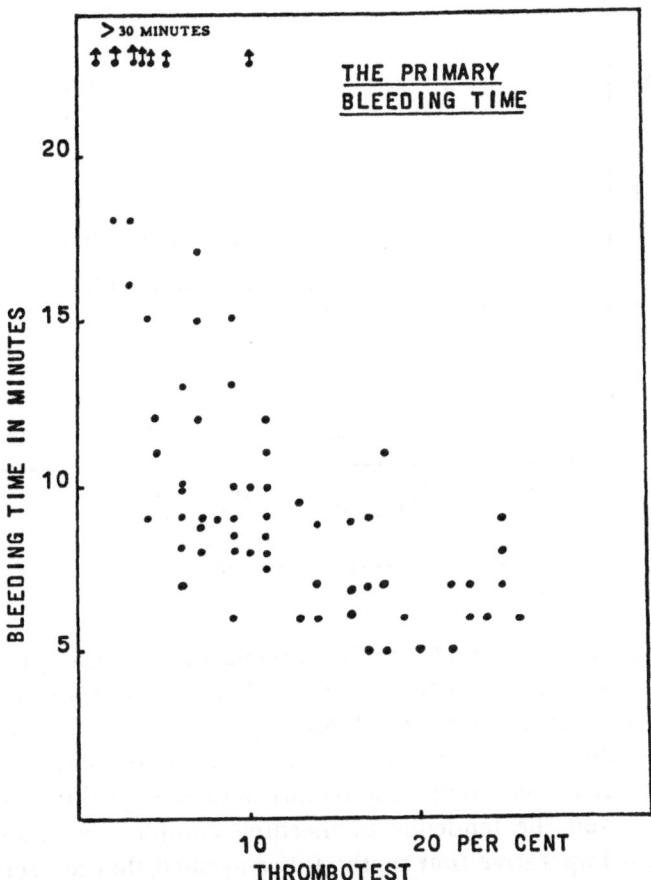

Fig. 2. The relation between the Thrombotest value and the bleeding time. All determinations were done in patients on long-term anticoagulant therapy, some with overdosage and
bleeding complications.

in 1963 (5) that anticoagulant therapy is associated with the occurrence
of an endogenous inhibitor, presumably a precursor of prothrombin.
This is the most important discovery made in this field in recent
years. Endogenous coagulation inhibitors are characterized by progressive reduction of activity by increasing dilutions of the test plas-

ma. The Thrombotest method has a dilution factor for whole blood in the final reaction mixture of only 1:6 and the same was true for our method for factor x estimation. We used charcoal-adsorbed ox plasma as being relatively free of factor x, but with residual prothrombin and

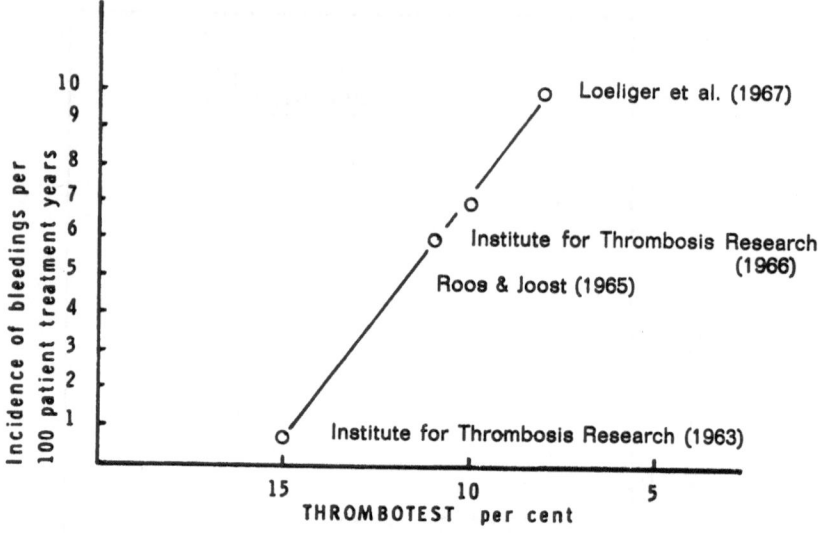

Fig. 3. The relation between the incidence of bleeding complications in large series and the mean Thrombotest value.

factor VII, and we used ox brain thromboplastin, which required a volume of test plasma similar to that used in Thrombotest. Both methods, therefore, are sensitive to the inhibitor.

During anticoagulant therapy the effect of the inhibitor adds to the effect of the reduction of clotting factors both as regarding antithrombotic effect and the tendency to bleeding complications; and consequently it is imperative that methods are applied that are sensitive to the inhibitor effect. The second point of importance is that the Thrombotest reagent, is meticulously standardized concerning all components of the reagent, and it is completely stable in the freeze-dried form in evacuated ampoules. Correlation curves for the method are based on the use of a standardized reference plasma of constant activity, and this provides for reproducibility of results for different batches and from one laboratory to another. These are important points concerning the general usefulness of a biological method.

The second main problem in anticoagulant therapy is the definition of therapeutic level. The recent studies of Loeliger and collaborators (7) seem to have answered the question why clinical results of therapeutic trials have been so inconsistent. The following diagram, which is from their paper (figure 4), demonstrates that low intensity of therapy is equi-

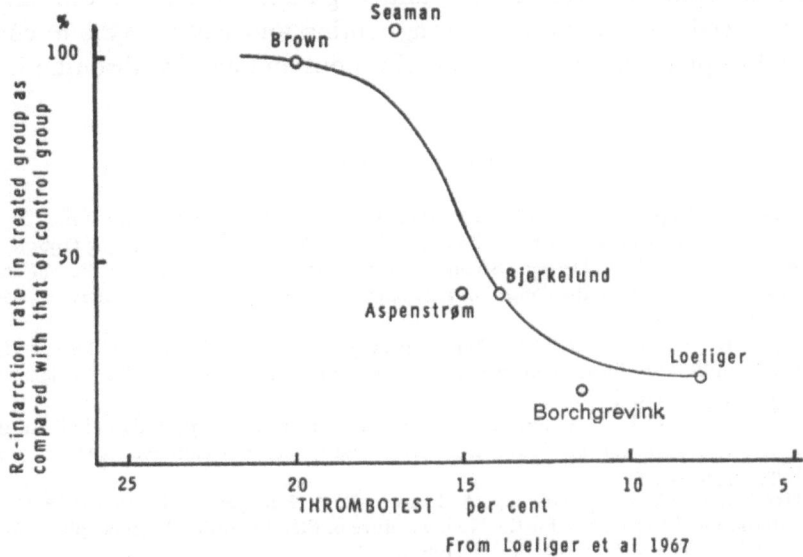

From Loeliger et al 1967

Fig. 4. The relation between the intensity of therapy as measured by the Thrombotest method and the re-infarction rate in survivors of myocardial infarction. From Loeliger and collaborators (7).

valent to no therapy, whereas high intensity has a highly beneficial effect. For many years, before convincing therapeutic results had been demonstrated, we preferred to play safe according to the rule of '*Nil nocere*' and aimed at a P & P level of about 20% and a Thrombotest level of 15%. Bleeding episodes were minimal and we obtained good results in venous thrombosis and also in angina pectoris, as demonstrated by the study of Borchgrevink (4). Loeliger informed me at an early stage of their studies that an intensity of 7-8% as measured by the Thrombotest method was associated with an acceptable low incidence of 10 bleeding complications per 100 treatment years. Since then we have been aiming at a level of 10% in arterial thrombosis and our incidence of bleeding complications has in later years been 7 per 100 treatment years. We are still using the level of 15% for the prevention of venous and intracardial thrombosis, particularly during the postoperative period and in rheumatic heart disease, and we have found that this intensity provides good protection under these circumstances.

In conclusion I would say that thanks to the very important contributions to this field from The Netherlands, anticoagulant therapy has ultimately been placed on a sound and strong footing and will in years to come defend its place in the prevention of venous and arterial thrombosis.

REFERENCES

1. Biggs, R., Report on the standardisation of the one-stage prothrombin time for the control of anticoagulant therapy. *Thrombos. Diathes. haemorrh.* Suppl. 17, 303 (1965).
2. Biggs, R., K. W. E. Denson, Second report on the standardisation of the one-stage prothrombin time for the control of anticoagulant therapy. *Thrombos. Diathes. haemorrh.* Suppl. 20, 345 (1966).
3. Biggs, R., K. W. E. Denson, Third report on the standardisation of the one-stage prothrombin time for the control of anticoagulant therapy. *Thrombos. Diathes. haemorrh.*, Suppl. 24, 445 (1966).
4. Borchgrevink, C. F., Long-term anticoagulant therapy in angina pectoris and myocardial infarction. A clinical trial between intensive and moderate treatment. *Acta med. scand.* Suppl. 359, 52 (1960).
5. Hemker, H. C,. J. J. Veltkamp, A. Hensen, E. A. Loeliger, Proc. Gleneagles Conf., International Committee for the Nomenclature of Blood Clotting Factors 1963. *Thrombos. Diathes. haemorrh.* Suppl. 13, 380 (1964).
6. Loeliger, E. A., A. Hensen, M. J. Mattern, H. C. Hemker, Factors II, VII, IX, and X in bleeding complications during long-term treatment with coumarin. *Thrombos. Diathes. haemorrh.* 10, 278 (1964).
7. Loeliger, E. A., A. Hensen, F. Kroes, L. M. van Dijk, N. Fekkes, H. de Jonge, H. C. Hemker, A double-blind trial of long-term anticoagulant treatment after myocardial infarction. *Acta med. scand.* 182, 549 (1967).
8. Owren, P. A., The coagulation of blood. Investigations on a new clotting factor. *Acta med. scand.* Suppl. 194,327 (1947).
9. Owren, P. A., A quantitative one-stage method for the assay of prothrombin. *Scand. J. clin. Lab. Invest.* 1, 81 (1949).
10. Owren, P. A., K. Aas, The control of dicumarol therapy and the quantitative determination of prothrombin and proconvertin. *Scand. J. clin. Lab. Invest.* 3, 201 (1951).

QUALITY CONTROL OF THROMBOTEST (TT)
AND NORMOTEST (NT)

H. STORMORKEN

Concerning reagents for the control of anticoagulant treatment, the work by the subcommittee of the International Committee for Haemostasis and Thrombosis under the chairmanship of Dr. Rosemary Biggs, Oxford, has shown that the requirements are not fulfilled by most preparations available (1). Since the same reagents are used for estimating coagulation activity in the near-normal range, such as in liver diseases, the same applies also in this case.

Table 1 is from the first report of the subcommittee (2). One normal blood sample and one sample from a patient on anticoagulant treat-

Table 1. Results obtained with different thromboplastin preparations, expressed in various terms.

Method	Clotting time of plasma sample in sec		Clotting time difference (sec)	Ratio Dindevan/ normal	% of normal	
	Undiluted normal	Dindevan			Saline dilution	Adsorbed plasma dilution
Geigy	16.4	24.8	8.4	1.50	32	28
Dade (rabbit brain)	12.5	20.8	8.3	1.76	31	24
Stayne (rabbit brain)	15.6	21.8	6.2	1.41	36	22
Difco (rabbit brain)	13.0	20.0	7.0	1.52	36	26
Simplastin	13.8	17.2	3.4	1.25	70	46
Acuplastin	15.7	26.2	10.5	1.77	24	19
Laboratory human brain	16.6	26.0	10.0	1.73	—	26
Thrombotest	38.5	80	41.5	2.1	14	21
II / VII / X	34.5	77	43.5	2.2	18	24
P & P	33	81	48.0	2.35	27	27

From: Biggs, R. (1).

ment were tested with ten different preparations. As can be seen, the results vary very considerably (14-70%).

Miale and Lafond (3) distributed one normal and one anticoagulated blood sample to 1177 different hospitals in the U.S.A.; the results were as illustrated in figure 1. With the normal, the results varied from 100 to 40 per cent and with the anticoagulant sample from 10 to 66 per cent.

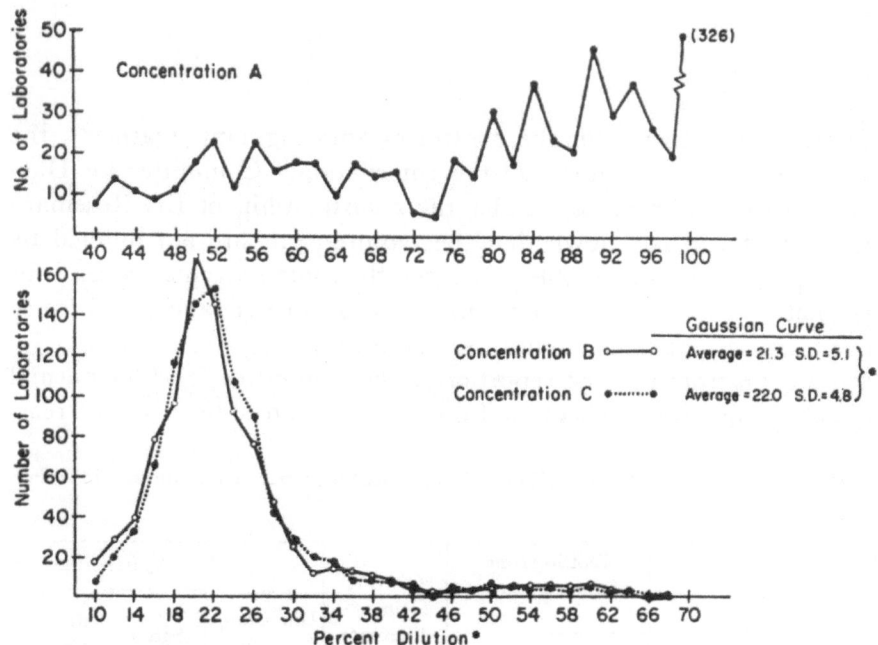

Fig. 1. Distribution of values reported for plasmas A, B, and C when values are given in 'percentage of normal' based on the dilution curve. From: Miale, J. B., D. J. Lafond, *Am. J. clin. Path.*, 47, 40 (1967).

It should be clear from this that in no other area of laboratory medicine is the situation equally bad, and that it must not be allowed to persist. In view of the fact that the drugs in question might be potentially lifesaving or fatally dangerous, the situation represents a shame for the medical profession. The use of such reagents, whether produced in local laboratories or commercially, without a rigorous quality control therefore must not continue.

The following requirements should be fullfilled for a laboratory test reagent:

1. Sensitivity of adequate degree to all factors influencing the final result.
2. Identity of subsamples within batches and from batch to batch.
3. Stability within a defined period of time.
4. Reproducibility both within one laboratory and between laboratories.

Sensitivity

The sensitivity of the preparations may be divided into general sensitivity and specific sensitivity. The general sensitivity represents the clotting time that the preparation gives with normal plasma. This should therefore be checked with normal standard plasma of constant activity; and to secure a reproducible sensitivity it is necessary to rigorously follow a detailed production procedure from the time the brain is taken out to the final product.

The specific sensitivity concerns the sensitivity of these preparations to each single factor taking part in the reaction. A main point in the production procedure is to avoid contamination of the reagent with these factors, because such contamination will decrease the sensitivity to the factor in question in the test plasma. By the specific way of producing the Thrombotest and the Normotest reagents, contamination of these factors is avoided. To make absolutely certain, the reagents have to be checked with plasmas deficient in each separate factor.

Identity

Since the reagent consists of more than one component, it is of course not only the thromboplastin component that needs to be exactly identical from test to test. Thus, the adsorbed plasma present must be manufactured in the same way throughout. It should be freed of barium sulphate, free of fibrinogen breakdown products, which may inhibit the coagulation process, and of course free of the factors to be assayed (II, VII, IX, X) and have a high content of factor V and reactive fibrinogen. Its ionic strength should also be carefully checked. Furthermore, the calcium concentration should be carefully considered, to obtain optimal calcium in the final reaction mixture. Identity also relates to the amount distributed in each ampoule after mixing the different components. Thus, each ampoule is continuously monitored by weighing, and all ampoules outside ± 2SD are discarded. Finally, identity is also affected by the freeze-drying procedure, but this procedure is more important for the following requirement.

Stability

Stability is mainly dependent on two factors, i.e. the freeze-drying procedure and the storage in evacuated sealed ampoules. A specific freeze-
drying procedure has therefore been worked out, taking into account
the freezing temperature, time, and the water content of the final preparation. By careful freeze-drying and storage in evacuated sealed
ampoules, stability is guaranteed for $1\frac{1}{2}$ years. We have, however, examples showing that five years old ampoules still give the same result as
they originally did.

Before a batch is released for sale, a representative cohort of ampoules
are tested for stability in four dilutions every week for three months in
two independent places. If there is any change during this time, the
batch is discarded, but this is a rare occurrence.

To do all these controls, a reliable standard plasma is required. This
represents the most intricate problem in the whole control procedure.
Production of such a plasma is extremely difficult, since one has to take
into account that the coagulation factors in question should represent
the normal level of an acceptably large population, and no activation
whatsoever should occur during the preparation. The problem of producing enough standard plasma to furnish with each batch, as would be desirable, has therefore not yet been solved. Each new batch has to be meticulously cross-checked against earlier preparations, which is very time
consuming. To overcome some of these difficulties, the producer has
established an 'original' or 'primitive' TT and NT standard. This consists of five batches which have undergone a very careful testing and
which have the sensitivity, identity, and stability necessary for such a
standard. All new batches are checked against these five, using four
blood samples representing the whole area between high and low activity. This primitive standard is stored under conditions securing stability for several years, and can therefore also serve as a back-check on
the standard plasma produced at any time. By this means, one has established a double control that should secure a preparation that is
constant. Consequently, results obtained with it may be compared from
place to place and from test to test. This is of great importance for comparing and evaluating clinical results. That the activity of this preparation reflects the normal level, has been shown in a population study
in Sweden, where it was demonstrated that among 214 normal persons
the distribution was normal with a mean of 98 per cent and a standard
deviation of 15 per cent.

Reproducibility

With a preparation fulfilling the above criteria, reproducibility is mainly dependent on: 1. the blood sampling, 2. a sharp endpoint, and 3. the skill of the technician and the accuracy of the automatic device, if used. It is necessary to follow strictly the instructions for blood sampling. If, for example, capillary sampling is not restricted to the first drop only, the results will be falsely high (short coagulation time), because thrombin formation will have started in subsequent drops. The endpoint is easy to read with both these reagents, and at this stage reproducibility depends on the skill and experience of the technician and the accuracy of any automatic device used.

REFERENCES

1. Biggs, R., *Thrombos. Diathes. haemorrh.*, Suppl. 2, (1963).
2. Biggs, R., *Thrombos. Diathes. haemorrh.*, Suppl. 17, (1965).
3. Miale, J. B., D. J. Lafond, *Am. J. Clin. Path.*, 47, 40 (1967).

INTRODUCTION OF THROMBOTEST AT
THE NETHERLANDS THROMBOSIS SERVICES

S. I. DE VRIES

I have been asked to explain in a few words why the Scientific Commit-tee of the Thrombosis Service of the Netherlands Red Cross has re-commended the use of Owren's 'Thrombotest' for the control of patients suffering from thrombo-embolic diseases and treated with indirect-acting anticoagulants.

The organization of the Thrombosis Services in The Netherlands is now almost twenty years old. In 1951, the first service was founded by Professor Jordan, Utrecht, who may be considered the father of the Thrombosis Service. In fact, this service was the first of this kind in the world.

Each local division has complete autonomy, and acts under the supervision of a physician, preferably an internist. He looks after the laboratory control of the patients and gives advice, either to the patient or his family doctor about the dosage of the drug and the frequency of the control. However, the medical director is not responsible for what happens if his advice is not followed. He never acts as the physician in charge of the patient. It is not his business to control whether the diag-nosis and the indication for treatment are correct or not. He does not examine the patient. Therefore, the advice given by the Thrombosis Service is primarily based on laboratory figures and refers only to the dosage of anticoagulants.

The autonomy of the medical director implies a free choice of the laboratory technique in his division, frequency of the controls, the se-lection of the anticoagulant, and the regulation of its dosage.

It will be clear that the Scientific Committee is actually an Advisory Board.

One of the various activities of our Committee has been to give ad-vice on laboratory control, particularly with respect to assay procedures.

One of the first things we did was to recommend the one-stage pro-

314

thrombin time according to Quick and to discard obsolete 'bed-side' methods. A simple manual was provided, containing the necessary details about reagents and how to perform the test. Although this alone meant considerable improvement, problems were still manifold. Some laboratories had human brain thromboplastin at their disposal; other services, however, used commercial preparations from different sources, with divergent sensitivity for the factors x and VII. Patients who travelled from one country or continent to another had to see a doctor every three weeks or even more often. Their dosage was determined in different laboratories using different thromboplastin preparations.

These shortcomings made it highly desirable to arrive at a standardized preparation. During the Congress of the European Society of Haematology at Copenhagen (1957) the same problem has been dealt with seriously and a project was devised for the distribution of a standardized human brain thromboplastin, but unfortunately nothing came out.

In The Netherlands, serious consideration was given to the preparation of standardized human brain thromboplastin to be put at the disposal of the Red Cross Thrombosis Services. Of the numerous difficulties encountered, we may mention the following:

a. The availability of large quantities is dependent on obtaining permission for autopsy from the family of the deceased, especially for the so-called complete autopsy, which includes the removal of the brain.
b. The length of the interval between death and autopsy may influence the autolysis of organs.
c. The possibility of delays in transportation make it necessary to keep a sufficiently large supply in stock.

During this period, Owren's Thrombotest became known in this country, and before giving further attention to the project of human brain thromboplastin we decided to investigate the possibilities of the introduction of the Thrombotest on a large scale.

Therefore, we had to take the following facts into account:

1. The reliability of the test, which means a great sensitivity of the reagent for the coagulation factors x and VII.
2. The test has to be carried out by people who are not skilled laboratory-workers.

3. The costs of introduction of the test, considered mainly from the point of view of the financial policy of the Thrombosis Services.
4. Finally, it had to be established that the Thrombotest meant a real improvement in the control of the patients under treatment, because this plea must be well-reasoned during negotiations with the authorities who would provide the financial support (health insurance).

After the results of a trial in two centres became known (The Hague and Leiden), our Committee decided unanimously to recommend the Thrombotest for the control of patients.

To summarize the favourable properties of Thrombotest, we may say that:

1. It is a great advantage that results are exchange able, both nationally and internationally. The still increasing tendency of people on this planet to travel from one end to the other has now become possible for those who are under 'long-term' treatment with anticoagulants.
   The already-mentioned international project has become a fact by the discovery of Thrombotest.
2. The Thrombotest can be learnt easily and is not difficult to perform by laboratory-workers who are not skilled coagulation technicians. Standardization of the reagent is not necessary; it has been done already by the firm, following a verification-chart added to each package. The reagent is stable. It can be shipped and held without deterioration. The test can be performed with both venous and capillary blood. The introduction of the Thrombotest involves neither the laboratory staff nor the purchase of expensive equipment.
3. Although in the beginning economic additions to problems seemed an obstacle because of the cost of the reagent, they have been overcome quite easily. Personally I have never considered this a serious matter. It is certainly not a reason for going back to other control methods.
4. Finally, I should like to make some brief remarks on the preference given to a special laboratory test for the safe control of patients. The prothrombin test according to Quick has always given satisfactory results. It would be incorrect and even unfair to call this test a second class one. The same holds true both for the P & P method

and the combined determination of the prothrombin activity and factor x.

The Thrombotest registers the reduction of factor x better than any other test does. With thromboplastin preparations of less sensitivity, deceptively shorter prothrombin times were obtained with the Quick test. For this reason, the Thrombotest is very important for the control of patients who undergo vascular surgery and are therefore treated pre-, per- and post-operatively with permanent anticoagulation. Safe per-operative anticoagulation requires many daily checks. It is the aim of the vascular surgeon to maintain values in the neighbourhood of 5 per cent Thrombotest activity. For the maintenance of low activities the Thrombotest is to be preferred to Quick's one-stage test.

We disagree with those who think the Thrombotest more difficult to perform than the Quick test or any other method.

The introduction of the Thrombotest has undoubtedly contributed to an extension of self-supporting thrombosis services in this country. The simple and reliable test has made possible the decentralization and the establishment of Thrombosis Services in small centres.

It is because of these various considerations that the Scientific Committee of the Thrombosis Service of the Netherlands Red Cross has decided to recommend the Thrombotest to their local sections as the control method of choice.

INTRODUCTION OF THROMBOTEST AT
THE AMSTERDAM THROMBOSIS SERVICE

J. E. JAPIKSE

After the foundation of the Amsterdam Thrombosis Service in 1953, the Quick test was used over a period of about 10 years for the determination of prothrombin activity in the follow-up of patients treated with anticoagulants. Thus, our experience with this method was ample and of long duration.

When we considered adopting Thrombotest around the end of 1963, we were of the opinion that this venture first required a long-term comparative study of the two methods.

During the next two years, both tests were routinely done in rapid succession on the same blood sample. From the results obtained in several thousand blood samples, a correlation curve was plotted (figure 1). It was found that the therapeutic zone of 10 to 30 per cent (Quick),

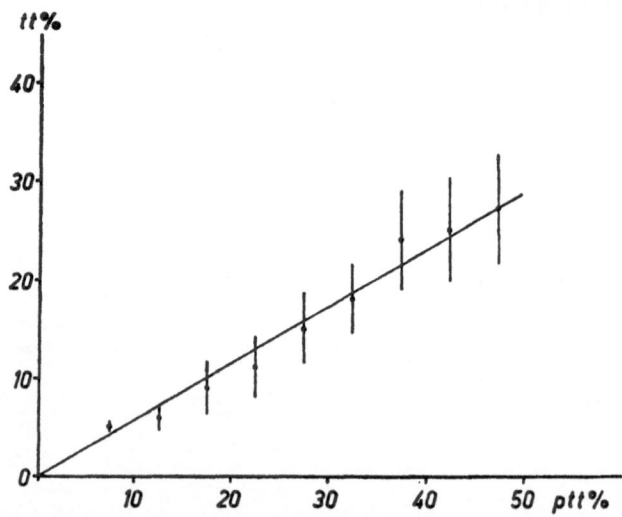

Fig. 1. Correlation curve obtained from a comparative study of Thrombotest (TT) and pro-thrombin time assay procedure performed with Roche thromboplastin (PTT).

introduced by Kettenborg, corresponded to a therapeutic zone of 6 to 18 per cent for Thrombotest. In the Amsterdam Thrombosis Service we have always aimed at lowering of the Quick test values to values ranging from 15 per cent to 20 per cent, thus corresponding to Thrombotest values ranging from 8 to 10 per cent. In our opinion, Thrombotest values above 10 per cent offer insufficient protection against the development of thrombotic processes.

In 1965 we switched to Thrombotest for all determinations. At present, this is the only test used. As regards the technical aspects, this transition did not give any serious difficulties. As regards the economic aspects, Thrombotest is certainly somewhat more expensive. Moreover, we have found that although the technical instruction for the Thrombotest may appear to be simple, the laboratory personnel must remain on the alert to avoid a variety of minor difficulties inherent in the test that can be responsible for erroneous results. There was no evident increase in the number of haemorrhages after the substitution of Thrombotest for the Quick test.

The frequency of serious haemorrhage may possibly have increased slightly, however. As far as can be seen, the frequency of recurrence remained unaltered. No difficulties whatsoever were encountered with respect to dosage.

THROMBOTEST VERSUS CONVENTIONAL THROMBOPLASTINS

E. A. LOELIGER

In a field in which men of basic research, clinical experience, and commercial interest join in discussion, we are badly in need of independent unprejudiced observers and arbiters. But who among us would dare to claim for himself that he is unbiased? I, for one, would not. We can, however, draw on experimental data that cannot be misinterpreted, to help us in clarifying misunderstandings and to lead us to relevant conclusions. The purpose of our contribution is to advise the clinician responsible for anticoagulant treatment, who must know how to obtain the most *reliable information* on the hypocoagulability induced by coumarin congeners. As you all know, the dosage of coumarin congeners, and hence the prognosis of thromboembolic disease, depends primarily on the reliability of this information.

Besides Thrombotest, there are at least ten different thromboplastin preparations in use for the control of coumarin-induced hypocoagulability, all of them hotly recommended by their producers and often fervently praised by the users. These criteria, however, are of less value than the following four parameters:

1. Specificity of test.
2. Sensitivity of reagent.
3. Reproducibility of results.
4. Simplicity of procedure.

Let us consider *specificity* first: Under the conditions of anticoagulant treatment, all reagents, Thrombotest as well as conventional thromboplastins, are meant to indicate the degree of depression of coagulability. As long as coagulation is not disturbed by other processes, alterations in coagulability depend solely on the action of the coumarin preparation. Both Thrombotest and other thromboplastins may therefore be called specific. But Thrombotest, since it reflects almost exclusively the

level of vitamin K-dependent factors, is certainly more specific than
any of the prothrombin time procedures, which in addition measure
factor v and depend on fibrinogen as well as several circulating anticoagulants. This difference in specificity, however, is of little importance
in practice, where Thrombotest and prothrombin times appear to produce comparable results, at least statistically (figure 1).

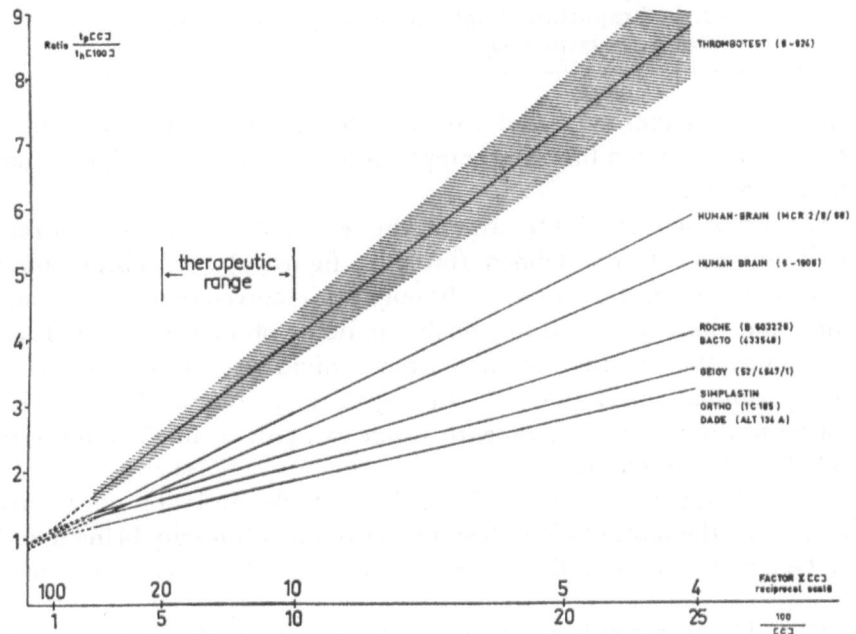

Fig. 1. Correlation between the factor II and x activity found in plasma of patients on long-
term anticoagulant treatment (x-axis; reciprocal scale) and the prolongation ratio of coagulation times calculated from values found for patients and normals (y-axis; ordinary scale).
The accentuated sectors cover the therapeutic range for patients without contra-indications
for long-term anticoagulant treatment.

More important is the *sensitivity of the reagent.* In this context sensitivity refers to the degree with which a reagent indicates changes in
coagulability. We must differentiate here between sensitivity with respect to the initial and to the prolonged (stable) effect of coumarin congeners. During the initial phase (table 1), the sensitivity of Thrombotest approaches that of human brain or Roche thromboplastin,
while Owren's P & P reagent considerably surpasses Thrombotest.
In sharp contrast, Geigy's thromboplastin preparation is exceptionally insensitive to the depression of coagulability (i.e. to factor VII

Table 1. Prolongation ratios of prothrombin times as assessed with different thromboplastin preparations during the initial phase of anticoagulant treatment.

Human brain thromboplastin	4-6
Thrombotest	5
Thrombokinase Lösung Roche	3.0
Bacto Aplastin	2.5
Ortho brain-thromboplastin or Simplastin	2.0
Thromboplastin Geigy	1.8

and *a fortiori*, factor IX), which can easily lead, in the first week of treatment, to unexpected bleeding complications in cases with relative contra-indication.

For prolonged (stable) treatment, the sensitivity of the different reagents is more clearly defined (table 1; figure 1) (2). Thrombotest is by far the most sensitive. Although this correlation is obtained from, and therefore holds for, pooled patients plasma, we know from experience that results obtained from individual plasmas display a closely similar correlation (2). In any case, recommendations with respect to the so-called therapeutic range can now be made in terms of an "absolute" standard.

There is ample statistical evidence that not all correlation curves are rectilinear, the most obvious deviations from rectilinearity being found for Geigy, Roche, and Bacto thromboplastin. This deviation is pro-

Table 2. The therapeutic range in terms of percentages of coagulation activity. On the left, the range to be aimed at by the large experience of the Thrombosis Service Leiden; and on the right, the range proposed by the different manufacturers.

	Therapeutic range (%)	
	according to experience	as proposed by manufacturer
Factors 11 and x	10 – 20	—
Thrombotest	5 – 10	7 – 20
MCR (Poller)	15 – 30	15 – 30
Roche	15 – 30	15 – 25
Geigy acc.	20 – 40	15 – 25
to		
Simplastin Quick	20 – 40	10 – 25
Ortho	20 – 40	12 – 20

bably due to factor vii-like substances contained in these preparations. Note that the correlation curves do not pass through the point defined by ratio 1 of the y-axis and [100] of the x-axis but higher (at a ratio of between 1. 025 and 1. 17). This is partially due to the factor vii-like activity of thromboplastin but also due to the fact that all reagents are to some extent sensitive to PIVKA (1, 3).

We may now proceed to the *reproducibility of results*. Reproducibility – apart from the technical error, sensitivity of the preparation, and stability of the reagent – depends on the manner of clot formation. Thrombotest times, although much longer than prothrombin times, are read with a better accuracy than most prothrombin times. A well-defined endpoint reading and the high stability of Thrombotest probably contribute to the good reproducibility of results. More important than easy readability and stability, however, is the fact that for Thrombotest, unlike conventional thromboplastin preparations, normality does *not* have to be assessed in order to express results as a percentage of normal. Each batch is carefully tested and provided with a reference curve by the manufacturer (table 2). This makes results obtained by the Thrombotest procedure more reliable than those obtained by any of the conventional prothrombin time assay procedures. The reproducibility of results is illustrated by the following example, in which the most and the least sensitive reagent are compared.

Table 3. The reproducibility of the results obtained in a given plasma with two tests for hypocoagulability (Thrombotest procedure and one-stage prothrombin time assay procedure using Simplastin).

	true value (%)	value found (%) (range)
Thrombotest	5	4.8 – 5.3
Simplastin	20	18 – 22.5

Lastly, with regard to the *simplicity of procedure*, we know from extensive experience that the various procedures under discussion do not differ substantially in this respect.

In conclusion, it may be said that at the present time, Thrombotest is the most sensitive reagent available and the Thrombotest procedure is the most accurate for the assessment of coumarin-induced hypocoagulability expressed as a percentage of normal.

REFERENCES

1. Loeliger, E. A., W. K. Taconis, J. J. Veltkamp, H. C. Hemker, Standardization of results obtained by different thromboplastin preparations. *Proc. Int. Conf. Int. Comm. Thromb. Haem., Princeton,* (1968), to be published.
2. Loeliger, E. A., Comparative study of different commercially available thromboplastin preparations. To be published.
3. Hemker, H. C., Kinetic aspects of the interaction of blood-clotting enzymes. III. Demonstration of the existance of an inhibitor of prothrombin conversion in vitamin K-deficiency. *Thrombos. Diathes. haemorrh.* 19, 346 (1968).

DISCUSSION

H. Booij (Amersfoort): I should like to ask Dr. Stormorken to comment on the statement he made about the use of only the first drop of blood for the Thrombotest. Such a procedure would limit us to only one determination per patient if we did not wish to become a nuisance to the patient.

Stormorken: It is our experience that when two tests are performed successively, a shorter coagulation time is found in the second test. We take blood samples from two different sites if we require two determinations. Highly trained technicians can, however, obtain two samples from the same site giving comparable results.

Owren: An important precaution might be mentioned: that no cotton wool should be used between the first and second tests as is often done for haemoglobin determinations. If cotton wool is used, it results in partially clotted blood in the second sample and abnormally high percentage values. Experienced technicians can obtain 2 or 3 samples in quick succession without appreciable shortening of the clotting time provided the bleeding is brisk and the collection is rapid. To take separate pipettes for each test is of course mandatory.

Loeliger: In the beginning, there seemed to be a need for duplicate determinations. All large Thrombosis Services have since abandoned duplicate tests; we know from experience that one determination is reliable because of the accuracy of the test.

Jordan: I should like to address a few remarks to Dr. Owren. The Thrombotest is related to the bleeding tendency in patients. You have changed your view on the cause of this observation. First you reported that factor IX sensitivity was important; later it seemed an especial sensitivity to factor x, and finally to Dr. Hemker's factor. Do you have any experimental evidence to support your current thesis?

Owren: Thrombotest was developed from clinical experience. In large clinical materials we found it to be better than other tests, and we have proposed changing explanations for this on the basis of steadily improving knowledge of the clotting mechanism. We might still have to modify our views, but I do hope that we are now very close to the final explanation of why Thrombotest is more sensitive to the specific changes produced by anticoagulants.

Loeliger: I think Dr. Hemker has found the reason for Dr. Owren's second view: although the production of factor x molecules is depressed during stable anticoagulant therapy to the same degree as that of factors ii, vii, and ix, their activity is lower. This is the result of the inhibitor (PIVKA) entering the circulation upon the action of the factor x molecule as an accelerator. All vitamin K deficiencies, whether naturally occurring or coumarin induced, will induce the appearance of this inhibitor. In the Thrombotest system it is directed primarily against factor x. Dr. Owren's assignment of an important role to factor x was therefore correct.

There is another point I should like to stress, and that is the factor vii sensitivity of Thrombotest, which is important in the prevention of bleeding complications. The levels of factors vii and ix run rather close together at the beginning of and, in case of abrupt changes, during anticoagulation therapy. So, indirectly, Thrombotest picks up variations in factor ix activity. If one uses a thromboplastin preparation that is insensitive to factor vii, factor ix is not, or at least is much less, reflected, which is the reason why unexpected bleeding complications may occur.

Haanen: Occasionally, Thrombotest values lower than 5 per cent are obtained. The correlation curve of Thrombotest stops at 5 per cent. I think it is of importance to know whether the value is 3 per cent or 4 per cent if one is attempting to adjust the dosage. Hence, we should ask the manufacturer to extend the correlation curve for values below 5 per cent.

Owren: Thrombotest times corresponding to values below about 3 per cent become difficult to determine exactly by manual methods. Exact reading can be obtained with automatic equipment. On request, we have extended the correlation curve down to 2.5 per cent. It has not been done routinely, because exact values at this very low range seem not to be important, since therapy has to be suspended in every case until the level again reaches about 5 per cent. If it is desired, however, I have no objection to extending the curve down to 2.5 per cent. It is important that Thrombotest should not be performed with twice the amount of plasma at these low levels in an attempt to obtain shorter coagulation times. By increasing the amount of test plasma the Thrombotest time will not be shortened accordingly, because of the inhibitor (PIVKA).

THERAPEUTIC LEVELS

THROMBOTEST LEVELS IN RELATION TO RECURRENCES AND BLEEDING COMPLICATIONS IN LONG-TERM TREATMENT OF PATIENTS SUFFERING FROM CORONARY HEART DISEASE

CORNELIA A. VAN DIJK, WILHELMINA B. DOMINICUS,
AND J. ROOS

Introduction

Although there are indications that a relatively high level of anticoagulation gives better clinical results, exact values are not known. The studies of many authors argue for lowering results obtained by Thrombotest to a 10 per cent level, perhaps with some difference between arterial and venous diseases.

Our work in a rather large thrombosis service (table 1) led us to wonder where the Thrombotest levels lie in patients with recurrent coronary heart disease at the moment of the recurrence. Unfortunately, we were not able to determine this level in more than half of a group of 314 cases, usually because the recurrence came to our knowledge too late. Nevertheless, the remaining material seemed sufficiently large.

Table 1. Figures from The Hague Thrombosis Service in 1967.

number of patients	10,750
number of thrombotests	179,040
number of patients with coronary heart disease	4,600
bleeding episodes (1 bleeding in 20 patient-treatment-years)	485

We do not examine the patients ourselves, but rely on the clinical data provided by 530 attending physicians. In the year under discussion, we tried to reach and maintain a Thrombotest value of between 110 and 130 seconds. To avoid reading errors, we did not convert this into percentage values. In this period we did not investigate the exact cause of bleedings, but in 16 per cent of the cases Thrombotest values lay above 160 seconds. In 1964, however, we did perform a specific investigation, and found that 60 per cent were caused by a local organic lesion (1).

We tried to eliminate the problem of our lack of familiarity with the patients themselves by choosing the least doubtful clinical parameter of all, death. Our aim was to find out whether in patients on long-term treatment with anticoagulants who had died of a recurrence of a coronary heart disease, there had been a difference in intensity or variability in the anticoagulation therapy as compared to a control group composed of living patients with the same disease. Under recurrence we also included the so-called sudden deaths (i.e. cases in which death occurred within a few minutes).

Material
In the year under analysis, 80 of our patients suffering from coronary heart disease were reported to have died because of a clinically diagnosed myocardial infarction. In addition, there were 80 so-called *mortes subitae*.

Of the 160 deceased patients, 63 were excluded, 49 of these on the basis of the criterion that the patient had received anticoagulation for a year and a half or longer, and 14 on other grounds (table 2). The

Table 2. Patients excluded on grounds other than by definition.

Reason for exclusion:	
temporary interruption of treatment	6
low dosage because of cerebral haemorrhage	1
incomplete data	1
uncooperative patient	1
no comparable control patient present	5

Table 3. Age distribution of the patients.

Age in years	Male	Female
40 – 49	2	—
50 – 59	24	2
60 – 69	30	9
70 – and older	23	7
total	79	18

control group of the same number of patients (97), was chosen at random from the files of patients suffering from coronary heart disease, such that it was identical to the group of deceased patients not only with respect to age and sex (table 3) but also to duration of therapy (table 4) and anticoagulant (table 5). Other important clinical conditions such as the degree of coronary disease, hypertension, and disturbance of heart rhythm, could not be taken into consideration. A significant difference was found between the two groups as to the frequency of recurrence and cardiac decompensation during the period investigated (table 6). Under recurrence in the context of clinical comparability of the two groups is understood clinical infarction as well as serious attacks of angina recorded at least three weeks before death.

For each patient, 6 of the 8 to 40 Thrombotest values obtained during the year preceding death or selection were chosen by taking the value of the first check of every two-month period. All Thrombotest data were assembled such that the information of each deceased patient was paired with that of an almost identical living patient.

Table 4. Number of patients by length of treatment.

$1\frac{1}{2}$ – 2	13
2 – 4	27
4 and more	57

Table 5. Number of patients by anticoagulant.

acenocumarine (Sintrom)	25
dicumarol (Dicumol)	47
ethyldicumarol (Tromexan)	1
phenprocoumon (Marcoumar)	24

Table 6. Clinical data of the patients.

	Deceased	Control
diabetes mellitus	11	6
decompensatio cordis	13	3
bleeding episodes	9	10
recurrences	13	2

Results

The intensity of anticoagulation in both groups, classified according to the drug used, is shown in figure 1. This curve is based on the combined results of all 582 Thrombotest values (6 × 97). The frequency in per cent is plotted against the Thrombotest activity in seconds. The Marcoumar curve is narrower, has a higher peak than that of Sintrom and Dicoumol, indicating that anticoagulation with Marcoumar was more stable. The apex of all the curves lies at approximately 110 seconds.

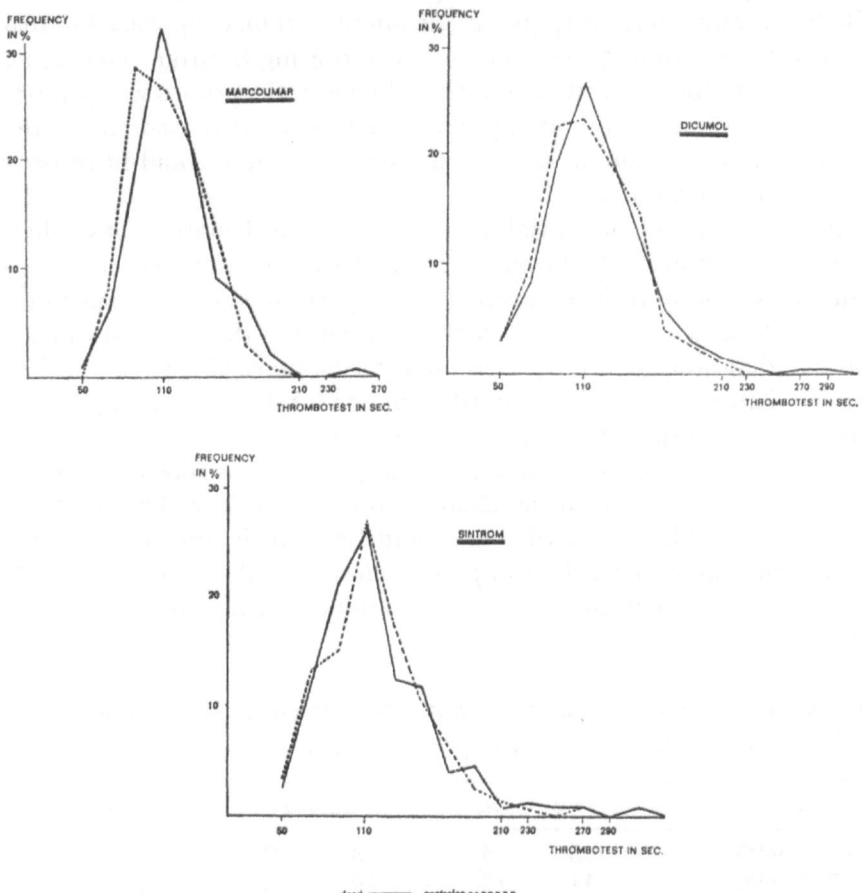

Fig. 1. Frequency distribution of the Thrombotest times (6 randomly sampled values per patient). The solid line refers to the deceased patients, the dotted line to the control patients.

We also evaluated the intensity of anticoagulation by considering the pairs: the mean of 6 values of a dead patient was calculated and compared with the average of the 6 values of the paired patient. The difference between these averages was as much as 67 seconds individually, but the grand mean for the two groups showed only a negligible dif-

ference. The differences between the grand means calculated for the
three different drug groups was 0.1 to 5.3 seconds, being far from significant either for the individual drugs or for the three combined (p=0.1).
The amount of anticoagulant used, a less important parameter in
measuring the intensity of anticoagulation, was virtually the same in
the two groups; however, 50 mg Dicoumol (1 tablet) appeared to display less effect than 3 mg Marcoumar and 4 mg Sintrom. Hence, no
difference in the intensity of treatment between the groups was demonstrated either as measured by Thrombotest or as measured by the
amount of anticoagulant drug used. However, there could have been
a difference in variability.

As a measure of the variability, the standard deviation was calculated from the individual average of the Thrombotest values. The calculation of the statistical parameters was performed on the logarithms
of the Thrombotest values, since it appeared that the frequency distribution diagram (figure 1) was almost symmetrical for logarithmic
values. Table 7 shows the standard deviation for the two groups, the frequency distribution of the standard deviation (y) being given in 7 different classes. Statistical analysis of the paired data showed that the
differences were far from significant. However, it is striking that the
average variability with Dicoumol and Sintrom is obviously greater
than with Marcoumar. It is apparent, however, that there is no important difference in intensity and variability between the groups as a
whole.

Table VII. Statistical data concerning stability of hypocoagulability as
induced by different coumarin preparations.

y	marcoumar		dicumol		sintrom	
0,02 — 0,05	5	5	3	10	2	4
0,06 — 0,09	11	13	18	13	7	5
0,10 — 0,13	6	6	9	12	7	6
0,14 — 0,17	1	—	13	9	3	6
0,18 — 0,21	—	—	1	2	5	1
0,22 — 0,25	1	—	2	1	1	3
0,26 — 0,29	—	—	1	—	—	—
Total	24	24	47	47	25	25
Median	0,08	0,07	0,11	0,10	0,12	0,12

Discussion and conclusion

This study was undertaken in an attempt to determine whether death due to recurrent infarction during anticoagulation therapy was due to sub-optimal anticoagulation. The best method seemed to be to compare the degree of anticoagulation in deceased patients with that of living patients on the same treatment. A drawback in every investigation done in patients of our Thrombosis Service is that we see the patients only for the check of the anticoagulation therapy, so that the clinical data are based not on our own observations but on those of other physicians.

We were unable to demonstrate any difference in stability and intensity of anticoagulation between the patients whose death was due to a recurrent infarction and the control group, notwithstanding the fact that the patients belonging to the deceased group showed more diabetes, cardiac failure, and recurrence of cardiac infarction in the case histories.

The conclusion must be that death due to recurrent infarction (sudden death included) in patients treated with oral anticoagulants for cardiac infarction is not correlated with low stability nor with low intensity of anticoagulant treatment.

Finally, the following already-known subsidiary facts were confirmed:
- Marcoumar gives significantly more stable anticoagulation than either Dicoumol or Sintrom.
- The quantity of Dicoumol required per day is, in terms of tablets, higher than that of Marcoumar and Sintrom.

Summary

Two groups of coronary heart disease patients treated with oral anticoagulants were studied with respect to intensity and stability of anticoagulant treatment as assessed by Thrombotest. One of these groups consisted of 97 patients who had died of a recurrence of the coronary disease (sudden death included); the other, or control, group was composed of living patients identical to the first group with respect to sex, age, anticoagulant drug, and duration of treatment. Although more symptoms of bad risk had occurred in the deceased group, no significant difference between the two groups as to hypocoagulability was found. The presumption that cardiac death is correlated with inadequate anticoagulation could not be confirmed.

REFERENCES

Roos, J., H. E. van Joost, The cause of bleeding during anticoagulant treatment. *Acta Med. Scand.* 178, 129 (1965).

THE UTRECHT DOUBLE BLIND TRIAL OF LONG-TERM ANTICOAGULANT TREATMENT AFTER MYOCARDIAL INFARCTION

O. J. A. TH. MEUWISSEN

A prospective double blind trial of long-term anticoagulant medication following myocardial infarction was carried out in Utrecht from May 1st 1964 to January 15th 1966. With the collaboration of all the Utrecht cardiologists, all their patients with acute myocardial infarction were included in this trial after a 4-month interval, to be distributed strictly at random over a phenprocoumon and a placebo group. Supplemental therapy and follow-up were identical in both groups. Of the total of 138 patients included in the trial, 68 received phenprocoumon and 70 were given a placebo. One patient in the phenprocoumon group died, and 8 patients in the placebo group. This difference is significant ($p < 0.01$). The difference in the number of reinfarctions was not significant (5 cases and 7 cases, respectively).

After January 15th 1966, when the difference between the two groups had become significant, all patients were further treated with phenprocoumon. Nevertheless, the difference in mortality continued through 1966, with 5 deaths in the original placebo group and only 1 death in the original phenprocoumon group.

Loeliger has shown the great importance of adequate dosage in long-term anticoagulant medication. In comparison of results of various studies, therefore, great importance must be attached to the mean level of hypocoagulability. However, the calculation of this level is a precarious undertaking. A primary disadvantage is the presence of an asymmetrical distribution of Thrombotest results: above the desired level, the range is from 15 per cent to 100 per cent Thrombotest, while below this level the range is only from 5 per cent to 1 per cent Thrombotest. This leads to a rise of the arithmetic mean Thrombotest level and consequently suggests a less favourable level of hypocoagulability.

If the mean dosage level is calculated, not on the basis of Thrombotest percentages but on the basis of clotting times determined, and if the arithmetic mean clotting time established is then expressed in Thrombotest percentage, then the asymmetrical distribution, which likewise characterizes the clotting times, leads to a low Thrombotest percentage, suggesting a very favourable level of hypocoagulability.

A second disadvantage lies in the fact that patients whose values lie above or below the desired level of hypocoagulability are likely to be more frequently examined in follow-up than patients who are firmly balanced at the desired level. Therefore, the frequency of follow-up on balanced patients and the frequency of follow-up on unbalanced patients are factors that partially determine the mean level of hypocoagulability if this is calculated as the mean of all Thrombotest results obtained. To avoid this second disadvantage we calculated, with the use of a computer, for each patient for each day between all successive follow-ups, the level of hypocoagulability as the mean of the preceding and the subsequent Thrombotest percentage (not the clotting time). On the basis of all these daily averages, we calculated the arithmetic mean level of hypocoagulability for the entire period of investigation and the entire material. The mean level of hypocoagulability thus calculated was 10.7 per cent Thrombotest.

As far as we know, this method of calculation has not been used by other investigators; even so, the problem of an asymmetrical distribution of Thrombotest results persists. Therefore, the level of hypocoagulability attained in the different trials is perhaps best compared on the basis of the mean dosage of anticoagulant used. This mean daily dosage can be calculated in a simple and identical way for all investigations. However, this mode of comparison, too, has some disadvantages, e.g. the dosage is dependent on dietary habits, climatological influences, and the patients' average age.

In our material the patients remained within the therapeutic limits, that is between 5 and 15 per cent Thrombotest during an average of 91 per cent of the entire period of investigation. The mean phenprocoumon dosage was 3.21 mg/day.

A total of 8 haemorrhages occurred in 7 patients (1 per 13 years of treatment). Overdosage played a role in only one case.

The results of our study are consistent with those of several other recently published investigations. The intensity of the hypocoagulability attained is probably of decisive importance.

The fact that in the original placebo group the results remained less favourable even after the switch to phenprocoumon, emphasizes the necessity of long-term treatment with adequate doses of anticoagulants following myocardial infarction.

THE LEIDEN DOUBLE-BLIND TRIAL OF LONG-TERM ANTICOAGULANT TREATMENT AFTER MYOCARDIAL INFARCTION

E. A. LOELIGER

It is beyond doubt that prevention of venous thrombosis requires institution of strong and well-balanced hypocoagulability (4, 5, 7, 9). But there is also some evidence that the same holds for arterial thrombosis (2, 8).

Complementary to the results obtained at Utrecht by Dr. Meuwissen and his co-workers, we have demonstrated in a recent double-blind study (6) that anticoagulant treatment, if continued for longer than one year after the occurrence of cardiac infarction, powerfully prevents re-infarction and other thrombotic cardiovascular complications, probably for an unlimited period of time. The mortality rate also appears to be lowered – much less but again significantly – if the group of patients suffering from atherothrombosis is considered as a whole, including intermittent claudication (3).

The basis for our results was provided by an intensive and stable anticoagulant treatment. The hypocoagulability aimed at, expressed in terms of Thrombotest, was 5 to 12 per cent.

Figure 1 shows the results achieved, here expressed as relative frequency of the hypocoagulability. The individual average Thrombotest values are compiled in classes of one per cent. Solid columns represent values found in the patients without contra-indications and hatched columns those found in the patients with contra-indications. As you can see, our aim to institute Thrombotest values between 5 and 12 per cent has generally been achieved. The geometric mean was about 8 per cent. This figure may remind you of the frequency diagram shown by Dr. van Dijk, who has compiled the results in terms of coagulation times. I can assure you that our figures, when translated into coagulation times, differ only slightly from those obtained at The Hague's Thrombosis Service. So it is evident that Leiden and The Hague both maintain

339

powerful anticoagulation in patients suffering from coronary heart disease.

For practical purposes, we have also translated our results into terms of other (commercially) available thromboplastins (table 1). For translation, the principle of Biggs' ratio method was used (1).

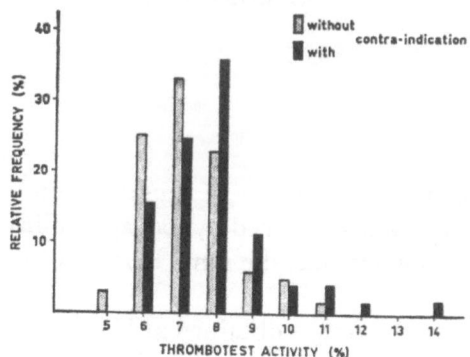

Fig. 1. Diagram of intensity and stability of hypocoagulability as measured by means of Thrombotest activity. The values are grouped in classes of 1 per cent. Solid columns represent values found in patients without contra-indications, and hatched columns those found in the patients with 'relative' contra-indications.

Table 1. Hypocoagulability to be aimed at in terms of different thromboplastin preparations. The percentages given for the different thromboplastin preparations are approximations, calculated from reference curves supplied by the manufacturer.

	mean (%)	range (%)
Thrombotest	8	5 – 12
Human brain (MCR)	24	15 – 36
Geigy (porcine lung)	32	20 – 48
Roche (rabbit lung)	24	15 – 36
Simplastin, Ortho, Dade (rabbit brain)	32	20 – 48

So much for arterial thrombosis. In active venous thrombosis, especially when it is a question of short-term treatment, we try to treat even more intensively, so that our general scheme, in terms of Thrombotest percentages, looks as shown in Table 2.

An exception is made for patients who are treated pre- per-, and postoperatively. For these cases we aim at 10 to 15 per cent.

Table 2. Therapeutic range, in terms of Thrombotest percentages

	without contra-indication	with contra-indication
Short-term treatment	4 – 8	8(–12)
Long-term treatment	5 – 10	8 – 12

We are aware that realization of these proposals demands experience in handling coumarin-congeners and Vitamin K_1; the tight supervision of the patient by experienced nurses may be considered a *conditio sine qua non.*

REFERENCES

1. Biggs, R., K.W. Denson, Standardization of the one-stage prothrombin time for the control of anticoagulant therapy. *Brit. Med. J.* 1, 84 (1967).
2. Borchgrevink, Chr. F., Long-term anticoagulant therapy in angina pectoris and myocardial infarction. A clinical trial between intensive and moderate treatment. *Acta med. Scand.* Suppl. 330, 1 (1957).
3. Hamming, J. J., A. Hensen, E. A. Loeliger, *The value of long-term coumarin treatment in peripheral sclerosis* (clinical trial). To be published.
4. Kuijer, P. J., C. H. W. Leeksma, Profylaxe van veneuze thromboembolische complicaties met behulp van anticoagulantia. *Ned. T. Geneesk.* 109, 1480 (1965).
5. Loeliger, E. A., personal experience.
6. Loeliger, E. A., A. Hensen, F. Kroes, L. M. van Dijk, N. Fekkes, H. de Jonge, H. C. Hemker, A double-blind trial of long-term anticoagulant treatment after myocardial infarction. *Acta med. Scand.* 182, 549 (1967).
7. Poller, L., J. S. Woothliff, The value of capillary Thrombotest method for the control of long-term anticoagulant treatment. *Thrombos. Diathes. haemorrh.* 8, 333 (1962).
8. Rozenberg, M. C., H. Kronenberg, B. G. Firkin, 'Thrombotest' and prothrombin time: A controlled trial. *Aust. Ann. Med.* 14, 3 (1965).
9. Sevitt, S., D. Innes, Prothrombin-time and thrombotest in injured patients on prophylactic anticoagulant therapy. *Lancet*, I, 124 (1964).

DISCUSSION

Roos: We think that many patients develop thromboses during surgery or immediately after surgery, and we therefore advise anticoagulant therapy during surgery. I should like to ask Dr. Owren for his recommendation as to Thrombotest values for such patients.

Owren: We think that it is advantageous to stabilize patients pre-operatively, because it is then easier to maintain therapeutic levels during and shortly after the operation. The dosage, however, has to be reduced for the first and second post-operative days. An injectable anticoagulant is preferred, because post-operative peroral therapy may be difficult. We have chosen 15 per cent Thrombotest as a therapeutic level post-operatively, because it appears to be sufficient for preventing early post-operative thrombotic processes. On the other hand, we have found that haemostasis as evaluated by the secondary bleeding time, our parameter for bleeding tendency, remains normal at this level. We have also found that tooth extractions at this level do not increase the bleeding. At a Thrombotest level of 10 per cent we have observed an occasional episode of excessive post-operative bleeding. We cannot say, however, that this bleeding was caused by the higher intensity of anticoagulation therapy. All we can say is that 15 per cent Thrombotest is a safe level for most operations except for those on the brain, medulla, and eye.

Loeliger: In Dr. Boerema's department (Amsterdam) per-operative levels of 5 to 10 per cent are aimed at. We aim at 10 to 15 per cent and descend slowly to 5 to 10 per cent post-operatively, when a *per primam* wound healing is to be expected.

Owren: There is no doubt that the prevention of venous thrombosis requires less intense anticoagulation than the prevention of arterial thrombosis. I believe that 10 to 15 per cent Thrombotest, as mentioned by

Loeliger, gives adequate protection against venous thrombosis in surgery.

Vreeken: Is there not another explanation for the results of long-term
anticoagulant therapy in arterial thrombosis or coronary heart disease?
Patients with unstable circulation often display unstable hypocoagulability and will therefore be checked more frequently than the patients
in the placebo group. Also, these patients will see their attending physicians more frequently. In general, patients who must return frequently tend to follow more accurately *all* the therapy prescribed (salt-poor
diet, less smoking, and better weight control). Differences between the
coumarin and placebo group may be due solely to this bias and unrelated to the anticoagulant therapy.

Loeliger: This could indeed have been the case. In our material, however, coumarin patients did not consult their physicians more frequently than the placebo-group patients because we included extra coagulation checks and advised visits to the doctor for the latter as well (all
patients had been treated beforehand for at least one year and were
checked at similar intervals during the trial and dosed with coumarin
or placebo according to the coumarin dosage known from the 'pre-
treatment' period). Moreover, only a few coumarin patients showed
unstable anticoagulation. So we think a possible bias, as rightly suggested by Dr. Vreeken, did not occur in our material.

De Vries: It seems that the patients require a certain amount of intelligence in order to follow the rules of treatment. I think that a score of
about 90 per cent within the therapeutic range is rather exceptionally
high. Is it possible that the patients have a higher intelligence than
normal?

Loeliger: I think that the mean I.Q of our patients is less than 100, but
the I.Q. of the nurses in our Thrombosis Services is excellent. Tight
supervision of the patient by the nurses is the main factor in the high
score of therapeutic values.

Owren: In arterial thrombosis we aim at a 10 per cent Thrombotest
level. In venous thrombosis we differentiate between prophylactic and
therapeutic levels. When we have to deal with a clinically established

venous thrombosis I do agree with Dr. Loeliger that intensive therapy should be applied, in terms of Thrombotest of 5 to 8 per cent. For primary prophylaxis, however, I am inclined to believe that 10 to 15 per cent is adequate as a rule. I may mention that a study in Oslo on anticoagulation in 700 cases of prostatectomies showed a reduction of post-operative thrombo-embolism from 8-10 per cent in non-treated patients to 0.8 per cent in the treated group. It is very likely, however, that higher intensity of anticoagulation might reduce or eliminate these residual cases of thrombo-embolism.

Loeliger: As a general contribution to the discussion, I would like to make the following remarks. Unsolved problems and differences of opinion will always be present in a scientific discussion; but, as I feel it, this is an important stimulus for further development. As far as the control of anticoagulant therapy is concerned, I can assure you that it was not because it differs principally from other tests that we chose Thrombotest for checking our patients. In fact, we started with Quick's one-stage assay procedure and used human brain thromboplastin for many years. We then had to change, because of supply problems, to a commercial thromboplastin preparation. We used the most sensitive preparation available at that time, which was made by Roche. Finally, for reasons so lucidly presented by Dr. de Vries, we switched once again, this time to Thrombotest. In all of the three periods mentioned, the frequencies of bleeding complications and thrombo-embolic recurrences was about the same, although we have no exact statistical evidence for this statement. Other experienced laboratories came to similar conclusions. By trial and error we have defined our therapeutic range of 5 to 10 per cent Thrombotest. Dr. Poller's course in Britain was quite similar; on the basis of his experience he recommends 15 to 30 per cent Quick value. This means that we both aim at the same optimal range (5 to 10 per cent Thrombotest = 15 to 30 per cent according to Quick when using Dr. Poller's thromboplastin), and even more important, the therapeutic results appear not to differ between the two centres.

VITAMIN K₁ THERAPY

J. VAN DER MEER

Introduction

Indirect anticoagulants of the 4-hydroxycoumarin type (coumarins) have been known for thirty years, but their clinical application was perfected only fifteen years ago, when vitamin K_1 became available as an antidote. Since then, vitamin K_1 has been increasingly used for this purpose, but exact information concerning the proper dosage is nevertheless not to be found in either the literature or the handbooks, which only refer in vague terms to doses lying between 1 and 50 mg. In an attempt to fill this need, we determined the intensity of the effect of vitamin K_1 in relative, i.e. coumarin-induced, vitamin K deficiency in man, with particular attention to:

1. The interval between the moment of oral or intravenous administration of vitamin K_1 and the onset of its effect, measured as increased coagulability of the blood.
2. The intensity of this effect in relation to the dose and manner of administration of vitamin K_1, as reflected by rate of change of the coagulability and the maximum level of coagulability reached.
3. The duration of the effect of vitamin K_1.

I. Methods

Although the main points have been published elsewhere (4), certain technical problems should be mentioned before the results of the investigation are discussed. The study was done in normal volunteer subjects and patients. Phenprocoumon was used as anticoagulant because it provides the most stable hypocoagulability (1, 2, 5) as a result of its slow turnover rate ($t\frac{1}{2}$ averaging about 4 days). The effect of coumarin and of vitamin K_1 was measured as the prothrombin time (according to Quick) and as the activity of factors II, VII, IX, and X in the blood. For coumarin-induced hypocoagulability in the normal subjects we aimed at a factor activity between 20 and 30 per cent, the patients' values usually lying between 10 and 25 per cent. All observations related to the effect of vitamin K_1 were made during uninterrupted administration of phenprocoumon. In the normal subjects we studied the effect of 1, 5, and 25 mg vitamin K_1 administered intravenously and 850 mg given orally (the latter divided over 1 week, 250 mg the first day and the rest in daily doses of 100 mg). The high oral dosage was intended to give maximum stimulation of the synthesis of the coagulation factors. The accuracy of the determinations was established, and proved to be on the same order of magnitude as that known for coagulation experiments (table 1).

Table 1. Accuracy of the coagulation determinations, expressed as the error of the coagulation time (c.v. = coefficient of variation) and the confidence interval for the coagulation-factor activities when the real value is 100%, 50% or 20%.

	c.v.	Real values and the relevant limits		
		100%	50%	20%
Factor II	4.1	75— 130	38— 65	15— 26
Factor VII	3.6	80— 125	40— 63	16— 25
Factor IX	6.6	53— 204	26— 102	11— 41
Factor X	> 4.7	<60—> 176	<30—> 88	<12—> 35

II. *The effect of vitamin K_1 in the normal subjects:*
The reaction to various doses of vitamin K_1 observed in volunteers is shown in the graph in figure 1.

1. *Onset of the effect*
The activity of the 4 factors of the prothrombin complex starts to rise about 2 hours after the oral administration of vitamin K_1; for intravenously administered vitamin K_1, this rise probably starts about 30 minutes earlier (figure 2).

2. *Intensity of the effect*
The initial rate at which the activity of the 4 coagulation factors in the blood increases was found, for the quantities used in this study, to be independent of the dose of vitamin K_1; there is no difference between the reaction rate after administration of 250 mg orally and 1, 5, and 25 mg intravenously (figure 1). The initial rate is therefore the same as the

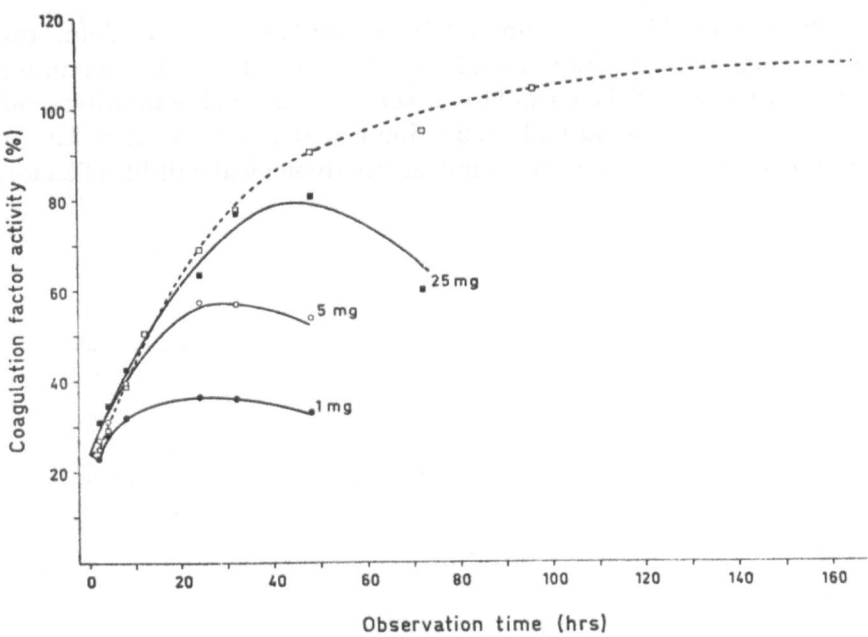

Fig. 1. Reaction of the coagulation factors after administration of vitamin K.₁ Solid lines = after intravenous administration; dashed line = after high oral dose. Each point represents the average of the values found for factors II, VII, IX, and X individually.

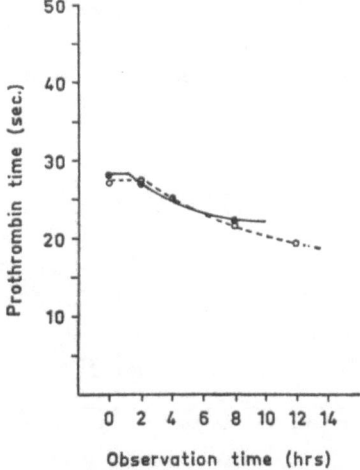

Fig. 2. Course of the prothrombin time after administration of vitamin K₁. Two hours after oral administration of 250 mg, no reaction can be distinguished (circles connected by dashed line). The start of the reaction to intravenous administration (averages of values found for 1, 5, and 25 mg vitamin K₁) can be estimated by extrapolation at about 1½ hr after administration (dots connected by solid line).

maximal rate. The latter can only be maintained by daily administration of high doses of vitamin K_1, however. Calculation of the maximum production rate of the coagulation factors gives a value showing good agreement with the normal production rate derived from data known for the normal turnover rate of the factors (biological half-life of factors

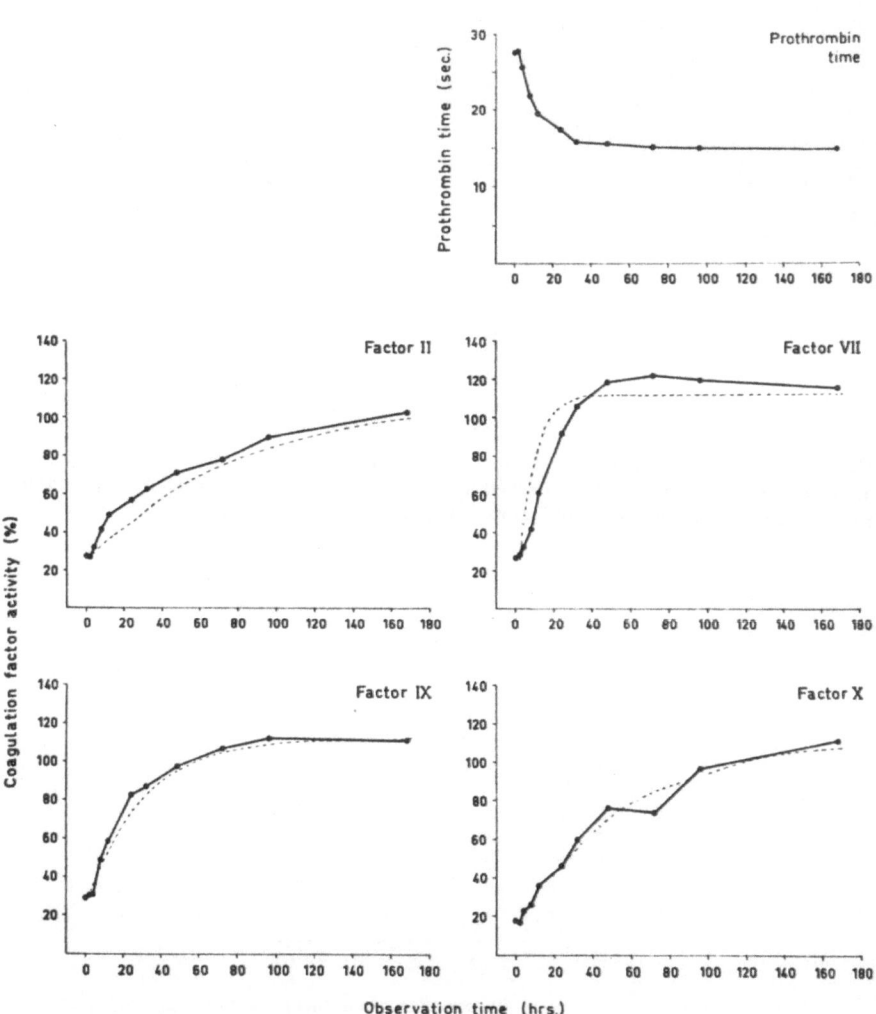

Fig. 3. Course of the prothrombin time and factor activities under maximal stimulation of coagulation-factor synthesis (250 mg vitamin K_1 followed by 100 mg daily). Dots connected by solid lines represent averaged values of 9 subjects. Dashed lines indicate increase in factor activities expected for normal synthesis.

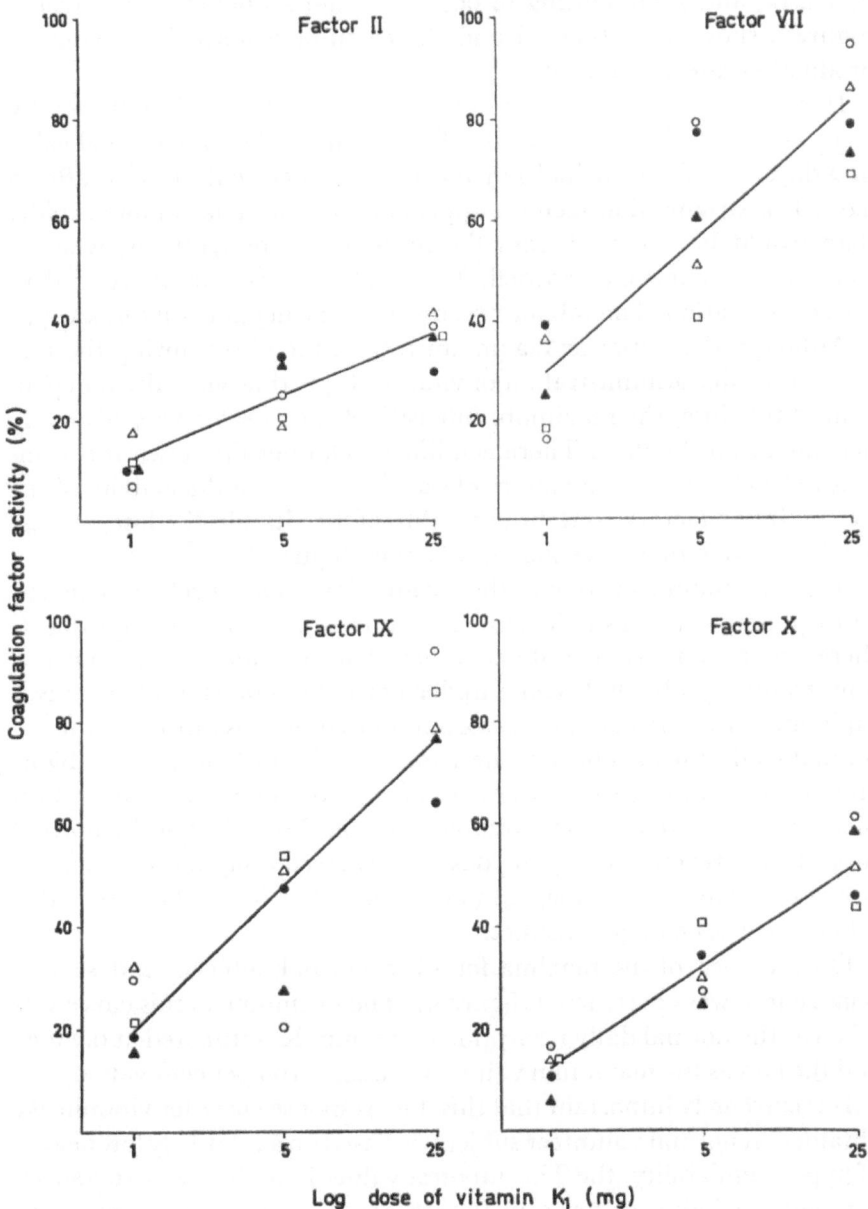

Fig. 4. Dose response relationship for the 4 coagulation factors separately. The maximum increase of the coagulation-factor activities in 5 normal subjects (ordinate) is plotted against the logarithm of the dose of intravenously administered vitamin K_1 (abcissa).

II, VII, IX, and X amounting to 60, 6, 20, and 40 hours, respectively). Figure 3 shows the observed and the calculated normal (maximum) production rates graphically.

It is clear that factor VII shows the most rapid synthesis, followed by factors IX, X, and II in that order. Factor VII reached the normal value in 2 days, but factor II had not reached 100 per cent activity after 7 days. It is striking that factor II appears to be synthesized more rapidly than would be expected from the normal rate of synthesis, whereas factor VII is somewhat retarded. This could conceivably be related to the accumulation of metabolic precursors in the hepatic cell (PIVKA) (3).

Although the initial or maximum rate of the effect during the first few hours after administration of vitamin K_1 is thus virtually independent of the dose, the maximum intensity of the effect is very distinctly dependent on the dose. There is a linear relationship between this intensity level (average maximum observed increase of the activity of the 4 coagulation factors) and the logarithm of the vitamin K_1 dose, at least for the reaction to intravenous application (figure 4).

The maximum elevation of the coagulation-factor level was reached 24 to 48 hours after a single dose of vitamin K_1, and in normal subjects there was no important difference between oral and intravenous administration, probably because under normal circumstances there is a rapid and virtually complete resorption of vitamin K_1 through the intestinal wall. But the effect of the 1 mg dose, for instance, was dubious after oral administration, whereas after intravenous administration there was a just barely measureable reaction. For a few of the normal subjects, the reaction to a 5 mg dose also showed a slight difference between oral and intravenous administration, but for higher doses this difference was no longer distinct.

On the basis of the maxima found in normal subjects, a dose response curve was constructed (figure 5). The beginning of this curve was taken as the normal daily resorption of vitamin K (estimated at 0.2 mg) and the end as the maximum values reachable (100 per cent values).

It is extremely important that this dose response curve for vitamin K_1 obtained in normal volunteer subjects is based on a relatively low degree of hypocoagulability, the Thrombotest values lying between 10 and 15 per cent averaging 12 per cent (which equals 20 to 30 per cent factor activity, averaging 24 per cent):

For the intensity of anticoagulation reached in the treatment of patients without contra-indications (5 to 10 per cent Thrombotest = 10 to

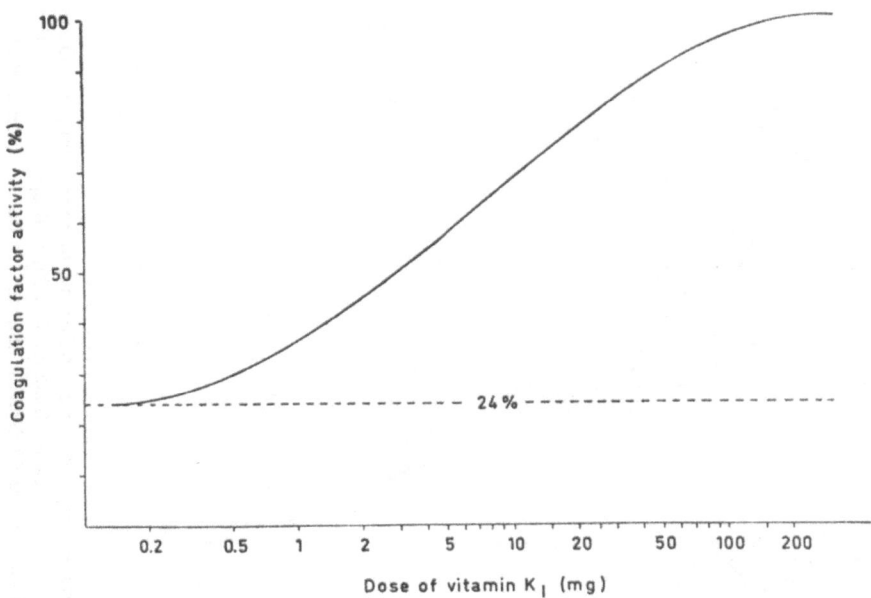

Fig. 5. Dose response curve for vitamin K₁ in phenprocoumon-induced hypocoagulability in normal subjects, based on the average maximum increases of the 4 coagulation factors after intravenous administration of 1, 5, and 25 mg doses.

20 per cent factor activity), the dosage required to achieve the same effect will be about twice as high.

3. Duration of the effect

The duration of the effect of vitamin K_1 was studied in relation to the dosage. In our normal subjects, for whom a normal metabolism may be assumed, it took about 3, 5, and 7 days after intravenous administration of 1, 5, and 25 mg, respectively, before the original hypocoagulability was again found.

Like the rate at which the clotting defect is corrected after administration of vitamin K_1, the duration of the effect of vitamin K_1 is to a high degree determined by the biological half-life of the factors of the prothrombin complex (figure 6).

III. Effect of vitamin K_1 in patients

1. Patients without manifest sickness

Patients who were not seriously ill reacted, in principle, in the same way as the normal volunteer subjects. The intensity of the reaction to a given

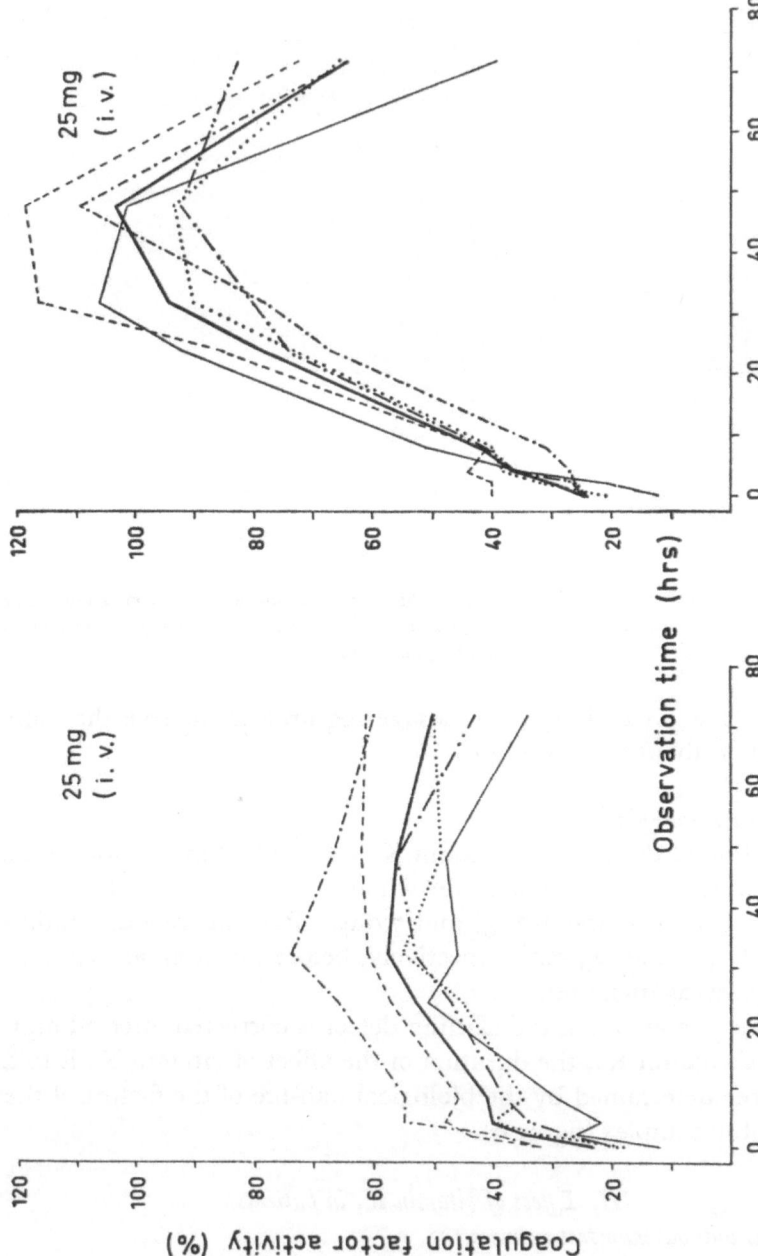

Fig. 6. Course of the activity of factors II and VII after intravenous administration of 25 mg vitamin K₁ to normal subjects during continued administration of phenprocoumon. After reaching its maximum within 24 to 48 hours, the activity drops according to the law of biological degradation (gradual decrease of factor II due to long half-life, and rapid decrease of factor VII due to short half-life).

dose was distinctly lower, however, since the patients had an appreciably more pronounced phenprocoumon effect or vitamin K deficency
(Thrombotest values 5 to 10 per cent). The difference in reaction between subjects and patients is clearly shown by figure 7.

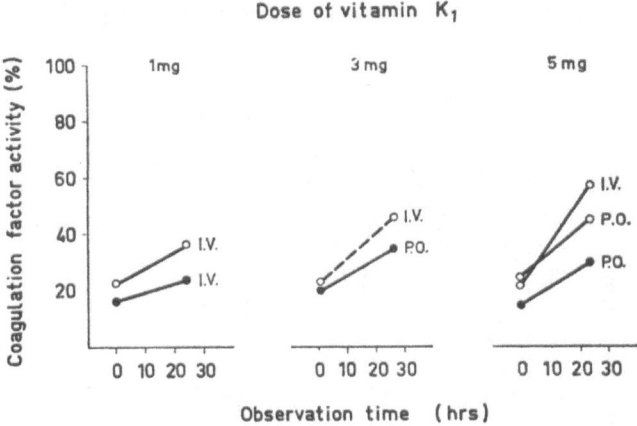

Fig. 7. Reaction over 24-hr period to vitamin K₁ in patients (dots) and normal subjects (circles).
The reaction of the subjects to 3 mg vitamin K₁ is derived from the dose-effect curve.

Even more distinct is the relatively more limited effect of vitamin K₁
in the treatment of patients with coumarin intoxication in whom doses
of 10 to 50 mg give distinctly less effect that in patients with a so-called

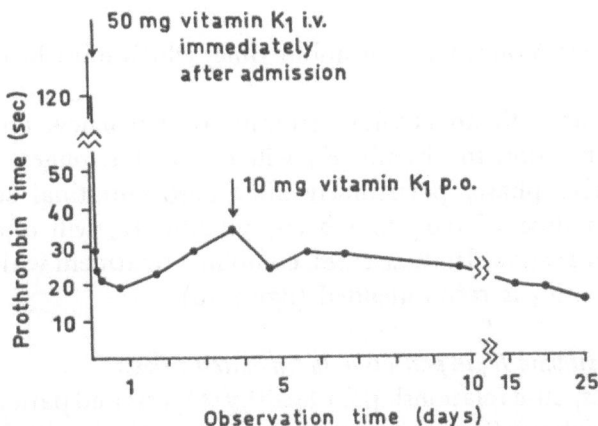

Fig. 8. Reaction to vitamin K₁, as shown by prothrombin-time values in a patient with
suicidal phenprocoumon intoxication. (Coumarin determinations in the blood demonstrated
that after admission the patient had taken no more coumarin).

therapeutically optimal hypocoagulability (Thrombotest values 5 to 10 per cent) (figures 8 and 9).

In cases of severe coumarin intoxication an initial dose of 20 mg vitamin K_1 should be given intravenously, after which the further dosage

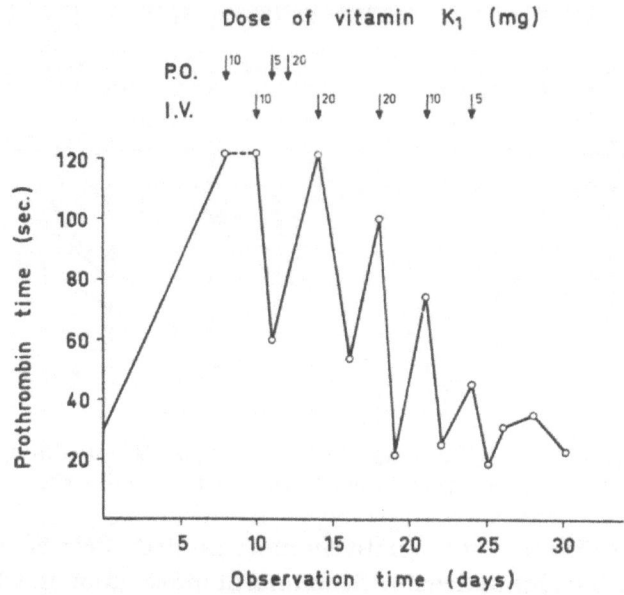

Fig. 9. Reaction to vitamin K_1 in a patient who erroneously took a tenfold dose of phenprocoumon for several weeks.

should be based on the prothrombin time, which must be determined daily.

In patients with an absolute vitamin K deficiency, on the other hand, the reaction to vitamin K_1 will be much stronger. E.g. in the post-operative phase, particularly after gastrointestinal surgery, an intravenous dose of 0.05 to 0.2 mg vitamin K_1 will often provide sufficient correction. In these cases, combined treatment with coumarin and vitamin K_1 is recommended (figure 10).

2. Effect of vitamin K_1 in patients with a manifest sickness

The dose response relationship for healthy subjects and patients without a manifest sickness (figure 5) does not hold for patients with fever, anaemia, hyperthyroidism, etc. Under these conditions the reaction to vitamin K_1 is in the first place much more rapid, because the rate of synthesis of the coagulation factors is often greatly accelerated. This can be seen from, for example, the course of the prothrombin time in the two patients with coumarin intoxication shown in figures 8 and 9, but it is also evident from the curves in figure 11.

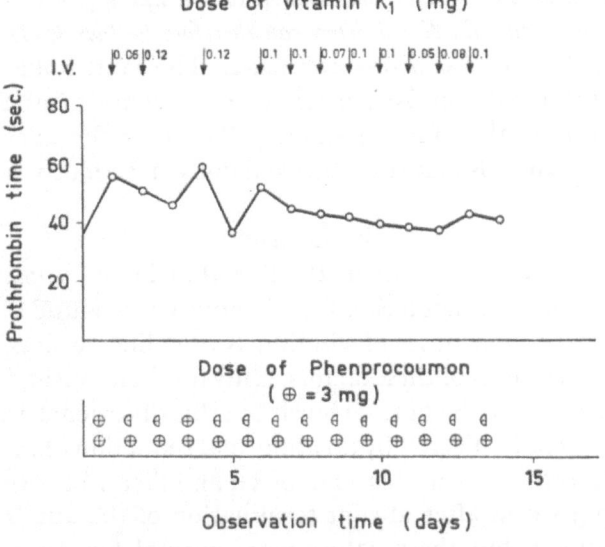

Fig. 10. Course of the coagulability of the blood, as expressed by the prothrombin time, in a patient suffering from a fat-resorption anomaly and treated with coumarin and vitamin K_1.

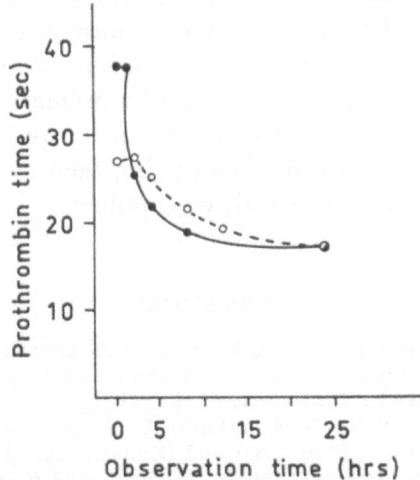

Fig. 11. Course of the prothrombin time after administration of high doses of vitamin K_1 in normal subjects (dashed line) and a seriously sick patient (solid line). Maximum rate of synthesis of the coagulation factors is assumed.

Determination of the reaction of the individual coagulation factors has shown that in normal subjects there is an average increase of the factor activity of 15 per cent within 8 hours after the administration of a high dose of vitamin K_1, whereas seriously sick patients show a similar rise within 2 hours. *The rate of the reaction to vitamin K_1 in cases of relative, coumarin-induced vitamin K deficiency can therefore be four times higher in seriously sick patients than in normal individuals.* The same holds for patients with an absolute vitamin K deficiency due to acholia (usually neoplastic obstruction of the biliary passages). To avoid the unexpected, the reaction to vitamin K_1 must be checked daily in seriously sick patients.

IV. Rebound?

In closing, we wish to point to the fact that in the *normal subjects* no overshooting of the coagulation factor activity was found after administration of very high doses of vitamin K_1 leading to maximal stimulation of the synthesis of these factors. Only the factor VII activity seemed to rise slightly above the normal level, but this divergence was not significant and was not reflected by an abnormal reduction of the prothrombin time. In *patients* a very high factor VII and factor IX activity was observed 2 to 3 weeks after abrupt termination of the administration of phenprocoumon, but these values were normal for the age-group to which these patients belonged. There is therefore no reason to fear a rebound hypercoagulability after administration of vitamin K_1 or after abrupt termination of coumarin in either normals or patients. The so-called rebound thrombosis must therefore have another explanation: either as an ordinary recurrence caused by premature cessation of the treatment (6) or as the result of the often severe hypercoagulability and strongly modified platelet functioning seen in cases of bleeding complications for which vitamin K_1 was applied.

REFERENCES

1. Brambel, E., G. L. Serra, Oral anticoagulant therapy and its control: Marcoumar (phenprocoumon), a new highly active anticoagulant and Konakion (phytomenadione), as an effective regulator. *Thrombos. Diathes. haemorrh.* 3, 271 (1959).
2. Clausen, J., P. Andresen, S. Gruelund, E. Harsløf, U. H. Andersen, J. Jørgensen, C. Mose, Über die Verwendung von Marcoumar und Dicumarol bei der Langzeitbehandlung (vergleichende Untersuchungen). *Thrombos. Diathes. haemorrh.* 6, 37 (1961).
3. Hemker, H. C., E. A. Loeliger, Kinetic aspects of the interaction of blood-clotting enzymes. III. Demonstration of an inhibitor of prothrombin conversion in vitamin K-deficiency. *Thrombos. Diathes. haemorrh.* 19, 346 (1968).

4. Meer, J. van der, H. C. Hemker, E. A. Loeliger, Pharmacological aspects of vitamin K$_1$. A clinical and experimental study in man. *Thrombos. Diathes. haemorrh.* Suppl. 29 (1968).
5. Rodman, T., B. H. Pastor, M. E. Resnick, Phenprocoumon, diphenadione, warfarin, and bishydroxycoumarin: A comparative study. *Amer. J. med. Sci.* 247, 655 (1964).
6. Sevitt, S., D. Innes: Evidence against 'Rebound' thrombosis after stopping oral anticoagulants. *Lancet* II, 974 (1963).

CHAPTER IV

THE ASSESSMENT OF LIVER FUNCTION BY BLOOD COAGULATION TESTS

BLOOD COAGULATION AND LIVER FUNCTION

E. A. LOELIGER

Nine of the ten proteins called coagulation factors because they are biologically active in blood coagulation, are produced by the parenchymal liver cell (13, 16). The exception is factor VIII, the bulk of which is synthesized elsewhere, probably in the cells of the reticuloendothelial system. The biosynthesis of four of the nine factors produced by the liver-cell is vitamin K dependent. These are factors II, VII, IX, and X, the factors of the so-called prothrombin complex.

Table 1. Physiological disappearance rate of the coagulation factors, according to various authors.

			approx. biol. t 1/2 (hrs)
Prothrombin complex	I	fibrinogen	100[5]
	II	prothrombin	60[4,7]
	V	proaccelerine	16[1]
	VII	proconvertine	6[4,7]
	VIII	A.H.F.	15[11]
	IX	Christmas factor	20[4,7,9]
	X	Stuart factor	40[4,7]
	XI	P.T.A.	60[1,2,15]
	XII	Hageman factor	60[17]
	XIII	F.S.F.	150[1]

Because liver cells and vitamin K have a central position in coagulation-factor synthesis, there seemed to be two ways in which coagulation tests could be helpful in clinical pathology:

1. for the assessment of the severity of liver-cell damage; and
2. for the differentiation between liver-cell damage and vitamin K- deficiency.

That both these expectations proved true we all know. As early as 1940, Koller developed the so-called *vitamin-K test*, which made differ-

361

entiation between liver-cell damage and vitamin K deficiency possible
(6).

A more exact correlation between liver-cell function, the action of
vitamin K, and blood coagulation has been found only recently, as will
appear from the following:

It is now rather well established that the *blood level of the enzymatic
coagulation factors*, particularly that of the prothrombin complex, directly *reflects the amount of functionally healthy liver-cell parenchyma* present, provided there is no vitamin K deficiency or overt intravascular coagulation. This correlation becomes perfectly comprehensible if we know
that *a.* as long as liver function is not hampered, the rates of production
and destruction of coagulation factors remain in balance, even under
severely pathological conditions; *b.* coagulation-factor synthesis is independent of the levels of these factors in the blood; and *c.* changes in
the production rate are followed closely by changes in blood levels.

ad a.: The blood levels appear to remain in the normal range even if,
in severe illness, there is a fourfold increase of the turnover rate, or,
in cases of hypothyroidism, a decrease to half the normal value occurs
(7, 10). It must be kept in mind, however, that under certain physiological conditions a significant elevation of the blood level may occur.
This holds for older age groups, and is even more pronounced (up to
more than 150 per cent of normal) in the last quarter of pregnancy. The
site of the metabolic change occurring under these conditions is not
known.

ad b.: We know from transfusion experiments that the blood level of
coagulation factors has no repercussions on the production rate, at least
as far as factors II, VII, IX, and X (8) and factor VIII (11) are concerned.
Coagulation-factor biosynthesis continues unabated even in case of prolonged transfusion of large amounts of these factors. We have also
learned that when the blood levels become reduced due to a shortage
of liver cells, the production rate per cell apparently does not increase.
Most convincing in this respect is the evidence provided by cases of
partial hepatectomy: the activity of the factors of the prothrombin complex decreases to a level roughly expected for the remaining liver tissue
and recovers normality only 4 to 6 weeks after the operation, a time-
lapse equal to the interval needed for liver-cell regeneration (12). Observations in patients suffering from chronic hepatitis corroborate the

view that the level of the coagulation factors in the blood likewise reflects the amount of morphologically more or less intact liver parenchyma (3,9). *ad c.*: Changes in liver function are observed to be closely followed by changes in blood coagulation when checked with a factor vII-sensitive test system (prothrombin time assay, using human brain thromboplastin; Normotest). This close parallelism is explained by the rapid turnover of factor vII, whose biological half-life is 6 hours or less.

We have found that the *coagulation-factor level* also has *prognostic value*, which may be added as circumstantial evidence of the important correlation between the coagulation-factor level and a functionally intact liver parenchyma. As long as the level of the prothrombin complex is above 50 per cent, the metabolic function of the liver is sufficient, even for major operations. A 20 to 30 per cent level is critical, and if the level drops below 15 per cent hepatic coma will soon follow, provided of course that vitamin K deficiency is not involved. The levels of fibrinogen and factor v, which must be assessed separately, give important additional information about the severity of liver-cell damage. The fibrinogen level seldom drops below 100 mg per cent (severe cases only), whereas in most cases the activity of factor v is lowered less than that of factors II, vII, IX, and X. If factor v activity decreases below 10 per cent, the prognosis of a hepatitis is bad; whereas subnormal, normal, or even increased values of factor v indicate a rather good prognosis.

Finally, as already mentioned, blood coagulation also occupies a place of paramount importance among the liver-function tests. By means of the well-known vitamin K test, i.e. assessment of the increase of activity of the factors of the prothrombin complex 24 hours after intravenous injection of 1 mg vitamin K_1 (14), a deficiency of vitamin K can be demonstrated. Less specifically and much more rapidly, however, vitamin K deficiency can also be diagnosed quite safely by means of coagulation tests disclosing the recently discovered coagulation inhibitor 'PIVKA', which enters the circulation in cases of vitamin K deficiency.

To sum up and conclude:
Damage to liver parenchyma can be easily and rapidly quantified by a factor vII-sensitive blood coagulation test. Shortage of vitamin K can be diagnosed within 24 hours by means of the well-known vitamin K test or almost immediately by means of coagulation tests sensitive to the circulating anticoagulant specific for vitamin K deficiency.

REFERENCES

1. Bowie, E. J. W., J. H. Thrompson, P. Didisheim, C. A. Owen, Disappearance rates of coagulation factors: transfusion studies in factor-deficient patients. *Transfusion*, 7, 174 (1967).
2. Britten, A. F. H., W. Salzman, Surgery in congenital disorders of blood coagulation. *Surg. Gyn. and Obstet.* 123, 1333 (1966).
3. Colombi, H., G. Thölen, G. Engelhart, F. Duckert, Y. Hecht, F. Koller, Blutgerinnungs-factoren als Index für den Schweregrad einer akuten Hepatitis. *Schweiz. Med. W'schr.* 97, 1716 (1968).
4. Esch, B. van der, E. A. Loeliger, De werking van coumarine-preparaten op de bloed-stolling bij hoge initiële dosering. *Verslag 3e Conf. Thrombosediensten Ned. Roode Kruis*, Zeist, p. 26 (1960).
5. Hart, H. C. H., De biologische halveringstijd van 131V-fibrinogeen. *Thesis* (1966).
6. Koller, F., Weitere Erfahrungen mit Vitamin K. Synthetische Vitamin K-Präparate - der Vitamin K-Test, eine Leberfunktionsprüfung. *Helv. med. acta* 7, 651 (1941).
7. Loeliger, E. A., B. van der Esch, H. C. Hemker, M. J. Mattern, The biological dis-appearance rate of prothrombin, factor VII, IX, and X from plasma in hypothyroidism, hyperthyroidism, and during fever. *Thrombos. Diathes. haemorrh.* 10, 267 (1964).
8. Loeliger, E. A., A. Hensen, M. J. Mattern, J. J. Veltkamp, P. F. Bruning, H. C. Hemker, Treatment of haemophilia B with purified factor IX (PPSB). *Folia Med. Neerl.* 10, 112 (1967).
9. Loeliger, E. A., Personal experience, not published.
10. Meer, J. van der, H. C. Hemker, E. A. Loeliger, Pharmacological Aspects of Vitamin K_1, A clinical and experimental study in man. *Thrombos. Diathes. haemorrh.* Suppl. 29 (1968).
11. Meyer, K., J. G. Eernisse, J. J. Veltkamp, H. C. Hemker, E. A. Loeliger, Treatment of haemophilia A with purified factor VIII obtained from human plasma by cryoprecipi-tation. *Folia Med. Neerl.* 10, 49 (1967).
12. Niléhn, J. E., I. M. Nillson, K. F. Aronson, B. Ericsson, Studies on blood clotting factors in man after massive liver resection. *Acta Chir. Scand.* 133, 189 (1967).
13. Olson, J. P., L. L. Miller, S. B. Troup, Synthesis of clotting factors by the isolated per-fused rat liver. *J. Clin. Invest.* 45, 690 (1966).
14. Pestalozzi, H., Die prognostische und differentialdiagnostische Bedeutung des Vitamin K-Tests. *Schweiz. Med. W'schr.* 88, 402 (1958).
15. Rosenthal, R. L., E. Sloan, PTA (Factor XI levels and coagulation studies after plasma infusions in PTA deficient patients. *J. Lab. Clin. Med.* 66, 709 (1965).
16. Straub, P. W., A study of fibrinogen production by human liver slices in vitro by an immunoprecipitin method. *J. Clin. Invest.* 42, 130 (1963).
17. Veltkamp, J. J., E. A. Loeliger, H. C. Hemker, The biological half-time of Hageman factor. *Thrombos. Diathes. haemorrh.* 13, 1 (1965).

THE THROMBOTEST DILUTION CURVE AND ITS DIAGNOSTIC SIGNIFICANCE

H. C. HEMKER

The appearance of a visible clot in a plasma mixture is the result of a set of interrelated biochemical reactions, each of which plays a specific role in the coagulation process. The situation is not unlike that in a factory, where several groups of workmen – each group having a circumscript and specific task – cooperate to produce a final product.

In such a factory the velocity of product formation is determined by the individual velocities of the separate groups. If, however, one group is much slower than the others, the over-all production velocity – and in the biochemical situation the reaction velocity – will be governed by the velocity of the slow group. This group has thus become *rate limiting*.

Fluctuations in the velocity of the rate-limiting group immediately show up as fluctuations of the over-all production velocity, whereas changes in the other groups, which are not rate-limiting, show up much less readily. It is therefore essential to know the location of the rate-limiting step if we are to understand the complete mechanism of end-product formation. In the Thrombotest reaction, any one of the three factors II, VII, or X can be rate-limiting, as is readily seen from the fact that plasmas congenitally deficient in these factors show very long Thrombotest times; but we have shown that where these factors are present in equal amounts (expressed in per cent), it is factor X that governs the over-all reaction rate (2). Where, however, the concentration of factor VII (or II) falls appreciably below that of factor X, factor VII (or II) will of course become rate-limiting.

To return to our analogy of the factory, it will be clear that once the rate-limiting group has been located, one would try to increase the capacity of this group. A moderate increase will speed up the over-all process very effectively, but an increase beyond reasonable proportions would simply make one of the other groups rate-limiting and would consequently have no further influence on the production velocity. In the same way, increasing the factor x concentration will increase the reaction velocity of a Thrombotest reaction, but to increase the factor x concentration to infinity would still leave us with a finite coagulation time.

It might, of course, be interesting to know what this coagulation time would be at infinite factor x concentration. Although it is physically impossible to estimate this coagulation time directly, it can be estimated by extrapolation in the so-called t-D plot (figure 1).

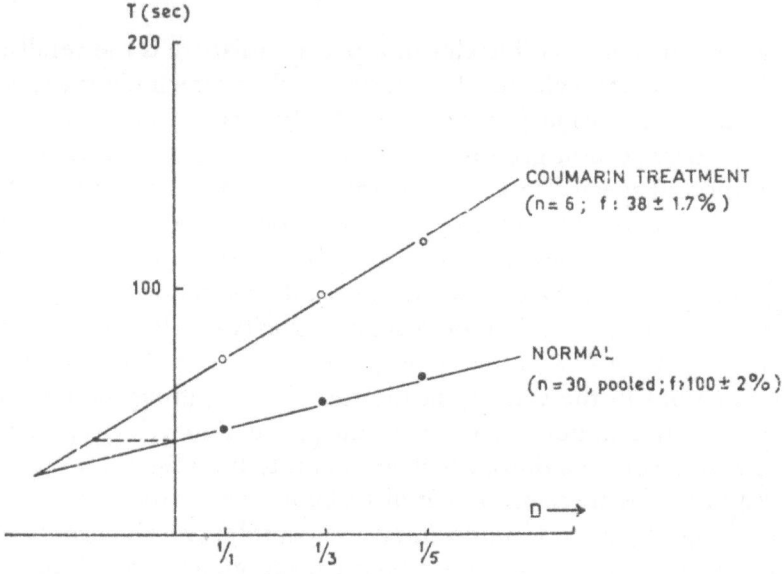

Fig. 1. *The t-D plot.* The lines were obtained from pooled plasmas. The 6 patients whose plasma provided the upper line (open circles) were under stable long-term steady-state anticoagulant treatment. n = number of cases; t = mean of the concentration of factors II, VII, and x in the individual plasmas.

The t-D plot is a graph in which the dilution ratio (D) of a plasma sample is plotted against the coagulation time obtained with that sample. The dilution ratio is defined as the ratio of the volume of the sample after dilution to that of the volume before dilution. Undiluted plasma thus would have a D equal to unity. It has been demonstrated that the t-D plot of the Thrombotest reaction, as well as that of most other tests of the Quick type, is a straight line (2). This enables us to determine the virtual coagulation time that will be obtained when D=0 by prolonging this straight line to the value D=0, i.e. to its intercept with the y-axis. It is easily seen that $D=0$ means an infinite concentration of the sample. This, however, immediately raises the question: what reactant in the sample is essentially the reactant whose concentration is extrapolated to infinity? It is clear that this must be the reactant(s) determining the coagulation time in the data from which the extrapolation is carried out. We have shown that in steady-state anticoagulation, factors II, VII, IX, and X have dropped to the same level (5). Moreover, as we have seen above, as long as the concentration (expressed in per cent) of these factors is equal, it is factor x that is rate-limiting. This holds for plasma from a steady-state anticoagulated patient as well as for its dilutions. *So t_{min} is the clotting time at infinite factor x concentration.*

Now, common sense tells us that if the Thrombotest time is determined by the factor x concentration, the coagulation time obtained with Thrombotest at infinite factor x concentration (t_{min}) must be the same no matter what sample provided the experimental data from which this minimal time was calculated. But, as occurs ever so often, common sense is misleading here, at least with respect to material from patients on anticoagulant treatment. In these cases t_{min} proved to be appreciably higher than was to be expected. We have shown that this phenomenon is caused by the presence of a competitive inhibitor protein in cases in which too little functional vitamin K is present. This inhibitor has been termed PIVKA (1, 3).

Calculations (whose discussion is beyond of the scope of this paper) show that the amount of inhibitor can be estimated by measuring the length of a horizontal line drawn in a t-D graph through t_{min} of normal plasma between its intercepts with the t-D line of the plasma to be estimated and the y-axis (3) (i.e. the dashed line in figure 1).

It has been shown (4) that the amount of inhibitor is indeed correlated with the presence or absence of vitamin K and not with the level of any of the known coagulation factors. The recognition of this inhibitor also explains the discrepancies between the results of various coagulation tests applied to blood from anticoagulated or vitamin K deficient patients.

A t-D plot based on a patient's plasma in principle gives us two kinds of information:

a. The slope of the curve, expressed as a percentage of the slope of a normal control, gives the amount of factor x present in the sample.

b. The length of the line *i* is related to the amount of PIVKA present, and can thus reveal the existence of vitamin K deficiency.

Unfortunately, however, the method of estimating *i* is very inaccurate when the concentration of factor x is above 50 per cent. Also, the method can only work satisfactorily in chronic cases, where the level of factor VII does not lie below that of factor x. A third drawback of the method is that the presence of other inhibitors occurring in isolated cases can obscure the results of the test. In spite of all these drawbacks, however, we have found the construction of t-D plots to be a useful routine procedure, since it has substantially deepened our insight into disorders of coagulation-factor synthesis in liver disease and vitamin K deficiency.

REFERENCES

1. Hemker, H. C., J. J. Veltkamp, A. Hensen, E. A. Loeliger, On the nature of prothrombin biosynthesis. *Nature* 200, 589 (1963).
2. Hemker, H. C., T. Siepel, R. Altman, E. A. Loeliger, Kinetic aspects of the interaction of blood clotting enzymes. II: The relation between clotting time and plasma concentration in prothrombin-time estimations. *Thrombos. Diathes. haemorrh.* 17, 349 (1967).
3. Hemker, H. C., J. J. Veltkamp, E. A. Loeliger, Kinetic aspects of the interaction of blood-clotting enzymes. III. Demonstration of the existence of an inhibitor of prothrombin conversion in vitamin K-deficiency. *Thrombos. Diathes. haemorrh.* 19, 346 (1968).
4. Hemker, H. C., P. W. Hemker, Kinetic aspects of the interaction of blood-clotting enzymes. IV: Kinetics of competitive inhibitor of clotting tests. *Thrombos. Diathes. haemorrh.* 19, 364 (1968).
5. Loeliger, E. A., B. van der Esch, M. J. Mattern, A. S. A. den Brabander, Behaviour of factor II, VII, IX, x during long-term treatment with coumarin. *Thrombos. Diathes. haemorrh.* 9, 74 (1963).

NORMOTEST IN THE EVALUATION
OF LIVER FUNCTION

P. A. OWREN

Because the four vitamin K dependent clotting factors (factors II, VII, IX, and X) are synthesized by the liver, clotting tests have been extensively used for the assessment of liver parenchymatous function and vitamin K deficiency. Prothrombin time methods are usually preferred because of simplicity. They are sensitive to three of the four factors involved: prothrombin and factors VII and X. The blood levels of these factors depend on the balance between synthesis and life-time in the circulation. The life-time may be reduced under certain conditions, but for practical clinical purposes this fact can be disregarded in liver diseases and the plasma concentration can be taken as an indirect measure of synthesis.

Endogenous coagulation inhibitors occur not only during anticoagulant therapy, as demonstrated by Hemker and collaborators (1), but also in certain diseases. The presence of such inhibitors might mimic defective synthesis and impaired liver function by influencing the clotting test used. For the control of synthesis as a measure of liver function, therefore, it is important to use methods which are insensitive to such inhibitors.

We have therefore developed a standardized method which is insensitive to all types of endogenous inhibitors except heparin. It is called Normotest, because it provides for accurate determinations also in the normal and near normal range. This range is of particular interest in liver diseases. The thromboplastin applied in this reagent has been purified in a way similar to that for Thrombotest, and the reagent is standardized and stabilized similarly.

The correlation curve for the Normotest method is steeper than that for Thrombotest and other methods in the higher concentration range, and thus provides for more accurate determinations between 50 and 100 per cent of normal (figure 1). For determinations above 100 per cent of normal, half the volume of the test sample can be used. The result read from the curve is then multiplied by 2. This procedure should not be applied for the Thrombotest method because the Thrombotest value increases on reduction of the test volume if endogenous inhibitors are present, as a result of the lowering of the inhibitor effect by dilution.

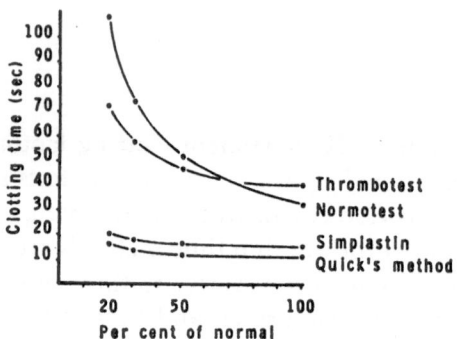

Fig. 1. Correlation curves for converting clotting time in seconds into per cent of normal. They are prepared by testing of serial dilutions of a normal standard plasma.

The liver has many and complex functions which are affected differently in different diseases, and consequently the various liver function tests are also influenced differently. A battery of tests are therefore often applied. We have tried to evaluate the merits of Normotest as compared with the most frequently used liver function tests, such as the determination of serum glutamic oxaloacetic (sGOT) and serum glutamic pyruvic transaminases (sGPT), serum bilirubin, the Thymol-turbidity test, the Bromsulphalein test, etc. (sGOT and sGPT was recorded in Karmen units which are twice the international U/1.)

Acute benign hepatitis
Normotest and Thrombotest give identical results, indicating that no inhibitor is present (figure 2). The degree of reduction in Normotest in such cases varies greatly, depending on the stage of the disease and its severity. Normotest, Thrombotest, and transaminases return to normal in about the same time of 2 to 6 weeks. Rapid rising of Normotest values is a good prognostic sign.

The prothrombin time test is not suitable for controlling the course of hepatitis, as illustrated in figure 3.

Severe, protracted and relapsing cases of hepatitis

We have controlled a number of such cases with the Normotest method, and the course of the disease seems to be well reflected in the Normotest values. Examples are given in figures 4 and 5. Of particular interest is the finding that during the period of slow recovery or improvement, the

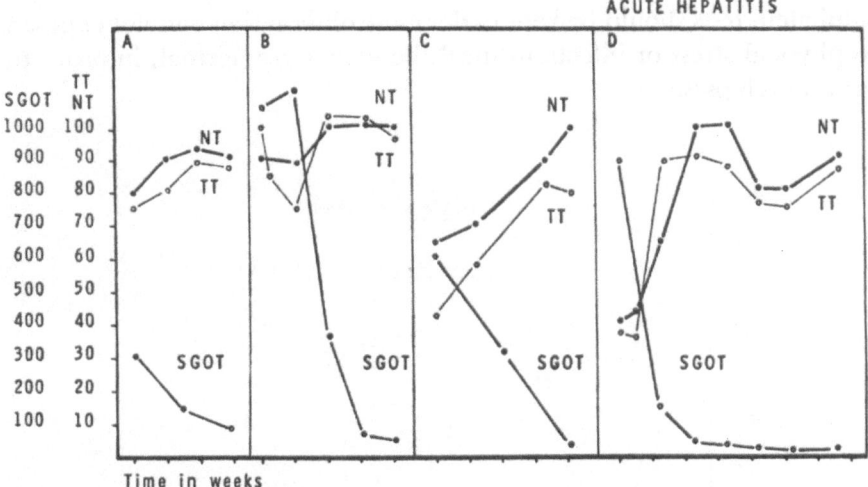

Fig. 2. Cases of acute benign hepatitis of different severity, but with complete recovery. SGOT and SGPT is given in Karmen units in this and the following figures. Upper limits of normal is 40, corresponding to 20 international U/l.

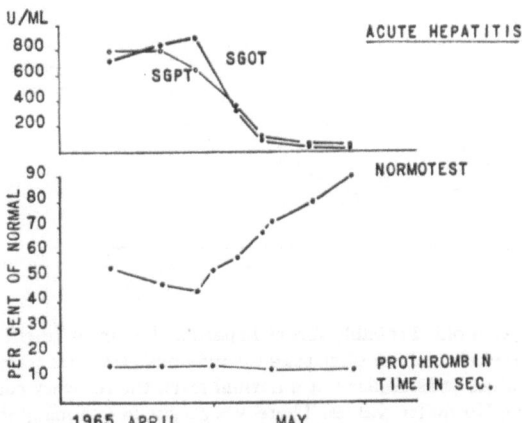

Fig. 3. The prothrombin time method is highly insensitive for determinations in the range above 40-50% of normal and consequently not appropriate for following the course of hepatitis.

transaminases usually return to normal at a stage when the Normotest values are still abnormal. Normotest seems to be more sensitive than the determination of transaminases in disclosing that recovery is not complete. The bromsulphalein test is also regularly abnormal at this stage of normal transaminase and abnormal Normotest values. This is reason to assume that patients with abnormal Normotest and bromsulphalein tests should be kept under close observation and not exposed to physical stress or infections until the values are normal, in order to prevent relapses.

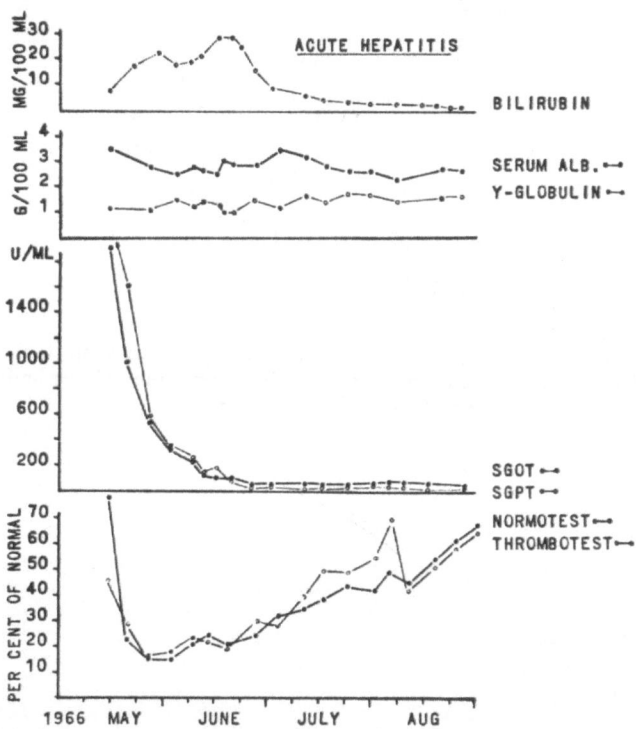

Fig. 4. Female, 23 years old. Probably serum hepatitis. The impairment of the synthesis of clotting factors appeared at a later stage than the maximal rise in transaminase values. After the transaminase values had stabilized at a normal level, the recovery could be followed by the slowly increasing Normotest values. There was no rise in gamma globulins and the thymol test was completely normal throughout. (Lack of antibody formation?) Serum albumin was moderately reduced (minimum 2.2 g/100 ml). Control October 30th: Serum albumin 4.7 g/100 ml. Thrombotest and Normotest gave about the same values, but for technical reasons Thrombotest showed greater fluctuations.

Chronic hepatitis

There is as a rule a good correlation between transaminases and Normotest, and both tests can be used to check on improvement or deterioration and for the evaluation of therapeutic effect, as illustrated in figure 6. In quiet periods the transaminases may return to normal, but the Normotest values usually remain at low values as a sign of defective hepatic function. A rise of transaminases often re occurs in such cases in association with exercise, alcohol, or intercurrent infections, but may again return to normal, whereas the Normotest values remain at an abnormally low level (figure 7).

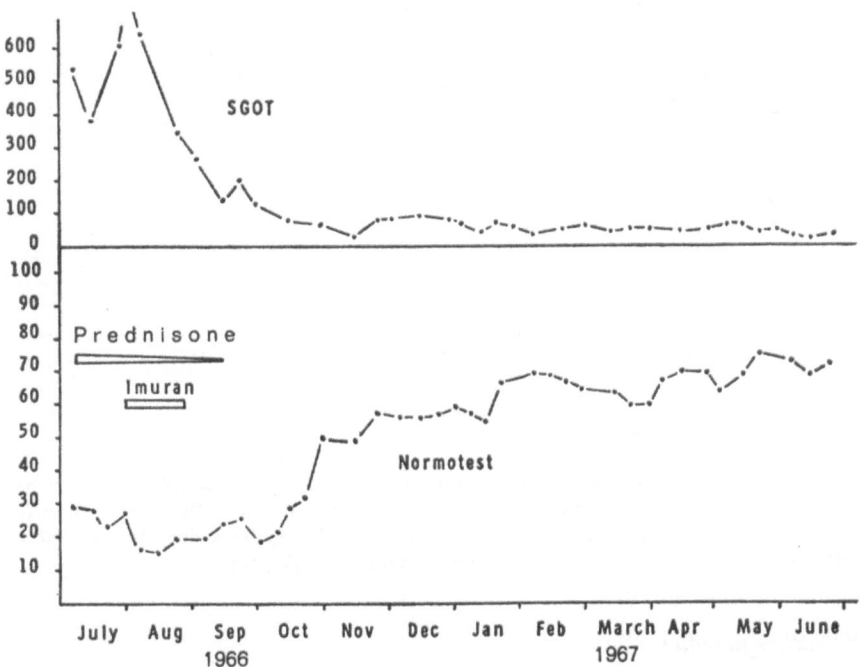

Fig. 5. Female 20 years. Acute hepatitis developing into chronic hepatitis. sGOT (and sGPT) reached normal values, but Normotest remained at an abnormal low level. The patient was dismissed from the hospital in June 1967, but was re-admitted after 2 months with a severe relapse and has developed chronic hepatitis.

Cirrhosis of the liver

It is well known that all liver function tests can be completely normal in cirrhosis of the liver, and this is also true for Normotest. In advanced

cases, however, lowered values are regularly found (figure 8). In such
cases the transaminases are either normal or only moderately increased,
but the bromsulphalein test has been positive in all advanced cases we
have observed so far.

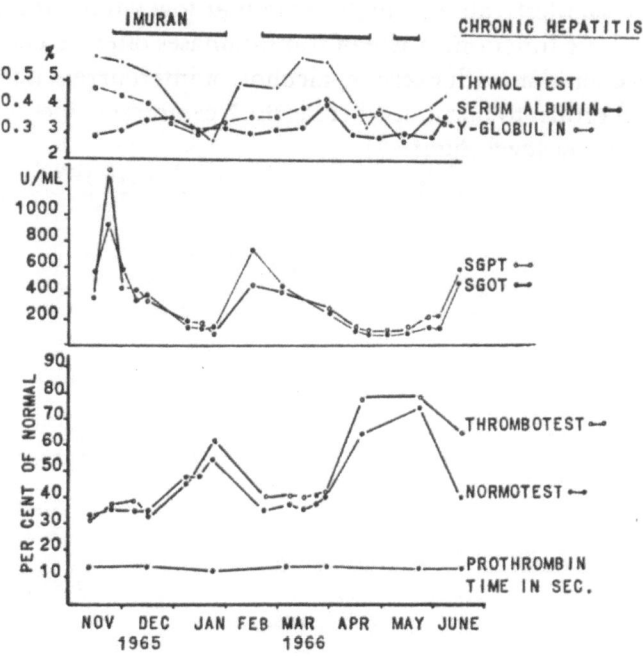

Fig. 6. Female, 18 years old. Infective hepatitis in April 1965, progressing to chronic hepatitis (post-hepatitis cirrhosis). Temporary improvements during Imuran therapy. Good correlation between falling transaminase values and increasing Normotest values. Imuran had to
be discontinued because of increasing anaemia and thrombocytopenia.

Obstructive jaundice

A difference is found between the values for Normotest and Thrombotest, similarly to the finding in patients on anticoagulant therapy.
Hemker, Van der Meer and Loeliger (2) first described the occurrence
of an endogenous coagulation inhibitor in obstructive jaundice, presumably pre-prothrombin, and suggested that the detection of this inhibitor could be used in differentiating between obstructive and parenchymatous jaundice.

Endogenous inhibitors

Inhibitors, probably of different types but producing significant differences between the Normotest and Thrombotest values, occur in certain diseases, particularly of the auto-immunological variety. The simultaneous application of Normotest and Thrombotest provides a sim-

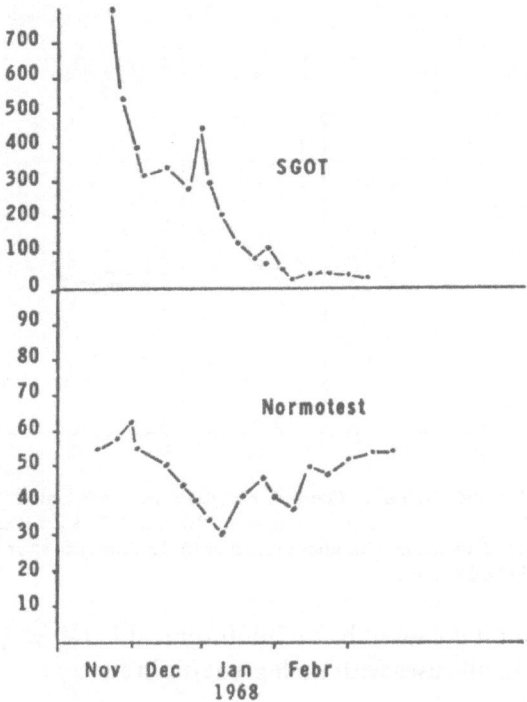

Fig. 7. Exacerbation in chronic hepatitis. sgot (and sgpt) decreased to normal values in a couple of months, but Normotest values remained at low levels as a sign of chronic liver disease.

ple screening for such inhibitors, which might have diagnostic importance. Inhibitors are found in some cases of prolonged or chronic hepatitis (figure 10). Lupoid hepatitis often displays this inhibitor symptom from the very beginning (figure 11), which gives a hint for correct diagnosis. The new type of factor ix deficiency, described by Hougie and Twomey (3) and which is associated with an endogenous inhibitor, is easily diagnosed by a marked difference between the Normotest and Thrombotest values. The three cases we have observed showed differences of 40 to 50 per cent between these two tests.

The greatest difference between the Normotest and Thrombotest values has been observed in cases of amyloidosis. We have seen five such cases during the last year, and all had normal Normotest values but Thrombotest values in the range of 20 to 30 per cent. The difference between the tests disappears on progressive dilution of the test sample,

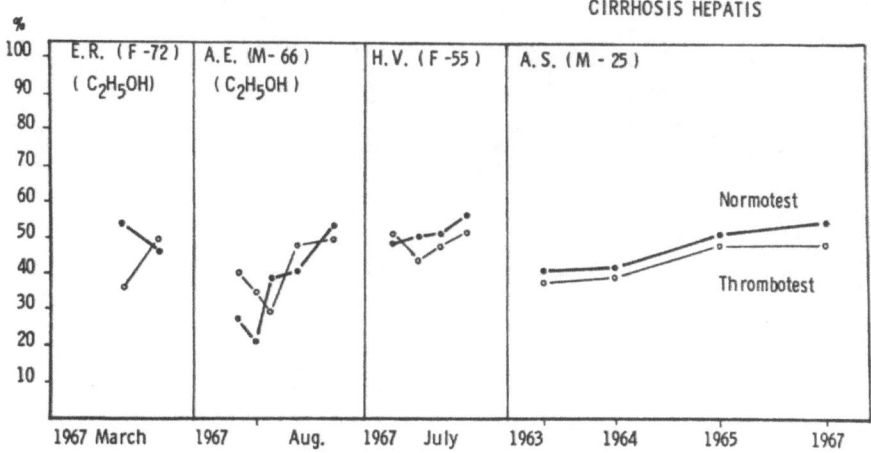

Fig. 8. Cases of hepatic cirrhosis. The first two cases were associated with alcoholism. In cases E.R. and H.V. transaminases were normal. In case A.E. SGOT was 822 Karmen units at admission, but fell to normal in about one month. In case A.S. SGOT and SGPT were moderately elevated at all checks.

suggesting that it is caused by an inhibitor (table 1). Amyloidosis should be suspected in all cases with such great differences.

Table 1. A case of amyloidosis. The influence of a highly effective inhibitor on the Thrombotest method disappears on progressive dilution of the test sample. Normotest is insensitive to this inhibitor.

Dilution of test plasma	Standard technique	I : 2	I : 4	I : 8
Thrombotest	23%	42%	72%	88%
Normotest	105%	94%	112%	112%

From the clinical experience of the last three years we might conclude that Normotest is a valuable test as a supplement to other liver function tests. It is particularly useful as a screening test for

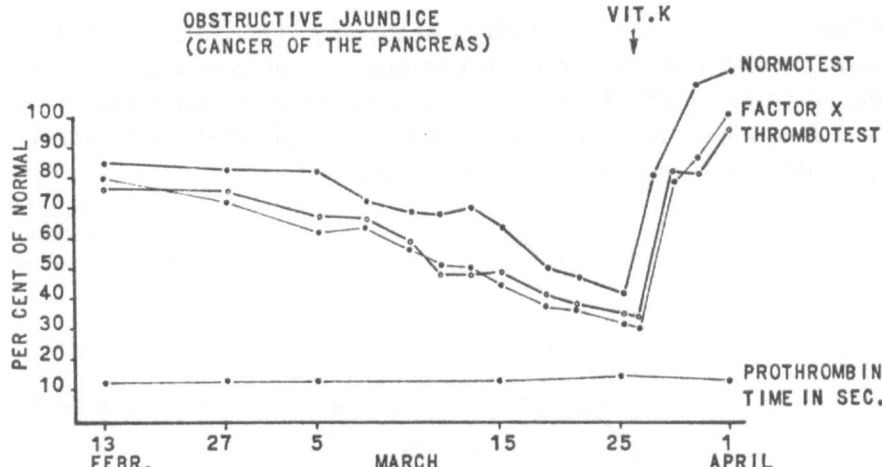

Fig. 9. Male, 60 years. Obstructive jaundice caused by cancer of the pancreas. Slowly decreasing Normotest values because of increasing vitamin K-deficiency. The administration of vitamin K produces a typical response, with Normotest values increasing to normal. Quick's prothrombin time test was not very useful for recording the effect of vitamin K. Prothrombin time methods require longstanding obstruction producing reduction of the 'prothrombin complex' to below about 30% in order to allow any definite conclusion from the vitamin K test. Thrombotest shows lower values than Normotest as a sign of inhibitor (pre-prothrombin).

Broms	6%		36%			4%
Thymol	0 10	0.16	0.36	0.28	0.19	0.14
Alb	4.6	3.2	4.1	3.7	3.8	3.9
Glob	1.6	2.1	3.2	2.8	2.0	2.1
SGOT	26	44	380	55	33	22
SGPT	34	38	370	58	37	22

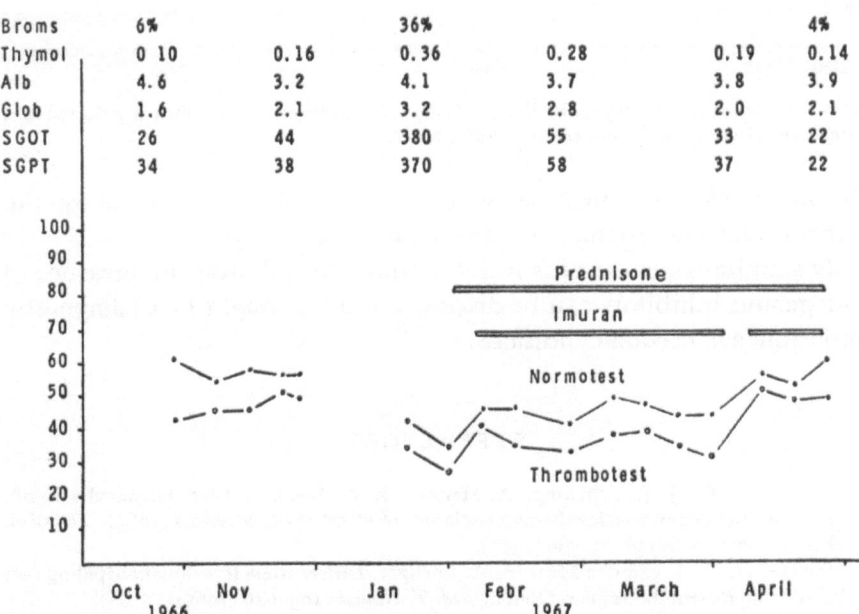

Fig. 10. Chronic hepatitis with a moderate difference between Normotest and Thrombotest, suggesting the presence of an inhibitor (SGOT and SGPT are given in Karmen units).

following the course and the effect of therapy. The Normotest values correlate well with the level of transaminases, but in certain instances the Normotest method seems to be *more sensitive in disclosing residual defects*. Normotest has the advantage of being simple, and it does not require the service of a biochemical laboratory.

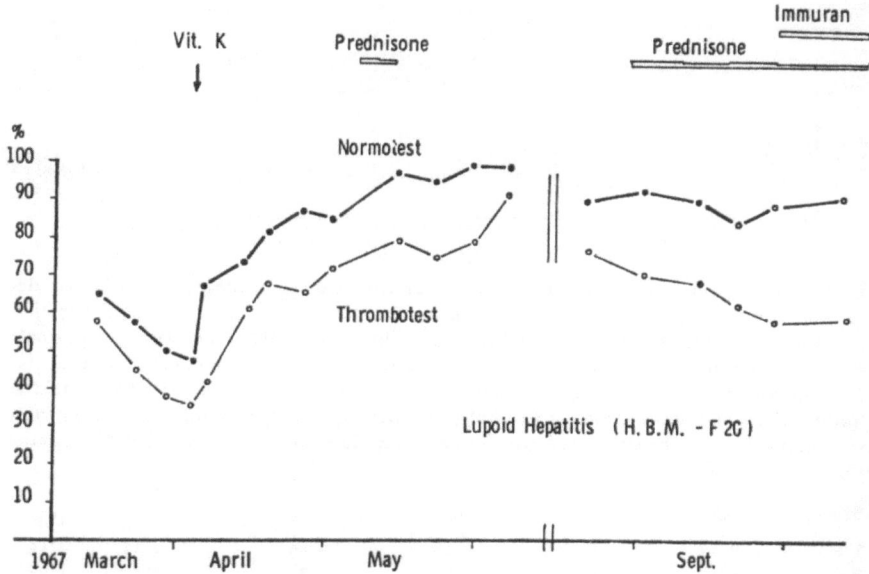

Fig. 11. A case of lupoid hepatitis. The presence of an endogenous inhibitor is reflected in a difference between the Normotest and Thrombotest values.

Normotest can of course be used as a general screening test for the extrinsic clotting system, for instance pre-operatively.

By simultaneous use of Normotest and Thrombotest the presence of endogenous inhibitors can be disclosed and this might be of diagnostic importance in certain conditions.

REFERENCES

1. Hemker, H. C., J. J. Veltkamp, A. Hensen, E. A. Loeliger, Proc. Gleneagles Conf., International committee for the nomenclature of blood clotting factors (1963). *Thrombos. Diathes. haemorrh.* Suppl. 13, 380 (1964).
2. Hemker, H. C., J. van der Meer, E. A. Loeliger, Differentiële leverfunctiebepaling met behulp van de trombotest van Owren. *Ned. T. Geneesk.* 109, 646 (1965).
3. Hougie, C. and J. J. Twomey: Haemophilia B_M: A new type of factor-IX deficiency. *The Lancet* I, 698 (1967).

CLINICAL EXPERIENCE WITH NORMOTEST

M. FISCHER AND H. W. PILGERSTORFER

In a study done in 1,966 patients hospitalized at the Cardiologic Clinic of the University of Vienna, Normotest and the one-stage prothrombin-time assay procedure (Quick test) were compared. The Quick test was done in the Coagulant Laboratory of the First University Clinic of Vienna, using acetone-dried human brain thromboplastin.

The Normotest was performed according to the manufacturer's pres-cription, with either an automatic pipette (according to Hartert) or normal glass pipettes. Reproducibility of the results of Normotest was good, even for different technicians and both kinds of pipettes.

The tests were performed with citrated blood, using 1 volume of 3.8 per cent sodium citrate and 9 volumes of venous blood from patients with the following diagnoses:

1. Cardiovascular diseases without heart failure; in these patients the test was performed as a screening procedure to eliminate potential bleeders before heart catherization and other diagnostic methods (67 patients; 41.4%).
2. Heart disease with congestive heart failure (32 patients; 19.3%).
3. Coumarin-treated patients with various diagnoses (39 patients; 23.5%).
4. Diverse diseases without a change of coagulability (28 patients; 15.8%).

Figure 1 shows that there was a good correlation between the results obtained by the Quick test (PTZ) and Normotest (NT). An analysis of variance was performed on 273 values obtained by the two techniques. The correlation was found to be linear ($y = 0.58 x + 20.91$ as intercept) and the regression line showed good adaptation to the values ($p < 0.01$). Although a greater deviation was seen for Normotest values, the corre-lation coefficient of 0.755 proved a significant positive correlation. In a small number of cases ($n = 21$) we investigated the correlation between results obtained with the Quick test, Normotest, coagulation-factor assay procedure (factors I, II, V, and X), and the partial thromboplastin time assay procedure. We found, as expected, a highly significant correlation between results of the Quick test and the activity of coagulation

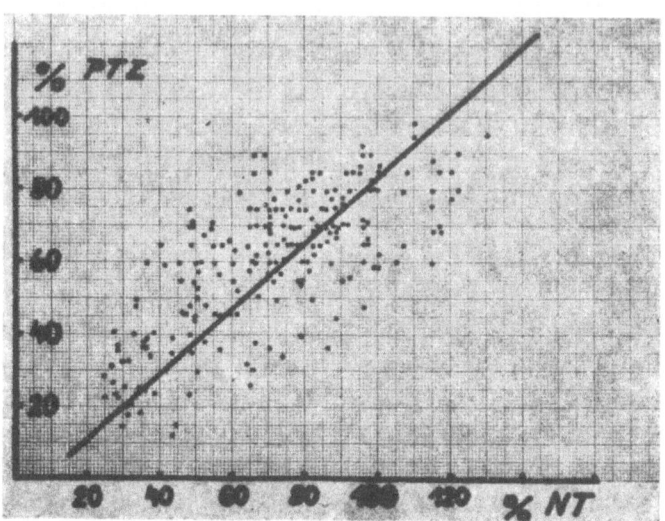

Fig. 1. Correlation between results obtained with Quick's one-stage prothrombin time assay procedure (PTZ) and Normotest (NT).

factors II, V, and X ($p=0.05$-0.001), whereas the Quick test results did not correlate with fibrinogen levels or partial thromboplastin times. Good correlation was also found between the results obtained with Normotest and factors II and X ($p=0.05$ and 0.01, respectively). Results obtained with Normotest did not correlate with factor V ($p=0.1$) and fibrinogen, or with the partial thromboplastin times.

In summarization of the foregoing, it may be said that in large series of patients we have observed good correlation between results obtained with Normotest and with the Quick test. Both correlate similarly with factors II and X (factor VII was not investigated). Normotest is insensitive to factor V. The conclusion must be that Normotest, in our hands, is not superior to Quick's one-stage prothrombin time assay procedure for screening disturbances of the extrinsic pathway of blood coagulation.

PRELIMINARY EXPERIENCE WITH NORMOTEST

J. J. VELTKAMP

When Normotest became available, we started to test the reagent itself for clotting factor activity. It contains, if any, less than 1 per cent of factors II, VII, and x. The amount of fibrinogen (150 mg%) and the factor v activity (25% of normal) are considered to be sufficient. Antithrombins are present in normal amounts.

Sensitivity of the reagent to depression of factors II, VII, and x was tested for each factor separately (figures 1-5). The correlation between the re-

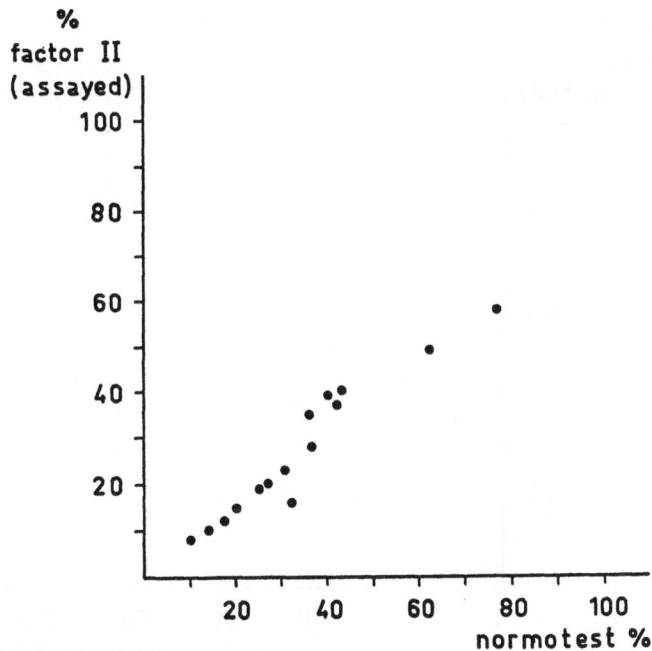

Fig. 1. Results obtained with a factor II one-stage assay procedure and Normotest on samples from a patient suffering from severe hypoprothrombinaemia who was treated by transfusion of concentrated prothrombin (see page 251).

sults of the specific factor assay and the Normotest value, although not
1, is satisfactory. A certain shift to the right is obvious for all three factors; this phenomenon is particularly pronounced in the factor VII correlation curve obtained for a patient suffering from congenital factor
VII deficiency and treated with Prothrombal (page 251). That the
curved correlation line is not due to the relatively high values of factors II and X induced by transfusion of the concentrated prothrombin
complex is shown by figure 4, in which the curve based on *in vitro*-
mixtures of normal plasma and plasma of the same patient shows almost the same shape. Normotest, hence, appears sensitive to all factors.

The sensitivity of the reagent to depression of the combined clotting
factors of the prothrombin complex as seen in liver diseases has not yet
been studied thoroughly, but seems to be generally satisfactory.

Another property of Normotest is a lack of sensitivity to PIVKA. Thir-
ty-four patients with coumarin-induced hypocoagulability displayed a
mean Thrombotest value of 13.3 per cent and a mean Normotest value

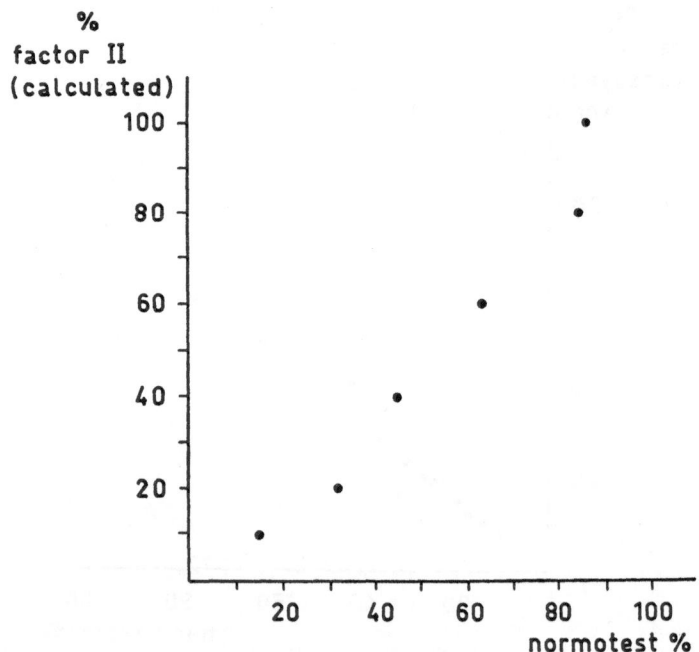

Fig. 2. Correlation between calculated factor II values as supposed to be present in plasmas
prepared by mixing normal pooled plasma (100% factor II) and congenitally factor II-defi-
cient plasma (about 1.5% factor II) and observed Normotest values.

of 28 per cent. The mean coagulation factor activity, assayed by the dilution-curve method (page 182) and classical one-stage assay procedures, approximated the mean Normotest value (table 1). The PIVKA insen-

Table 1. Results obtained with different coagulation factor assay procedures performed on blood and plasma from coumarin-treated patients.

n = 34	Thrombotest	Normotest	II + VII + IX + X
Blood (individual)	13.3%	28%	—
Plasma (individual)	12%	22.4%	—
Plasma (mixture)	*29%	*28%	29%

* assayed with dilution-curve method

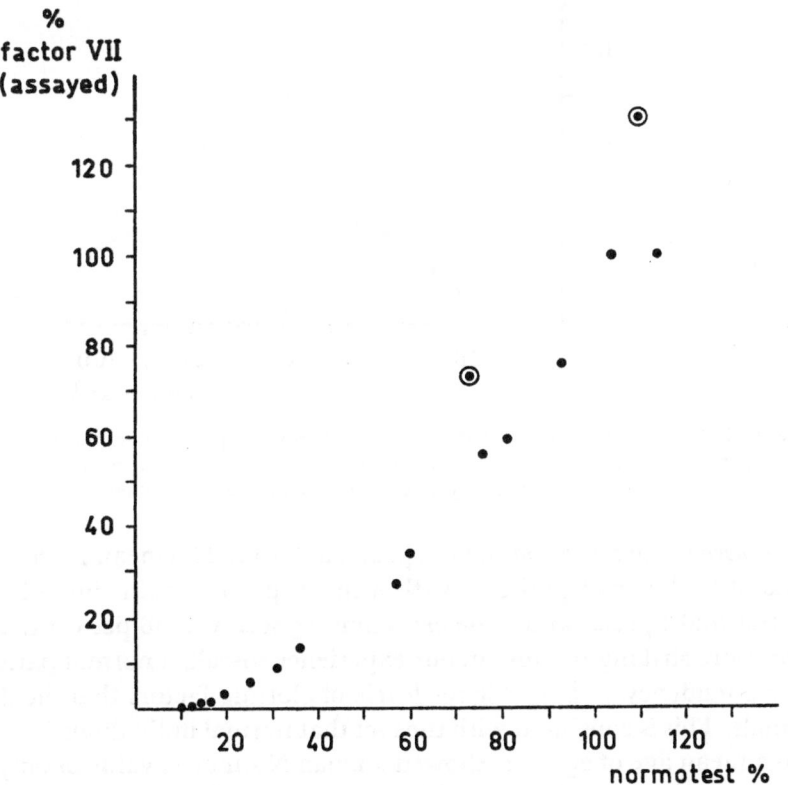

Fig. 3. Correlation between results obtained with a factor VII one-stage assay procedure and Normotest on samples from a patient suffering from severe hypoproconvertinaemia (about 1.5% factor VII) who was treated by transfusion of concentrated factor VII.
⊙ = during transfusion.

sitivity of Normotest originates from the relatively low PIVKA sensitivity of human brain material and, in addition, the dilution. This is
clearly demonstrated by the results given in table 1 for individual plasma, which is diluted in a ratio of 1:26. Whole blood is diluted 1:42.

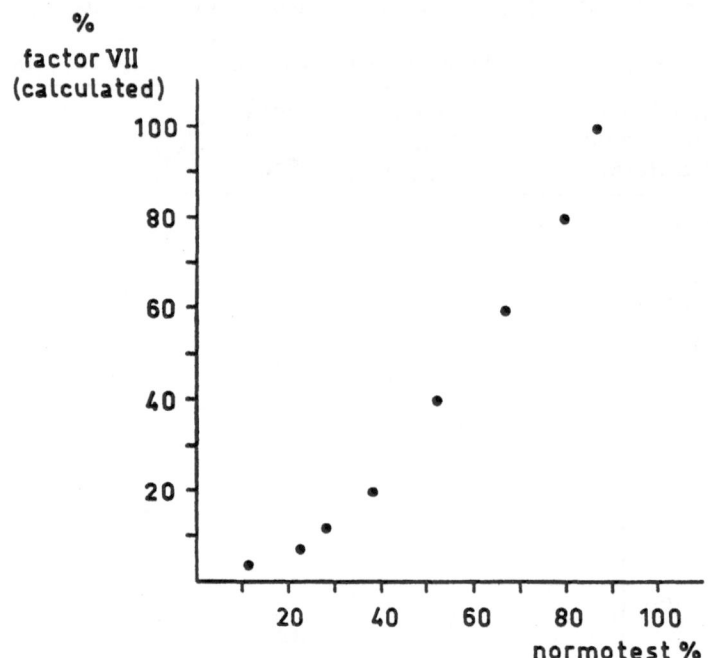

Fig. 4. Correlation between calculated factor VII values as supposed to be present in plasmas prepared by mixing normal pooled plasma (factor VII = 100%) and congenitally factor
VII-deficient plasma (activity about 1.5%) and observed Normotest values.

The normal value of Normotest is a problem for us. The mean Normotest
value of 84 'normal patients' with a mean prothrombin time of 12.8
sec. (normal 14 sec.) and none exceeding 15 sec., was 88 per cent. This
is the more striking because in our experience so-called normal patients
show a tendency to have higher levels of clotting factors than healthy
normals. This is consistent with the fact that normal individuals (n=30)
with a mean age of 29 years showed a mean Normotest value of only 80
per cent. Plasmas of these normals were also tested with the Normotest
reagent, and the percentage 'coagulation activity' was read on a standard reference curve, prepared with deep-frozen normal plasma from
30 normals (mean age 30 years, sex ratio 1:1). The mean Normotest

value in these normals was again 80 per cent rather than the 100 per cent expected by definition. This discrepancy cannot be caused by differences in age or sex, because the pooled group had the same composition as the 30 normals separately, or by technical factors such as calcium concentration, pipetting, etc. The only difference is that the pooled plasma had been stored for some months at -20°C and some activation of factor VII may have occurred.

Finally, it may be mentioned that Normotest seems to be sensitive to small changes in distilled water. We use only small bottles kept at +4°C.

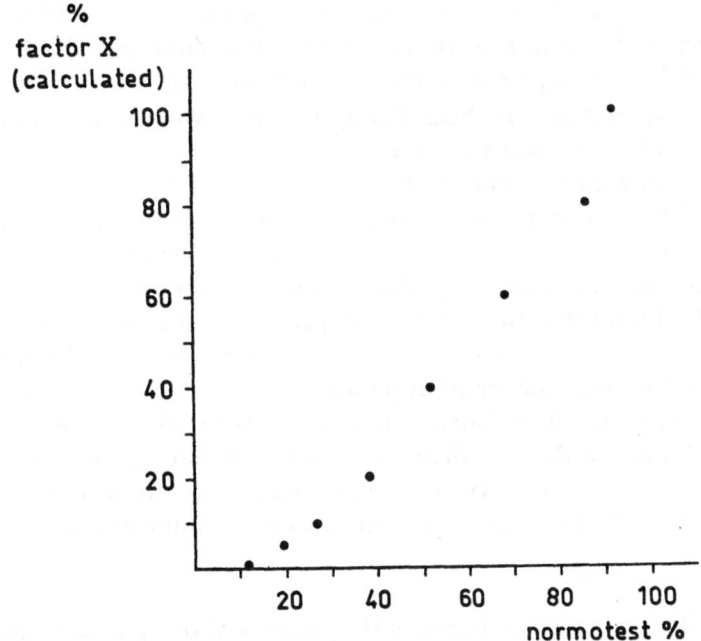

Fig. 5. Correlation between factor x as supposed to be present in artificially factor x-deficient plasmas prepared by mixing normal pooled plasma (100% factor x) and factor x-deficient plasma (about 2% factor x) and Normotest performed on the same samples.

DISCUSSION

Mannucci (Milan): I would like to know whether there are any differences between the P & P test and Normotest. As far as I know, the only difference is that higher plasma dilutions are tested in Normotest. We have compared three one-stage assay procedures in patients with liver disease. These tests were: 1. Prothrombin Time, 2. P & P test, and 3. Partial Thromboplastin Time. We included the Partial Thromboplastin Time because it theoretically covers a wide range of clotting factors – all factors except VII and XIII.

We found that the Partial Thromboplastin Time assay procedure was the least sensitive, and we suspect that this is not because it does not measure factor VII but rather that it is sensitive to factor VIII, which is often strongly increased in patients with liver disease.

We also found that the P & P assay procedure was the most sensitive test. Results were nearly always normal in patients with mild hepatitis and mostly clearly abnormal in patients with liver cirrhosis, also when the results of other liver function tests were only slightly pathologic.

In the study of three patients suffering from haemophilia B with an abnormal type of factor IX, we found abnormal Thrombotest values. The mother of one of these patients also had abnormal Thrombotest values.

Owren: We were unable to study the parents of our patients suffering from haemophilia B and displaying the inhibitor phenomenon, but we did study one cousin and he also had a normal Normotest and a low Thrombotest value. Concerning the relation to the P & P method, the Normotest can largely be looked upon as a standardized P & P method, in which the thromboplastin preparation has been standardized according to the same requirements as for the ox brain thromboplastin used in the Thrombotest method, in which factors II, VII, IX, X and intermediate clotting products are completely eliminated. Hence, whether or not the P & P method and Normotest give the same results will depend on the preparation of the human brain thromboplastin for the P & P test. After 10 years of experience with the P & P method in more than 100,000 tests we found that the reagent varied too much from batch to batch when the human brain thromboplastin was prepared by the usual laboratory procedure.

It is true, as has been mentioned, that the high dilution of the test plasma in the Normotest method reduces the effect of inhibitors. By comparing three preparations of Thrombotest made with ox brain, human brain, and rabbit brain thromboplastins respectively, we found, however, that with identical techniques giving identical dilutions of the test plasma, the ox brain preparation was far more sensitive to the effect of the PIVKA-inhibitor than the human brain and rabbit preparations. Concerning the normal range for Normotest, I would particularly mention the study of Dr. Tryding at Kristianstad, Sweden of 214 persons (110 men and 104 women) who had been thoroughly examined for the absence of disease. The mean Normotest value was 98 per cent with a standard deviation of 15 per cent.

Loeliger: Factor VII is still one of the most intricate factors in blood coagulation. Although we started our investigation of factor VII almost 20 years ago, the factor VII problem is not yet settled. Factor VII is very labile. In the plasma of a large percentage of females who are taking the pill, a many hundredfold increase of factor VII is found after storage at 4^0C for 12 to 16 hours. We also know that the mean value of factor VII assessed from freshly drawn normal plasma is slightly elevated in females taking the pill. This could be one of the possible explanations for the puzzling fact that Dr. Veltkamp did not find a mean of 100% for normals. To Dr. Fischer: In laboratories acquainted with coagulation tests and hence experienced in the prothrombin time assay procedure, a good correlation of the results with those obtained by Normotest is expected. Most of the smaller laboratories, however, are not experienced and often work with home-made or less adequately standardized commercial preparations. We hope that Normotest will turn out to be as well standardized as Thrombotest, because then Normotest will give more reliable results than Quick's one-stage procedure, at least in less well-trained hands.

Stormorken: None of our normal subjects was taking the pill during our studies.

Unidentified: Is it not possible that during preparation of a normal plas-

ma pool from a large number of normal persons, some degree of contact
activation may occur? In our laboratory also the mean normal Thrombotest value is lower than 100% as assessed by our normal plasma pool.
Is it not possible that the reason why the Leiden group has found lower
normal values of Normotest is that they have higher contact activation
of the normal reference plasma than the Norwegian group?

Veltkamp: Contact activation will certainly be reflected in the results
obtained by Normotest. So your supposition may indeed be true.

Hemker: Thrombotest is also sensitive to contact activation. The rectilinear correlation between Thrombotest times and dilution of plasma
tested is only obtained if one works in the absence of glass activation.
Thrombotest times are significantly shortened by glass contact.

Owren: Virtually all coagulation tests are sensitive to contact activation
by glass. This is the main problem in the preparation of a standard reference plasma. We would like to have a plasma preparation which can
not be activated by glass and which can still be used as a reference standard. The contact activation can be prevented by small amounts of
heparin, but we have found such plasmas to be unreliable as standard.
Attempts to make a stable plasma by removing factors xi and xii have
also been unsuccessful.

Hemker: The solution of the problem may be found by using Hageman
factor deficient plasma as a standard.

Unidentified: The Standardization Groups (Biggs and Denson) proposed
a ii-vii-x-reagent. Why has it not been used here?

Owren: The ii-vii-x-reagent is a copy of Thrombotest that is prepared
in a quite similar way.

Loeliger: Concluding, I may be allowed to stress, that, as far as Normotest is concerned, we are still slightly dissatisfied. For experienced laboratories it is not needed. I think, however, that it may be a successful
reagent for the smaller laboratories, which certainly need a test for the
assessment of the prothrombin complex as reliable as Thrombotest has
proven to be.

INDEX OF SUBJECTS

absolute standard for thromboplastins 322
accuracy of results 199
- bleeding time 199
- coagulation factor assay procedures (II, VII, IX, X) 200
- general considerations 199
- prothrombin time 199
- recalcification time 199
acetylsalicylic acid (Aspirin ®) 218
A-chain, thrombin (a.a. composition) 19
activated
- coagulation factor (general) 124
- factor X (types) 124
activation
- of factor VII by the 'pill' 387
- of factor XIII, by trypsin, reptilase, papain 14
activator of factor X 48
adenosin diphosphate, platelet 149
adhesion, platelet 149
adsorption of factors XI and XII 73
agar noble (Ouchterlony technique) 228
aggregation, platelet 149
alpha granules, platelet 148
amino
- acid sequences (of the chain-fragments of fibrinogen) 8
- black staining 194
amniotic fluid embolism therapy 220
amyloidosis, diagnostic value of Normotest 376
anaphylatoxins 101
animal factor VIII preparation 221
antibodies against coagulation factors, use of 50
anticoagulant treatment
- control by thromboplastins 320
- control by Thrombosis Services 284
- control by vitamin K 285
- coumarin congeners 320

- discussion on control 342
- therapeutic range 340
antifibrinogen reaction with fibrinogen films 74
antifibrinolytics in haemorrhagic diathesis 240
antihaemophilic factors A and B, hereditary defects 206
antithrombin III 115
- deficiency, treatment 222
arthritis (gouty) 97
aspirin, in treatment of thrombocytopathy, therapy 218
automatic clot timer, according to Schnittger 173
autoprothrombin C 40

bacteriolysis 100
B-chain, thrombin a.a. composition 19
binding sites (prothrombinase) 114
biological half-life time of coagulation factors 361
biopsy, contra-indications for 216
bleeding complications 300, 304
bleeding factor, hereditary defects 206
bleeding time
- Ivy 155
- secondary according to Borchgrevink 157
bloodcoagulation and liver function (general considerations) 361
blood smear, preparation of 159
bone biopsy, 216
Borchgrevink, determination of factor V 184
bovine thrombin, primary structure 19
Boyden-technique 230
break-down products of fibrin(ogen)
- qualitative assay procedure 228
- quantitative assay procedure 228
- quantitative assay procedure according

to Merskey 230
bronchoscopy and biopsy 217
buffer, Michaëlis 179

capillary blood in Thrombotest 325
capillary microscopy 154
carbohydrates in factor VII 85
carriership
 - of haemophilia A and B, factor VIII and
   factor IX values in 277, 278
 - in haemophilia A and B, genetic counselling 275
 - of haemophilia A and B, individual
   change based on factor VIII and IX
   assay 277, 278
case history, in the investigation of haemostasis 153
C.I. esterase inhibitor 102
circulating anticoagulants
 - reflected by Normotest and Thrombotest 375
 - treatment 221
cirrhosis of the liver, laboratory findings 208
citrated blood 159
Clauss, fibrinogen determination,
 - technique 186
 - correlation curve 187
clot retraction 192
clotting factor, consumption 55, 58
clou hémostatique 149
coagulated blood 159
coagulation
 - defects, treatment of, general considerations 218
 - factor, general: activated 124
 - factor, see factor
 - factors, biosynthesis 361, 362
 - systems, enzyme kinetic evaluation 104
 - tests in liver disease 361
coagulometer 173
 - according to Schnittger 173
collection of blood 158
commercial phospholipid preparations 172
comparison between different coagulation
   tests in liver disease 386
complement system 99
 - biological effects 100
complex formation between factors VIII and
   IX 50
complexon blood 158
concentrate of prothrombin complex, preparation and clinical use of 251, 258

concentrated prothrombin complex
 - clinical use 253
 - dosage scheme 253
 - preparation of 252
consumption of factors IX and XI 80
contact
 - activation 73
 - activation and its influence on Normotest and Thrombotest 388
 - activation of normal plasma 388
 - factors, triggered by enzyme systems 94
 - product, adsorbed and free 119,120
 - product (CP), action on factor VII and
   IX 121
correlation curve
 - in factor I assay procedure 187
 - of Thrombotest 326
coumarin induced hypocoagulability 283
 - loading dose 283
 - maintenance dose 283
 - therapeutic range in 284, 322
cryoprecipitate
 - experience with freeze-dried material
   271
 - experience with large-scale production
   271
 - general considerations 239, 260

defibrination syndrome 223
degradation products of fibrin(ogen)
 - qualitative assay procedure 228
 - quantitative assay procedure 228
 - quantitative assay procedure, according
   to Merskey 230
degranulation, platelet 150
deoxycholate, solubilization with tissue
   thromboplastin 85
derivative, hypothesis of prothrombin 136
desorption of activation product 73
diagnosis, laboratory 205
diagnostic value of blood coagulation tests in
   liver disease 363
diffuse intravascular clotting (DIC), pathogenesis treatment 225
di-isopropyl phosphorofluoridate inhibition
   of thrombin 18
dilution ratio 105
discussion
 - on anticoagulation control 297, 325,
   342, 386
 - on blood coagulation tests in liver
   disease 386
disulfide, next page

– bonds in fibrinogen 9
– knot of fibrinogen 8
dose-response curve for vitamin K
– in patients 350
– in volunteers 350
drug-induced
– haemorrhagic diathesis 153
– thrombocytopathy 218
duplicate readings of Thrombotest 325
dystrophie thrombocytaire hémorrhagipare 208

EACA 97, 158
electron microscopy of blood platelets and haemostatic plug 148
endogenous inhibitors, reflected by Normotest and Thrombotest 375
enzyme
– cascade 54
– cascade, alternative hypothesis 52
– kinetic evaluation of coagulation systems 104
– systems, triggered by contact factors 94
esterase activity of factor VII 92
evolution of clotting factors 134
experimental error
– see accuracy of results
– in assay of factor II, VII, IX and x 346
extrinsic
– coagulation system 83
– system, initial reactions 86

factor I, assay procedure 186
factor II, see prothrombin
factor V 41
– activation 45, 128, 184
– plasma devoided of 184
– reversible activation 125
– role in prothrombinase 35
factor va, molecular weight 128
factor VII
– activation in the intrinsic system 79
– bovine, molecular weight 85
– calcium binding 83
– carbohydrate portion 84
– in dicumarol treatment 84
– esterase activity 92
– activation, by contact product, non enzymatic 121, 122
– role in intrinsic system 77
– sensitivity of thromboplastins 323
– serum, physico-chemical properties 83

– stabilization 93
– and tissue thromboplastins 83
factor VIII
– activation in vivo 122
– assay procedure according to Veltkamp 175, 176
– effect on thrombin 49
– experimental error of assay 276
– high potency preparations 239
– normal value 276
– reversible activation 125
– substitution with animal products 221
– values in carriers of haemophilia A 276
factor IX
– activation by tissue thromboplastin 77
– activator 58
– concentrates, general considerations 239
– experimental error of assay 276
– normal values 276
– values in definite carriers 276
factor x
– activation 24
– activator 48
– activator, formation of 54
– tissue factor 93
– ways of activation 123
factor x, xa 40
factor XI 58
– assay procedure according to Veltkamp 175, 176
– consumption 66
– free plasma 174
factor XII 58
– activation, mechanism 68
– activation of plasminogen 62
– activation, pseudo-reversibility 60
– assay procedure according to Veltkamp 175, 176
– mode of action of 62
– proteolytic properties 62
– -factor XI, complex formation 66
factor XIII
– activation 13
– assay procedure, qualitative aspect 192
– mechanism of action 14
factors v and xa, bound to phospholipid 29
factors VII and x, fingerprints of (dansylated) tryptic peptides 22
factors VIII, IX and x, interaction 48
factors VIII, IX, XI and XII, assay technique

for 173
factors VII and X terminal amino acids, 22
factors VIII, IX and XII free plasma 173
factors XI and XII, adsorption 73
factors XII and XI, interaction of 63
Feissly, platelet count 166
fibrin
 – clot 7
 – isolation of crosslink 15
 – solubility 13
 – stabilizing factor 13
fibrinogen
 – abnormal 12
 – assay procedure 186
 – Detroit 12, 16
 – dimer, molecular weight 10
 – electron-microscopic picture 11
 – in disulfide bonds 9
 – film 73
 – foetal 16
 – hereditary defect 206
 – interfaces, adsorption 73
 – Paris, Zürich, Baltimore, Louvain 17
 – reactions with antifibrinogen 74
 – treatment with cyanogen bromide 7
fibrin(ogen) degradation products (FDP) 224
 – action on haemostasis 224
 – clearance rate 225
 – qualitative assay 228
 – quantitative assay procedure 228, 230
fibrinolysis 94
 – kinin activity 99
 – as measured by thrombelastography
   162
fibrinopeptide(s) 7
 – chains, digestion with thrombin 7
 – structural features 11
filipin 89, 128
filter paper for bleeding time test 155
forms for diagnostic laboratory investigations 201, 202, 203, 204
formula for replacement therapy in haemophilia 238
four factor concentrate
 – dosage scheme 253
 – preparation and clinical use of 252,
   253, 258
frequency of coumarin-treated patients 236
FSF, hereditary defects 206

gamma globulin, prophylaxis of serum
   hepatitis 219

general considerations
 – on blood coagulation and liver function
   361
 – on treatment of haemorrhagic diathesis
   236
genetic counselling 275
Glanzmann-Naegeli, disease of 205
glass tubes, for recalcification time assay
   procedure 169
glycine-ethyl ester in fibrinogen incorporation 13
gout 97

haematocrit 169
haemophilia 82
 – general considerations on replacement therapy 237
 – A, treatment with cryoprecipitate 261
   (see also cryoprecipitate)
 – A, treatment, dosage scheme 238
 – A and B, genetic counselling 275
 – B, and Thrombotest 386
 – B, circulating anticoagulant reflected
   by Thrombotest 375
 – B, treatment with coagulation factor
   concentrates 251
haemostatic plug 149
haemostasis
 – laboratory investigation 153
 – mechanism of 143
Hageman factor 94
Hardisty-Caen, trombocytopathy 208
heparin
 – in treatment of diffuse intravascular
   coagulation 225, 239, 240
 – titration or assay 190
hepatectomy, partial and blood coagulation
   362
hepatitis
 – acute, laboratory findings in 208
 – chronic, laboratory findings in 208
hereditary
 – angioneurotic oedema 102
 – coagulation factor defects 206
hexadimethrine 94
 – bromide 95, 96
high potency factor VIII preparation 239
Horowitz, assay of PTA 174
human brain thromboplastin
 – in anticoagulant control 297
 – preparation of 178, 294
hyperfibrino(geno)lysis 224
 – per-operative treatment 220

immune
- haemolysis 100
- phagocytosis reaction 100
indication, laboratory investigation of haemostasis 152
inflammatory
- effusions 97
- reaction 94
inhibition
- by DFP (tissue factor) 92
- by excess substrate (prothrombinase)
113
inhibitor
- induced by coumarin congeners (PIVKA)
assay procedure 183, 184
- of fibrinolysis 158
- sensitivity of human brain thromboplastin 297
- sensitivity of Thrombotest 326
interactions, prothrombin, factors x and v,
phospholipids 24
interpretation of coagulated blood 171
intrinsic
- coagulation factor assay procedure 176,
177
- pathway, mechanism of 121
- pathway, role of platelets 121
- system, role of factor VII 77
investigation of transported blood 198
Ivy bleeding time 155

K₁, see vitamin
kallikrein inhibitor 102
kallikreinogen 96
kaolin
- light (BDH) 173
- or celite activated p.t.t. 173
K-complexon 158
kidney biopsy of 216
kinin
- formation 94
- -like activity 101
kinins 96

laboratory
- advice 216
- diagnosis 205
- investigation indications for 152
large membrane aggregates in thromboplastin 126
leucocyte migration 96
leucotaxins 101

Lineweaver-Burk plot 105
lipid-protein complexes, inhibition by filipin
91
liver biopsy 216
liver function as assessed by coagulation
tests, general considerations 362
loading dose of coumarin 283, 322
long-term anticoagulant treatment, discussion of 343
Lyon hypothesis, lyonization 276
Lüdin, platelet counting 166

maintenance dose
- of coumarin 283
- for stabilized anticoagulation 334
Manchester
- Comparative Reagent 290, 297
- Standard Reference Scheme 290
Mancini technique 228
mean daily dose for acenocoumarin, dicou-
marol and phenprocoumon 334
mechanism
- of haemostasis 143
- of intrinsic pathway 121
Merskey technique 230
Michaëlis buffer 179
microfibrills, platelet 148
microtubules, platelet 148
Milstone, phospholipid according to 175
Mitochrondria, platelet 148
mixed plasma thrombelastography 165
mixer for test tubes 169
model reaction(s) 104
monoinositophospholipid, influence on prothrombinase 37
Morbus Weil, therapy 221
morphology of the process of haemostasis
148

native blood 161
natural inhibitors, role of 55
needles for venapuncture 158
normal pooled plasma
- as standard references for factors II, V,
VII, IX, X, XI and XII 173, 174
- as standard reference for factor VIII 173,
174
- as standard reference for Normotest
and Thrombotest 388
Normotest
- assay procedure 181
- in cirrhosis 373

– clinical experience with 379
– compared to other liver function tests 370
– as compared to prothrombin time in liver disease 386
– constitution 381
– in the control of liver function 369
– correlation to Quick-test 379, 380
– in hepatitis 370, 371
– in hypoproconvertinaemia 383
– in hypoprothrombinaemia 381
– in liver disease 386
– normal value 384
– in obstructive jaundice 374
– sensitivity to endogenous inhibitors 375
– sensitivity to factors II, VII, and X 381
– sensitivity to PIVKA 382, 387
– standardization of 387
– standardization of normality 297, 387
N-terminal of fibrinogen 7

observation
– of clot retraction 193
– of coagulated blood 171
Ouchterlony technique 194, 228
Owren's human brain thromboplastin 178

papain 18
paraproteinaemia, treatment of 221
partial thromboplastin time (p.t.t.) 171
– in liver disease 386
permeability-producing factor 95
per-operative
– anticoagulant treatment 341
– hyperfibrino(geno)lysis, treatment of 220
phagocytosis reaction, immune 100
phospholipid
– adsorption 39
– binding of Ca-ions 34
– charge requirements in coagulation 35
– preparation 175
– preparation, commercial 175
– protein complexes 89
– prothrombin, bound to factors V and x_a 29
– titration curves 33
pill, activation of factor VII by oral contraceptive 387
PIVKA 367
– assay of 184
– sensitivity of human brain thrombo-

plastin 294
– sensitivity of thromboplastins 297
plasma
– congenitally deficient of factors VIII, IX and XII 173
– devoided of factor V 184
– devoided of factor XI 174
– normal 174
– to be investigated, preparation of 174
– thromboplastin antecedent 58
– thromboplastin antecedent, factor XI 94
– transglutaminase and factor XIII 15
plasmin 102
plasminogen,
– activated Hageman factor 94
– activation by factor XII 62
plastic, polystyrol crystal tubes 158
platelet
– count 166
– morphology, electronmicroscopy 148
– poor plasma, preparation 173
– stickiness 73
– transfusion 217, 218, 242
– transfusion, general considerations 237
Platelin 172
polyene antibiotics 128
pooled plasma, see normal pooled plasma
post-operative bleeding complications, treatment of 220
P & P method 303, 304
– in liver disease 386
prevalence of coumarin-treated patients 236
primary hyperfibrino(geno)lysis 224
primary structure of (bovine) thrombin 19
proaccelerin, hereditary defects 206
proconvertin, hereditary defects 206
prognostic value of blood coagulation tests in liver disease 363
prokinins 96
protamin sulfate, dilutions for heparin assay 190
protein
– induced by vitamin K absence or antagonists (PIVKA) 284
– phospholipid complexes 89
Prothrombal
– clinical use 253
– dosage scheme 253
– preparation 252
prothrombin
– activation 19, 42
– bovine, N-terminal 18

- complex 42
- complex, assay of 181
- complex, separation of factors 135
- definition 40
- factors v and x, phospholipids, inter-actions 24
- hereditary defect of 206
- influence of Ca-ion concentration 39
- labelled 130
- residual 137
- time (p.t.), assay procedure 178
- time, in anticoagulant control 322, 387
- time in liver disease 386
Prothrombinase 40, 45
- density characteristic 26
- dependence offormation on concentrations of lipids and proteins, factors v and x_a 27
- influence of monoinositophospholipid 37
- inhibitor by excess substrate 113
- formation of 131
PT, see prothrombin time
PTA, hereditary defects 206
PTT, see partial thromboplastin time
puncture 216
purification of factor XII 59

quality control of Thrombotest and Normotest 309
Quick's prothrombin time 178
rebound hypercoagulability, in treatment with vitamin K_1 356
recalcification
- assay technique in assessing factor VIII, IX, XI and XII 173
- thrombelastography 164
- time assay procedure on plasma 171
- time assay procedure on whole blood 169
release reaction, platelet 149
replacement therapy in haemophilia, general considerations 237
reproducibility of results obtained with different thromboplastin preparations 323
residual serum prothrombin in factor VII deficiency 77
retractilité du caillot 192
role of platelets in intrinsic pathway 121
Rümke technique, see Mancini technique
Rumpel and Leede 154
Russel's viper venom, 24, 128

salycylic acid 218
screening deficiency of intrinsic coagulation factors 177
Scribner shunt 222
secondary hyperfibrino(geno)lysis 224
sensitivity of Normotest 369, 372, 381
serine esterases, tertiary structure 136
serum, aspect of – after retraction of clot 193
smear, preparation of blood smear 159
solution of trasylol, EACA, and thromboplastin 158
Soulier-Bernard thrombocytopathy, 208
spleen puncture, biopsy 216
stability of anticoagulation, comparison of coumarin preparations 333
stabilization of factor VII by tissue factor 87
stabilized anticoagulation, prolongation ratios of prothrombin times 321
standard reference plasma for Normotest and Thrombotest 311, 388
standardization
- of Normotest 387
- of Prothrombin time 322, 387
- of Thrombotest 387
staphylocoagulase-reacting factor (CRF) 284
steady-state kinetics, validity in coagulation 106
sterols 128
Stuart Prower, hereditary defects 206
substitution therapy in haemophilia, general considerations 237
substrate specificity of thrombin 12
sudden death and non-sudden death 331
surface activation, Hageman factor 58
surgery investigation of haemostatic functions 216
synovial fluid 97
synthetic phospholipid 127

tachostyptan 172
tanned red-cell haemagglutination inhibition immunoassay (TRCHII) 230
T-D plot 366
tertiary structure of serine esterases 136
theorem of Bayes 278
therapeutic level
- to be aimed at, general scheme 341
- in anticoagulant treatment, discussion 342
- at the Hague Thrombosis Service 330
- at the Leiden Thrombosis Service 339
- at the Utrecht Thrombosis Service in

terms of Thrombotest value 336
- in oral anticoagulant treatment 307
- pre-, per- and post-operatively 341
- in terms of mean daily dose 336
therapeutic range 284
- in terms of different thromboplastin preparations 322, 340
thrombelastography
- in circulating anticoagulants 163
- in haemophilia 163
- in Hageman-factor deficiency 163
- on mixed plasma 165
- in PTA deficiency 163
- on recalcified citrated plasma 164
- technique 160
- in vitamin K-deficiency 163
thrombin 7
- activates factor XIII 13
- effect on factor VIII 49
- formation, platelet 150
- inhibited with di-isopropylphosphorofluoridate DFP 7, 18
- -like activity, adsorbed onto glass from factor XII-containing plasma 75
- N-terminal amino acids 19
- and prothrombin, structure 18
- specificity 18
- specificity of action 11
- time 189
- 'Roche' 187
thrombocythaemia, prolonged bleeding time 157
thrombocyte
- count (Feissly-Lüdin) 167
- transfusion 218, 242
thrombocytopathy 205
thrombocytopenia, prolonged bleeding time 156
thrombocytosis 168
Thrombofax 172
thrombopathy, see thrombocytopathy
thrombophilia, treatment of 221
thromboplastin
- human brain, preparation of 178, 294
- large membrane aggregates 126
- lipid composition 83, 134
- lipid parts 126
- protein 126
- species specificity 126
- time 178
Thrombosis Service 286
thrombosthenin, platelet 148

Thrombotest
- assay procedure 181
- capillary blood 325
- as compared to other conventional thromboplastin preparations 320
- correlation curve 326
- experience at the largest thrombosis service (Amsterdam) 318, 319
- dilution curve 182, 365
- duplicate readings 325
- factor IX sensitivity 326
- factor X sensitivity 326
- and factor VII activation 387
- in haemophilia B 386
- history of 300
- introduction at the Netherlands Thrombosis Services 314
- kinetics of 104
- PIVKA sensitivity 326
- sensitivity to endogenous inhibitors 375
- standardization of normality 297, 387
tissue
- factor, inhibition by DFP 92
- thromboplastin, activation of factor IX 77
- thromboplastin, and factor VII 83
- thromboplastin, separation 125
- thromboplastin, solubilization with deoxycholate 85
transported blood for laboratory investigations 197
trasylol as a constituent of the inhibitor-solution 158
treatment
- of diffuse intravascular coagulation 220
- of haemophilia A 261
- of haemophilia B 251
- of haemorrhagic diathesis 217
- of thrombocytopathy 217, 218
- of thrombocytopenia 217, 242
- of vitamin K deficiency 219, 345
- Von Willebrand disease 218

uraemic thrombocytopathy, therapy 218
urea solubility test 192

vaccinostyle 155
vascular permeability 95
Veltkamp's intrinsic coagulation factor assay 176, 177
venapuncture technique of 158
veronal acetate buffer (Michaëlis) 179
viscous metamorphosis in platelets 150

vitamin K (and K1)
– deficiency, therapy, general 345
– deficiency, laboratory findings 210
– deficiency, general considerations 236
– test 363
vitamin K_1 345
– difference in effectiveness between oral and intravenous administration 350
– dosage in cases of vitamin K_2-deficiency 354
– dose response relationship in patients 350
– dose response relationship in volunteers 350
– duration of effect 351
– maximum elevation of coagulation factors after a single dose 350
– maximum effect in patients 350
– maximum effect in volunteers 350
– intoxication 353, 354
– onset of effect 346

Weil's disease 214
whole blood recalcification 169
Willebrand, Von – disease 218

X-chromosome 276